MEDICAL RADIOLOGY
Diagnostic Imaging

Editors:
A. L. Baert, Leuven
K. Sartor, Heidelberg

Springer
*Berlin
Heidelberg
New York
Hong Kong
London
Milan
Paris
Tokyo*

C. I. Bartram · J. O. L. DeLancey (Eds.)
S. Halligan · F. M. Kelvin · J. Stoker (Assoc. Eds.)

Imaging Pelvic Floor Disorders

With Contributions by

C. I. Bartram · J. T. Benson · J. O. L. DeLancey · A. V. Emmanuel · D. S. Hale · S. Halligan
F. M. Kelvin · H. K. Pannu · E. Rociu · J. Stoker · K. Strohbehn · C. J. Vaizey

Foreword by

A. L. Baert

Introduction by

J. O. L. DeLancey

With 163 Figures in 192 Separate Illustrations, 19 in Color and 7 Tables

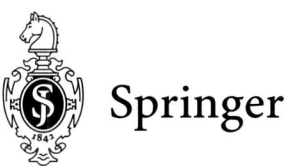

Springer

Editors:

CLIVE I. BARTRAM, FRCS, FRCP, FRCR
Consultant Radiologist, St. Mark's Hospital
Northwick Park
Harrow, Middx. HA1 3UJ, UK
and
Professor of Gastrointestinal Radiology
Imperial College Faculty of Medicine, London

JOHN O. L. DELANCEY, MD
Norman F. Miller Professor of Gynecology
Department of Obstetrics and Gynecology
L 4000 Women's Hospital
1500 E. Medical Center Dr.
Ann Arbor, MI 48109-0276, USA

Associate Editors:

STEVE HALLIGAN, MD, MRCP, FRCR
Intestinal Imaging Centre, Level 4V,
St. Mark's Hospital, Northwick Park
Harrow, Middx.HA1 3UJ, UK

FREDERICK M. KELVIN, MD
Department of Radiology
Methodist Hospital of Indiana
Clinical Professor of Radiology
Indiana University School of Medicine
1701 North Senate Boulevard
Indianapolis, IN 46202, USA

JAAP STOKER, MD, PhD
Department of Radiology
Academic Medical Center
University of Amsterdam
P.O. Box 22700
1100 DE Amsterdam, The Netherlands

MEDICAL RADIOLOGY · Diagnostic Imaging and Radiation Oncology
Series Editors: A. L. Baert · L. W. Brady · H.-P. Heilmann · F. Molls · K. Sartor

Continuation of Handbuch der medizinischen Radiologie
Encyclopedia of Medical Radiology

ISBN 3-540-66303-7 Springer-Verlag Berlin Heidelberg New York

Library of Congress Cataloging-in-Publication Data
Imaging pelvic floor disorders / C. I. Bartram, J. O. L. DeLancey (eds.) ; S. Halligan, F. M. Kelvin, J. Stoker (assoc. eds.) ; with contributions by C. I. Bartram ... [et al.] ; foreword by A. L. Baert.
     p. ; cm. -- (Medical radiology)
   Includes bibliographical references and index.
   ISBN 3540663037 (alk. paper)
   1. Pelvic floor--Imaging. 2. Urinary incontinence--Iamging. 3. Fecal incontinence--Imaging. I. Bartram, Clive I. II. DeLancey, John O. L. III: Series.
   [DNLM: 1. Pelvic Floor--anatomy & histology. 2. Diagnostic Imaging. 3. Intestinal Diseases--diagnosis. 4. Urogenital Diseases--diagnosis. WP 155 I31 2003]
   RC946 .I525 2003
   616.3'0754--dc21   2002034509

This work is subject to copyright. All rights are reserved, whether the whole or part of the material is concerned, specifically the rights of translation, reprinting, reuse of illustrations, recitations, broadcasting, reproduction on microfilm or in any other way, and storage in data banks. Duplication of this publication or parts thereof is permitted only under the provisions of the German Copyright Law of September 9, 1965, in its current version, and permission for use must always be obtained from Springer-Verlag. Violations are liable for prosecution under the German Copyright Law.

Springer-Verlag Berlin Heidelberg New York
a member of BertelsmannSpringer Science+Business Media GmbH

http//www. springer.de
© Springer-Verlag Berlin Heidelberg 2003
Printed in Germany

The use of general descriptive names, trademarks, etc. in this publication does not imply, even in the absence of a specific statement, that such names are exempt from the relevant protective laws and regulations and therefore free for general use.

Product liability: The publishers cannot guarantee the accuracy of any information about dosage and application contained in this book. In every case the user must check such information by consulting the relevant literature.

Cover-Design and Typesetting: Verlagsservice Teichmann, 69256 Mauer

21/3150 – 5 4 3 2 1 0 – Printed on acid-free paper

Foreword

A major breakthrough in the understanding of pelvic floor disorders has been achieved by the introduction of MRI into clinical research. Indeed, this cross-sectional non-invasive technique not only provides superior depiction of the pelvic anatomy but also yields unique dynamic information due to the rapid acquisition of images.

Imaging, and especially MRI, is nowadays increasingly utilised in clinical practice for patients suffering from pelvic floor dysfunction, and it is imperative that all radiologists involved in the care of these patients be fully informed about the rapidly emerging potential of radiologic imaging in handling these problems.

This book is the fruit of a collaborative effort by radiologists and surgeons. Professor Clive Bartram and Professor John DeLancey have been involved in research into pelvic floor disorders for many years and are well known worldwide for their pioneering work in this complex field.

The editors have been successful in engaging a number of experts with outstanding qualifications as contributors to the different individual chapters of this superb book, which provides a comprehensive overview of our current knowledge on pelvic disorders.

I am confident that this splendid volume will meet with great interest from radiologists and all other clinicians involved in the care of the large and increasing group of patients suffering from incontinence and utero-vaginal prolapse. I sincerely wish it the same success with readers achieved by the previous volumes published in this series.

Leuven ALBERT L. BAERT

Preface

Over the past decade there has been considerable research into pelvic floor disorders, often involving imaging, which has led to an increased utilization of imaging in the evaluation of these disorders. This has also been due to dramatic improvements in image quality, most notably in MRI with greatly improved anatomical definition, and the rapid acquisition of images for dynamic studies. Imaging has been able to yield answers where it was previously unable to do so. Functional disorders are particularly difficult to investigate, as there is usually no pathological change on which to base a gold standard for diagnosis. Perhaps because of this, much of the research has been collaborative in nature with clinicians and radiologists learning from each other, and gradually pushing forward areas of certainty. This spirit of interaction between clinicians and radiologists has been a guiding light for this book.

    A difference between imaging and clinical investigation is that imaging is not restricted in the same way that a surgeon's approach would be to a repair, as with MRI the entire pelvic floor is visualized at once. The boundaries of urogynecology and coloproctology that exist for the clinician do not limit the radiologist, who may frequently see abnormalities outside the remit of their referring group, but lack the expertise to be certain of what is wrong or its significance. Conversely, clinicians may not understand reports involving descriptions of abnormalities outside their particular field. Damage and functional disorders of the pelvic floor are not subject to any such limitation. Many patients with fecal incontinence have urinary incontinence and uterovaginal prolapse, so that the entire pelvic floor is dysfunctional. For this reason we should view the pelvic floor globally, and resist compartmentalizing symptoms and treatment. This poses the greatest problems for surgical management, but whatever group is involved a team approach will be required with a degree of shared knowledge. Both clinicians and radiologists have contributed to this book. The book starts with a detailed anatomical MR-based review of the anatomy. This is followed by an overview of how the pelvic floor works and then by chapters, both clinical and imaging, on investigation and treatment. The emphasis is radiological, and the book is intended mainly for radiologists, but is hopefully of sufficient breadth to be of interest to the clinician wishing to understand imaging of functional disorders throughout the pelvis in greater detail.

Harrow	Clive I. Bartram
Ann Arbor	John O. L. DeLancey

Introduction

Why a Book on Imaging and Pelvic Floor Disorders?

J. O. L. DeLancey

What should this new field of pelvic floor imaging be? What portents do these pictures hold for improving treatment for women and men who suffer from pelvic floor disorders? How can making images of the structures and their movements increase the success of current treatments and help in devising new treatments for these common problems? Definitive answers to these questions lie in the future, but the enormous potential for imaging to change our understanding and treatment of pelvic floor disorders is real.

The pelvic floor, in its limited sense, refers to the levator ani group of muscles, but the term also includes a more complex structural apparatus that spans the opening in the pelvis, closing its canal. It includes not only the levator ani muscles that close the pelvic canal, but also the connective tissues that support the pelvic organs by connecting them to the pelvic walls. The sphincters and viscera that comprise the excretory and reproductive organs are supported in the pelvis. The nerves and blood vessels that coordinate, control, and supply these structures play a central role in controlling the complex interactions of the urinary, intestinal and reproductive tracts. This entire tension-based structural apparatus must hold the organs of the pelvic floor in equilibrium. It must maintain this equilibrium while subjected to the considerable forces imposed by large transient tenfold increases in abdominal pressure during a cough, for example, and also support the weight of the abdominal organs 16 hours a day without fatigue or failure.

No-one pays any more attention to their normal pelvic floor function than they do to the beating of their heart or the action of their lungs. However, unlike these relatively simple activities of heart and lung, expelling gaseous intestinal contents from an opening in the bottom of a viscus containing liquid and solid, permitting the passage of a seven-and-a-half-pound infant through a small opening, coordinating contraction of the bladder and relaxation of the urethral sphincter only at socially acceptable times, and allowing men and women to enjoy sexual intercourse are complex pelvic floor activities that science does not completely understand. That the pelvic floor functions at all should be a marvel more remarked upon than the fact that it sometimes fails in the tasks that it carries out faultlessly hundreds of thousands of times over the years.

Great strides have been made in understanding the function of the pelvic floor's muscles and organs through the advent of miniaturized pressure transducers and the ability to record and store their data for analysis beginning in the 1960s. These recordings have allowed us to gain insights into what was different in the function of normal women and women with pelvic floor dysfunction. Has a sphincter become weak? Is it powerless to increase its squeeze in times of need? Does it respond at appropriate times? Are critical reflexes intact? Similarly, electromyography has helped disclose the state of neural control needed to coordinate these complex functions. This has been especially true in understanding the role of vaginal birth in pelvic floor dysfunction, but it has also helped in understanding age-related changes and the deterioration in function that occurs over the expanding life-span.

But what about the structure of the muscles, ligaments, sphincters and nerves? The pelvic floor, after all, is a three-dimensional mechanical apparatus that has a complex job description. What parts break? What structural arrangements are more prone to injury or deterioration? How does nerve dysfunction or muscle weakness influence the alignment of the different parts. These are structural questions that require us to look at the spatial arrangement of the elements of the pelvic floor and to assess their interdependent actions and reactions. Displacement of an organ may place it below where a muscle can support it. Break a connection between a muscle and its attached connective tissue and the normal muscle contraction can no longer cause an effect.

One of the primary problems in understanding pelvic floor function and dysfunction is that the involved structures are invisible. No one can see the muscles, ligaments and sphincters while they function during day-to-day life. Understanding the complex capabilities of the human hand would be very difficult with its complex structural arrangement if we did not see it every day. The first use of imaging in the investigation of pelvic floor function concerned studying the motions of the organs to make them visible. Although we could not see them as they functioned during their normal activities, it was possible to watch certain actions in a laboratory, although under unnatural conditions. These studies allowed some hypotheses to be generated, usually about the measurable angles between parts of the organs or the gross displacements of specific parts of the pelvic floor.

These contrast studies, however, did not allow us to actually see the pelvic floor structures: the muscles, ligaments, sphincters and nerves. Speculating about the reasons for these motions and abnormal appearances has been an enjoyable game for many years. Countless theories have been put forth. Definitive scientific experiments to decide which theory is correct have not been carried out, largely due to a lack of tools that would permit proper experiments to be performed. If we thought that a specific ligament was broken in women with stress incontinence, then carrying out a study where normal women and women with stress incontinence were studied to see if the ligament was broken in the stress incontinent women would resolve this question quickly. Because X-rays cannot see the ligament, because cadaver continence is not known, and because operating on live continent women is not ethical, proper studies could not be carried out.

The advent of soft tissue imaging with ultrasound and MR has changed this situation. It is now possible, for example, to see that a symptom of fecal incontinence and physiologic abnormality of a low anal closure pressure is caused by a structural break in the anal sphincter. This is no longer a matter of speculation or inference. Pictures of intact sphincters and of separated sphincters are decisive. Admittedly, there are instances where distinguishing between normal and abnormal is difficult, but this should not cloud the importance of the fact that in the majority of instances, a sphincter is either obviously normal or abnormal. Other studies identifying damage to the levator ani muscles and endopelvic fascia are following this lead and evolving rapidly.

What will the ability to see the structures of the pelvic floor allow us to do that we cannot do now? It is possible to see the motions of pelvic floor structures with real-time ultrasound and dynamic MR. This, of course, has been possible with contrast and fluoroscopy. There is the advantage that the walls of the organs and the abdominal contents can be seen more easily with MR than with fluoroscopy, but the unnatural supine position is a limitation. However, simply being able to see the nature of these conditions with all the structures visible will likely stimulate interested observers to better understand the nature of these problems and to formulate new hypotheses that fall closer to the truth than our current understanding. Whether or not imaging studies disclose important problems such as enterocele that might not be picked up on physical examination or in the operating room, and whether this disclosure improves the outcome of treatment, can now be evaluated.

The ability to see breaks in the structures comprising the pelvic floor is the radically new capability of advanced soft-tissue imaging. For example, it is possible to see injuries to the levator ani muscle in women with pelvic organ prolapse. It is the opinion of the author that this damage will prove to be an important determinant of operative failure. Being able to accurately assess this muscle damage will allow us to study the outcome of surgery in women with and without muscle damage. Once the results of these studies are known, new treatments, and techniques for injury prevention, can be devised. One of the often-overlooked advantages of imaging is its creation of a permanent record of the structures that can be re-examined later when new findings become available, and also that one person's images can teach generations of interested physicians and scientists.

Over the last century, imaging has changed medical care. Who would now depend on physical examination to diagnose a broken bone, without an X-ray? Who would depend on an X-ray to diagnose a placenta previa, without an ultrasound scan?

This book assembles our nascent understanding of pelvic floor imaging. We have chosen not only to include information about emerging imaging modalities and results, but also to consider the basic functional anatomy of the pelvic floor and clinical topics such as physiologic assessment of the lower urinary tract and gastrointestinal tracts. We include clinical material for radiologists so that they can see the context within which imaging technique selection and interpretation fall. We know that some imaging information may seem obvious to radiologists, but is new to clinicians.

Contents

1 The Anatomy of the Pelvic Floor and Sphincters
J. Stoker 1

2 Functional Anatomy of the Pelvic Floor
J. O. L. DeLancey 27

3 Innervation and Denervation of the Pelvic Floor
J. T. Benson 39

4 Imaging Techniques (Technique and Normal Parameters)
S. Halligan, F. M. Kelvin, H. K. Pannu, C. I. Bartram,
E. Rociu, J. Stoker, K. Strohbehn, A. V. Emmanuel 45

    4.1 Evacuation Proctography
        S. Halligan 45

    4.2 Dynamic Cystoproctography: Fluoroscopic and MRI Techniques
        for Evaluating Pelvic Organ Prolapse
        F. M. Kelvin and H. K. Pannu 51

    4.3 Ultrasound
        C. I. Bartram 69

    4.4 Endoanal Magnetic Resonance Imaging
        E. Rociu and J. Stoker 81

    4.5 Urodynamics
        K. Strohbehn 89

    4.6 Anorectal Physiology
        A. V. Emmanuel 101

5 Urogenital Dysfunction
D. S. Hale, F. M. Kelvin, K. Strohbehn 107

    5.1 Surgery and Clincal Imaging for Pelvic Organ Prolapse
        D. S. Hale 107

    5.2 Urinary Incontinence: Clinical and Surgical Considerations
        K. Strohbehn 125

6 Coloproctological Dysfunction
  S. Halligan, C. J. Vaizey, C. I. Bartram 143

  6.1 Constipation and Prolapse
      S. Halligan 143

  6.2 Faecal Incontinence
      C. I. Bartram 159

  6.3 Surgical Management of Faecal Incontinence
      C. J. Vaizey and C. I. Bartram 165

Subject Index 171

List of Contributors 175

1 The Anatomy of the Pelvic Floor and Sphincters

J. Stoker

CONTENTS

1.1 Introduction 1
1.2 Embryology 1
1.2.1 Cloaca and Partition of the Cloaca 2
1.2.2 Bladder 2
1.2.3 Urethra 3
1.2.4 Vagina 3
1.2.5 Anorectum 3
1.2.6 Pelvic Floor Muscles 3
1.2.7 Fascia and Ligaments 3
1.2.8 Perineum 4
1.2.9 Newborn 4
1.3 Anatomy 4
1.3.1 Pelvic Wall 4
1.3.2 Pelvic Floor 6
1.3.3 Bladder 9
1.3.4 Urethra and Urethral Support 12
1.3.5 Uterus and Vagina 16
1.3.6 Perineum and Ischioanal Fossa 18
1.3.7 Rectum 19
1.3.8 Anal Sphincter 20
1.3.9 Nerve Supply of the Pelvic Floor 25
References 25

The anatomy of the pelvic floor is described in an integrated manner, with special attention to the connections between structures that are crucial for a proper function of the pelvic floor. Apart from line drawings, T2-weighted magnetic resonance imaging (MRI) is used to illustrate normal anatomical structures.

The structure of the pelvic floor and its attachments to pelvic bones are an evolutionary adaptation to our upright position, which requires greater support for the abdominal and pelvic organs overlying the large pelvic canal opening. The initial evolutionary step was the development of a pelvic girdle, as found in amphibians, which were the first vertebrates adapted to living on land. The second was adaptation of the pelvic floor muscles. Pelvic organ support in early primates was controlled by contraction of the caudal muscles pulling the root of the tail forward against the perineum. With the gradual introduction of upright posture this mechanism became inadequate, and further adaptive changes occurred with the caudal muscles becoming more anterior, extra ligamentous support (coccygeus and sacrospinous ligament), and the origin of the iliococcygeus muscle moving inferiorly to arise from the arcus tendineus levator ani with some associated changes in the bony pelvis (Lansman and Robertson 1992). Partial loss of contact of the pubococcygeus with the coccyx led to the development of the puboviscerealis (puborectalis).

1.1 Introduction

The pelvic floor supports the visceral organs, is crucial in maintaining continence, facilitates micturition and evacuation, and in women forms part of the birth canal. This multifunctional unit is a complex of muscles, fasciae and ligaments that have numerous interconnections and connections to bony structures, organs and the fibroelastic network within fat-containing spaces. A detailed appreciation of the pelvic floor is essential to understand normal and abnormal function. The embryology of the pelvic floor is included to help explain certain anatomical features.

J. Stoker, MD, PhD
Department of Radiology, Academic Medical Center, University of Amsterdam, P.O. Box 22700, 1100 DE Amsterdam, The Netherlands

1.2 Embryology

The embryology of the pelvic floor and related structures remains unclear and new concepts are continually being introduced, e.g. the fusion of the urogenital septum and cloacal membrane (Nievelstein et al. 1998). This brief overview may be supplemented by more detailed texts (Arey 1966; Hamilton and Mossman 1972; Moore and Persaud 1998).

1.2.1
Cloaca and Partition of the Cloaca

The earliest stage in the development of the pelvic floor, comprising the urogenital, anorectum and perineal regions, is the invagination of the yolk sac 4 weeks after fertilization to form the foregut, midgut and hindgut. A diverticulum, the allantois, develops from the hindgut. The part of the hindgut connected to the allantois is called the cloaca (Figs. 1.1, 1.2). The cloaca is joined laterally by the nephric (later mesonephric) ducts. At the angle of the allantois and hindgut there is a coronal rim of endoderm and mesenchyme proliferation – the urogenital septum (or cloacal septum), which develops from the sixth week (Fig. 1.1). The septum grows in the direction of the cloacal membrane while fork-like extensions produce lateral cloacal infolding. At the margins of the cloacal membrane, mesenchyme migrates from the primitive streak to form lateral (genito- or labioscrotal) folds and a midline genital tubercle (precursor of the phallus) (HAMILTON and MOSSMAN 1972). By the seventh week, the urogenital septum divides the endodermal lined cloaca in a larger anterior urogenital sinus (including the vesicourethral canal) continuous with the allantois, and a smaller posterior anorectal canal (BANNISTER et al. 1995). The nodal centre of division of the cloacal plate is the future perineal body.

1.2.2
Bladder

The cylindrical vesicourethral canal is a part of the primitive urogenital sinus superior to the opening of the mesonephric ducts. The canal has a dilated upper portion and a relatively narrow lower part, representing the primitive bladder and urethra. The upper part of the bladder is continuous with the allantois, which regresses early on into the urachus, a fibrous cord attached to the apex of the bladder and the umbilicus. The mucosa of the bladder primarily develops from the endodermal lining of the vesicourethral canal, the bladder musculature from the surrounding splanchnic mesenchyme, and the ureteric orifices from dorsal outgrowths of the mesonephric ducts. During the developmental process the mesonephric ducts are absorbed into the bladder wall and contribute to the trigone (BANNISTER et al. 1995).

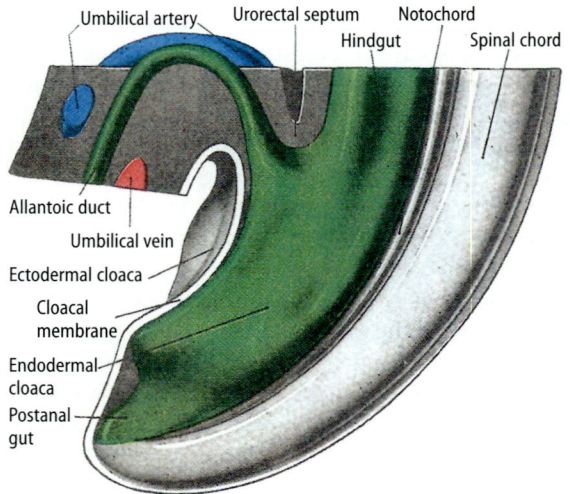

Fig. 1.1. The tail end of a human embryo, about 4 weeks old. Reprinted from BANNISTER et al. (1995, p. 206), by permission of Churchill Livingstone

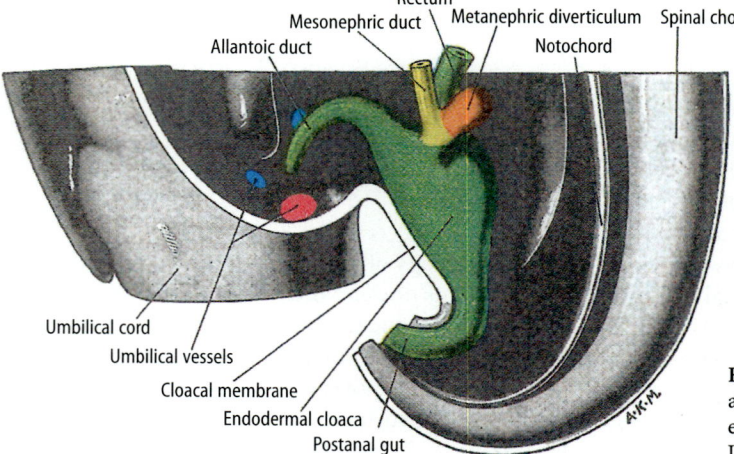

Fig. 1.2. The caudal end of a human embryo, about 5 weeks old. Reprinted from BANNISTER et al. (1995, p. 207), by permission of Churchill Livingstone

1.2.3
Urethra

In women the urethra is derived mostly from its primitive counterpart, whereas in men this develops into the superior part of the prostatic urethra extending from the internal urethral orifice to the entrance of the common ejaculatory ducts. In men the mesonephric ducts also contribute to the proximal urethra. The connective tissue and smooth muscle develop from the adjacent splanchnic mesenchyme. Striated muscle fibres form around the smooth muscle, initially anterior, and later encircling the smooth muscle. The epithelium of the remainder of the prostatic and the membranous urethra in males is derived from the endoderm of the urogenital sinus. Fusion of the urogenital swellings with primary luminization gives rise to the penile urethra, whereas the glandular part of the urethra is formed through secondary luminization of the epithelial cord that is formed during fusion of the arms of the genital tubercle, i.e. the glans. In both fusion processes, apoptosis plays a key role (VAN DER WERFF et al. 2000). The consequence of fusion of the urogenital swellings is that their mesodermal cores unite on the ventral aspect of the penile urethra, where they differentiate into the integumental structures.

1.2.4
Vagina

The paramesonephric ducts play a major role in the development of the uterus and vagina. The uterus is formed from the cranial part of the paramesonephric ducts, while the caudal vertical parts of the paramesonephric ducts fuse to form the uterovaginal primordium (BANNISTER et al. 1995). From this primordium part of the uterus and the vagina develop. The primordium extends to the urogenital sinus and at the dorsal wall of the urogenital sinus an epithelium proliferation develops (sinovaginal bulb), the site of the future hymen. Progressive proliferation superiorly from the sinovaginal bulb results in a solid plate in the uterovaginal primordium, which develops into a solid cylindrical structure. It is not clear whether this epithelium is derived from the urovaginal sinus or paramesonephric ducts. Subsequent desquamation of central cells establishes the central vaginal lumen. The tubular mesodermal condensation of the uterovaginal primordium will develop into the fibromuscular wall of the vagina. The urogenital sinus demonstrates relative shortening forming the vestibule.

1.2.5
Anorectum

The rectum develops from the posterior part of the cloaca, with regression of the tail gut (MOORE and PERSAUD 1998). The upper two-thirds of the anal canal is endodermal from the hindgut; the lower one-third is epithelial from the proctoderm. The proctoderm is formed by mesenchymal elevations around the anal membrane, which originate from the primitive streak and migrate between the ectoderm and endoderm. The dentate line represents the junction of these epithelial and endodermal tissues and is the site of the anal membrane. Inferior to the dentate line is the anocutaneous line where there is a transition from columnar to stratified keratinized epithelium. At the outer verge, the anal epithelium is continuous with the skin around the anus. The arterial, venous, lymphatic and nerve supply of the superior two-thirds of the anus is of hindgut origin, compared to the inferior one-third, which is of proctodermal origin.

1.2.6
Pelvic Floor Muscles

The pelvic floor comprises several muscle groups of different embryological origin, some developing from the cloacal sphincter and others from the sacral myotomes (HAMILTON and MOSSMAN 1972). The urogenital septum divides the cloacal sphincter into anterior and posterior parts. The external anal sphincter develops from the posterior part, and the superficial transverse perineal muscle, bulbospongiosus and ischiocavernosus from the anterior part (MOORE and PERSAUD 1998; HAMILTON and MOSSMAN 1972), thus explaining their common innervation by the pudendal nerve The levator ani muscle and coccygeus muscle develop from the first to the third sacral segments (myotomes) (HAMILTON and MOSSMAN 1972).

1.2.7
Fascia and Ligaments

The fascia and ligaments of the pelvic floor arise from the mesenchyme between and surrounding the various organ rudiments (HAMILTON and MOSSMAN 1972; AREY 1966). The mesenchyme may develop into either nondistensible or distensible fascia (e.g. the visceral peritoneal fascia of the pelvic viscera) (LAST 1978). Fascial tissues arise from condensations of areolar tissue surrounding the branches of the iliac vessels and hypogastric plexuses to the viscera (LAST 1978). Genital ligaments (e.g. in females broad ligament) develop from loose areolar tissue precursors originating from the mesenchymal urogenital ridge (AREY 1966). The vagina and uterus develop from paired paramesonephric ducts. These ducts, with their mesenterium attached to the lateral wall, migrate and fuse medially, carrying the vessels that supply the ovary, uterus and vagina. Tissue around these vessels condenses into the cardinal and sacrouterine ligaments that attach the cervix and upper vagina to the lateral pelvic walls. Fusion of the embryological cul-de-sac creates the single layered Denonvilliers' fascia in men (VAN OPHOVEN and ROTH 1997).

1.2.8
Perineum

As the cloacal membrane disappears, a sagittal orientated external fissure between the labioscrotal folds develops, except where the urogenital septum is fused. This fold, covered by encroaching ectoderm and marked by a median raphe, is the primary perineum (AREY 1966). Later in development of male embryos, the perineal raphe becomes continuous with the scrotal raphe, the line of fusion of the labioscrotal swellings. The perineal body, the tendineus centre of the perineum, is formed at the junction of the urogenital septum and the cloacal membrane.

1.2.9
Newborn

The pelvic anatomy is almost complete at birth, although some changes occur from birth to adulthood. These relate to organ maturation as well as responses to other effects, such as respiration and an increased intraabdominal pressure. Notable are the pelvis changing from its funnel shape in newborns, and the straight sacrum becoming curved (LANSMAN and ROBERTSON 1992), and nerve endings at the dentate line as part of the continence mechanism developing after birth (LI et al. 1992).

1.3
Anatomy

The pelvic floor is attached both directly and indirectly to the pelvis. Its layers, from superior to inferior, are the endopelvic fascia, the muscular pelvic diaphragm, the perineal membrane (urogenital diaphragm) and a superficial layer comprising the superficial transverse perineal, bulbospongiosus (bulbocavernous) muscle and ischiocavernous muscles. The pelvic floor is traversed by the urethra and anal sphincters, and in women the vagina. As the majority of patients with pelvic floor disorders are women, emphasis will be on the female anatomy.

Most of the MRI figures in this chapter were obtained at a field strength of 1.5 T with phased array coils, and a few with an endoluminal coil (used either endovaginally or endoanally), as indicated in the legend. All are T2-weighted images (turbo spin-echo sequences), where the bony pelvis exhibits a relatively hyperintense marrow with hypointense cortex. Fascia, tendons and striated muscles have a relatively hypointense signal intensity. Smooth muscles (e.g. internal anal sphincter) are relatively hyperintense. Fat and most vessels are relatively hyperintense.

1.3.1
Pelvic Wall

The bony pelvic wall is the site of attachment of pelvic floor structures. Pelvic floor structures attach directly to bone at the pubic bones, ischial spines, sacrum and coccyx and indirectly by fascia. The muscles attached directly to the bony pelvic wall are the primary components of the pelvic diaphragm: the anterior part of the levator ani (the anterior part of the pubococcygeus muscle, including the puboviceralis) and the coccygeus muscle. The periosteum of the posterior surface of the pubic bone at the lower border of the pubic symphysis is the site of origin of the pubococcygeus and pubovisceralis muscles (Figs. 1.3, 1.4). The tip of the ischial spine is the origin of the coccygeus muscle (Figs. 1.3, 1.4), which inserts into the lateral aspect of the coccyx and the lowest part of the sacrum. The sacrospinous ligament is a triangular shaped ligament at the posterior margin of the coccygeus muscle, separating the sciatic notch in the greater sciatic foramen, containing the piriformis muscle and pudendal nerve, and, together with the sacrotuberous ligament, the lesser sciatic foramen, which transmits amongst others the internal obturator tendon muscle and the pudendal nerve (Fig. 1.3).

The internal obturator muscle forms the major constituent of the pelvic sidewall (Fig. 1.5). It originates from the obturator membrane (covering the obturator foramen), the margins of the obturator foramen and the pelvic surfaces of the ilium and

The Anatomy of the Pelvic Floor and Sphincters

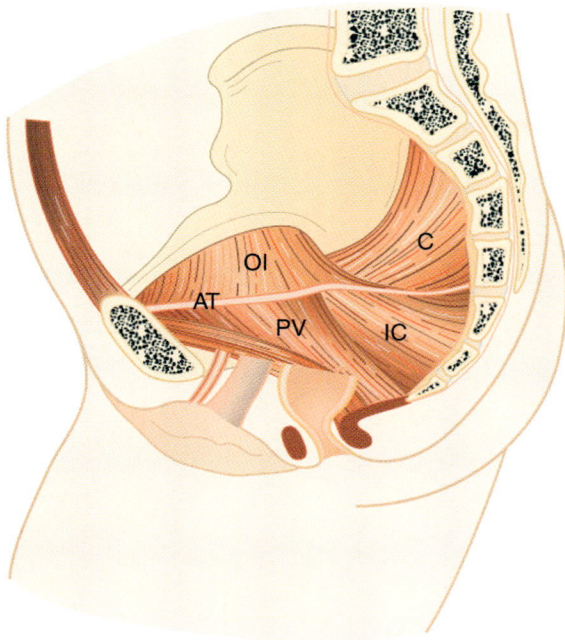

Fig. 1.3. Diagram of the levator ani showing the pubovisceralis (*PV*), iliococcygeus (*IC*), coccygeus (*C*), and the arcus tendineus (*AT*) arising from the obturator internus (*OI*) fascia

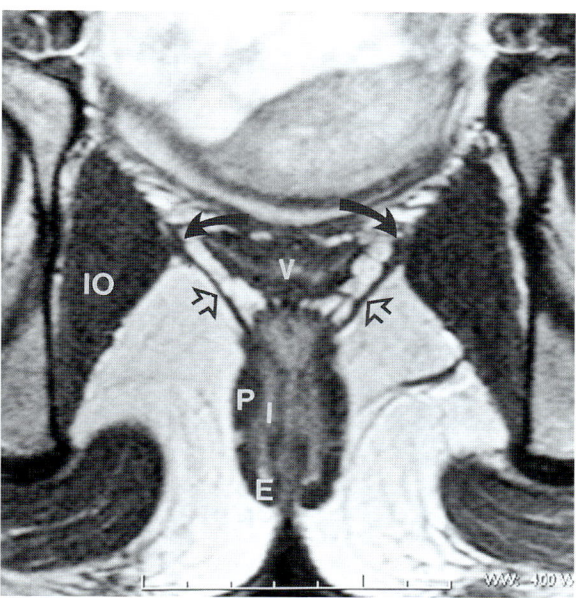

Fig. 1.5. Coronal oblique T2-weighted turbo spin-echo parallel to the axis of the anal canal in a woman (*I* internal anal sphincter, *E* external anal sphincter, *P* puborectalis, *V* vagina). The iliococcygeus (*open arrows*) inserts into the arcus tendineus levator ani (*ATLA, curved arrows*) formed from fascia over the internal obturator muscle (*IO*)

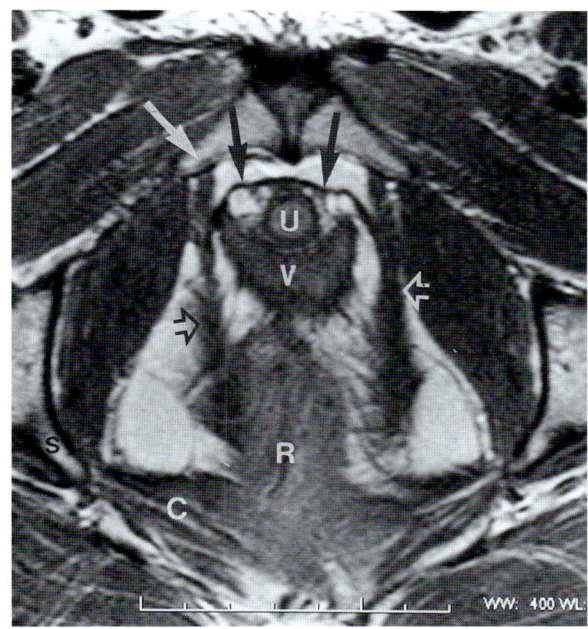

Fig. 1.4. Axial oblique T2-weighted turbo spin-echo. Note the attachment of the pubovesicalis (*black arrows*) to the levator ani (*open arrows*) (*U* urethra, *V* vagina, *R* rectum, *S* ischial spine, *C* coccygeus). Note the attachment of pubococcygeus to pubic bone (*white arrow*)

ischium (Tobias and Arnold 1981). The obturator tendon inserts into the greater trochanter of the femur. A tendineus ridge of the obturator fascia, the arcus tendineus levator ani, forms the pelvic sidewall attachment for the levator ani (Figs. 1.6, 1.7, 1.8). The piriformis is a flat triangular shaped muscle arising from the second to fourth sacral segments inserting into the greater trochanter of the femur. It lies directly above the pelvic floor and is the largest structure in the greater sciatic foramen (Fig. 1.3). The sacral plexus is formed on the pelvic surface of the piriformis fascia. The fascia of the pelvic wall is a strong membrane covering the surface of the internal obturator and piriform muscles with firm attachments to periosteum (Last 1978).

1.3.1.1
Tendineus Arcs

The arcus tendineus levator ani and the arcus tendineus fascia pelvis are oblique sagittal orientated linear dense, pure connective tissue structures at the pelvic sidewall. These structures have well-organized fibrous collagen, and are histologically akin to the tendons and ligaments of the peripheral musculo-

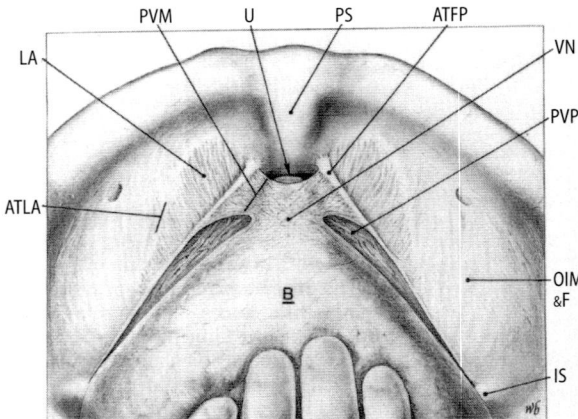

Fig. 1.6. The space of Retzius drawn from a cadaveric dissection. The pubovesical muscle (*PVM*) is shown passing from the vesical neck (*VN*) to the arcus tendineus fasciae pelvis (*ATFP*), running over the paraurethral vascular plexus (*PVP*) (*ATLA* arcus tendineus levator ani, *B* bladder, *IS* ischial spine, *LA* levator ani, *OIM&F* obturator internus muscle and fascia, *PS* pubic symphysis, *U* urethra). Reprinted from CARDOZO (1997, p. 36), by permission of the publisher Churchill Livingstone

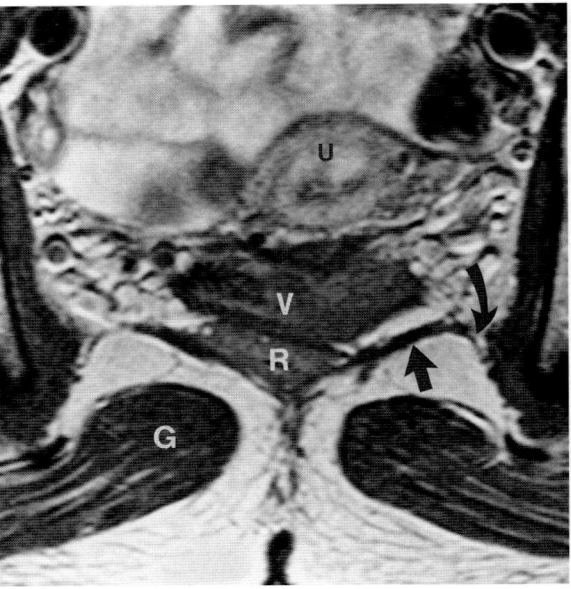

Fig. 1.7. Coronal oblique T2-weighted turbo spin-echo posterior to the anal canal of a woman. The iliococcygeus part of the levator ani muscle (*black arrow*) has its origin at the arcus tendineus levator ani. The lateral part of the iliococcygeus is relatively thin and membranous (*curved arrow*) (*R* rectum, *V* vagina, *U* uterus, *G* gluteus maximus)

skeletal system. The arcus tendineus levator ani is a condensation of the obturator fascia, extending to the pubic ramus anteriorly and to the ischial spine posteriorly. Most of the levator ani muscle arises from it (Figs. 1.5, 1.6, 1.9).

The posterior half of the arcus tendineus fascia pelvis joins with the arcus tendineus levator ani, whereas the anterior half has a more inferior and medial course than the arcus tendineus levator ani (Fig. 1.6) attaching to the pubis close to the pubic symphysis (DELANCEY and STARR 1990) (Fig. 1.10).

These tendineus arcs are reinforced by a four stellate-shaped tendineus structure originating from the ischial spine (MAUROY et al. 2000), including the tendineus arcs, sacrospinous and ischial arch ligaments. The latter is the transition between the fascia of the piriform muscle and the pelvic diaphragm. These tendineus arcs form the attachment for several structures: the levator ani muscle, endopelvic fascia (anterior vaginal wall), pubovesical muscle and other supportive structures.

1.3.2
Pelvic Floor

The pelvic floor comprises four principal layers: from superior to inferior, the supportive connective tissue of the endopelvic fascia and related structures, the pelvic diaphragm, the perineal membrane (urogeni-

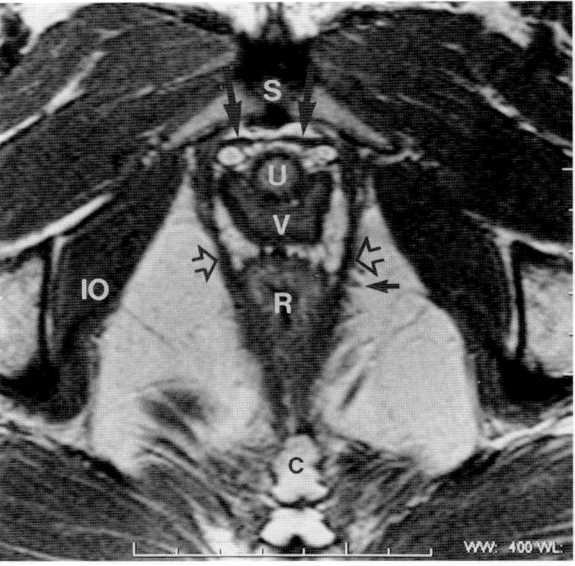

Fig. 1.8. Axial oblique T2-weighted turbo spin-echo in a woman (*black arrows* pubovesical muscle, *U* urethra, *V* vagina, *R* rectum, *S* pubic symphysis, *IO* internal obturator muscle, *C* coccyx, *open arrows* transition between the pubococcygeus (anterior) and iliococcygeus (posterior), at the borders of the urogenital hiatus). Note fibres of the iliococcygeus extending towards the pelvic sidewall (*small solid arrow*)

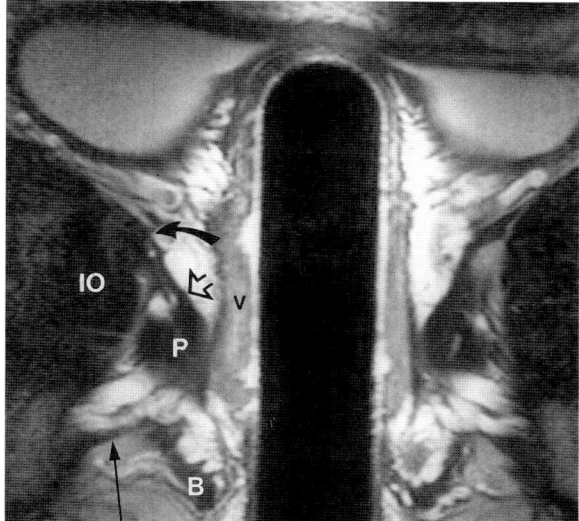 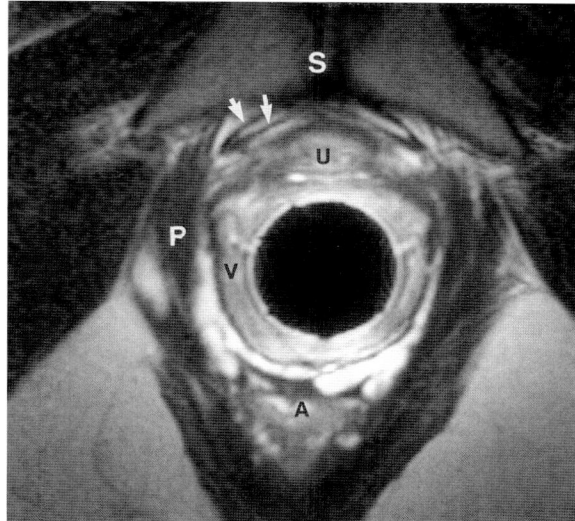

Fig. 1.9. Endovaginal coronal oblique T2-weighted turbo spin-echo parallel to the vaginal axis (*V* vaginal wall, *B* bulbospongiose muscle, *long arrow* perineal membrane, *P* pubovisceralis. The levator ani (iliococcygeus) (*open arrow*) has its origin from the arcus tendineus levator ani (*curved arrow*) formed from the fascia of the internal obturator muscle (*IO*). Note the attachment of the lateral vaginal wall to the pubovisceralis. Reprinted with permission from TAN et al. (1998)

Fig. 1.10. Endovaginal axial oblique T2-weighted turbo spin-echo in a woman (*S* pubic symphysis, *small arrows* arcus tendineus fascia pelvis, *U* urethra, *V* vaginal wall, *A* anus, *P* puborectalis). Reprinted with permission from TAN et al. (1998)

tal diaphragm) and the superficial layer (superficial transverse perineal muscle, bulbospongiosus and ischiocavernous muscles). The pelvic floor is given active support by the muscular contraction and passive elastic support by fascia and ligaments.

1.3.2.1
Supportive Connective Tissue (Endopelvic Fascia)

The connective tissue of the pelvis and pelvic floor is a complex system important for the passive support of visceral organs and pelvic floor. The connective tissue comprises collagen, fibroblasts, elastin, smooth muscle cells, and neurovascular and fibrovascular bundles (NORTON 1993; STROHBEHN 1998). The connective tissue is present in several anatomical forms (e.g. fascia, ligaments) and levels, constituting a complex meshwork (DE CARO et al. 1998). The diffuse layer and less well-defined aggregations of connective tissue is the endopelvic fascia. Well-defined, specialized aggregations that are named ligaments.

1.3.2.1.1
Endopelvic Fascia

The endopelvic fascia is a continuous adventitial layer covering the pelvic diaphragm and viscera. This expansile membrane is covered by parietal peritoneum. The structure of the endopelvic fascia varies considerably in different areas of the pelvis. For example, primarily perivascular connective tissue is present at the cardinal ligaments with more fibrous tissue and fewer blood vessels at the rectal pillars. The endopelvic fascia envelops the pelvic organs, including the parametrium and paracolpium, giving support to the uterus and upper vagina. Ligamentous condensations within this fascia are primarily aggregations of connective tissue surrounding neurovascular bundles.

1.3.2.2
Pelvic Diaphragm

The levator ani muscle and coccygeus are the muscles of the pelvic diaphragm. The pelvic diaphragm acts as a shelf supporting the pelvic organs (Figs. 1.7, 1.8). It has been described as a basin based on observations at dissection when the muscles are flaccid or surgery without normal tone. However, the constant muscle tone of the levator ani and coccygeus muscles by type I striated muscle fibres combined with fascial stability, results in a dome-shaped form of the pelvic floor in the coronal plane, and also closes the urogenital hiatus. This active muscular support prevents the ligaments becoming over-stretched and damaged by constant tension (DeLancey 1994a).

1.3.2.2.1
Coccygeus Muscle

The coccygeus arises from the tip of the ischial spine, along the posterior margin of the internal obturator muscle (Figs. 1.3, 1.4). This shelf-like musculotendinous structure forms the posterior part of the pelvic diaphragm. The fibres fan out and insert into the lateral side of the coccyx and the lowest part of the sacrum. The sacrospinous ligament is at the posterior edge of the coccygeus muscle and is fused with this muscle. The proportions of the muscular and ligamentous parts may vary. The coccygeus is not part of the levator ani, having a different function and origin, being the homologue of a tail muscle (agitator caudae).

1.3.2.2.2
Levator Ani Muscle

The iliococcygeus, pubococcygeus, and pubovisceralis form the levator ani muscle, and may be differentiated by their lines of origin and direction (Fig. 1.8). The iliococcygeus muscle and pubococcygeus muscle arise from the ischial spine, the tendineus arc of the levator ani muscle and the pubic bone.

The second and third sacral segments, mainly via direct branches and probably also the pudendal nerve, innervate the levator ani muscle. The coccygeus muscle is supplied by the third and fourth sacral spinal nerves.

The iliococcygeus arises from the posterior half of the tendineus arc (Fig. 1.7) inserting into the last two segments of the coccyx and the midline anococcygeal raphe. An accessory slip may extend to the sacrum (iliosacralis). The anococcygeal raphe extends from the coccyx to the anorectal junction and represents the interdigitation of iliococcygeal fibres from both sides (Last 1978). The iliococcygeus forms a sheet like layer and is often largely aponeurotic.

The pubococcygeus arises from the anterior half of the tendineus arc and the periosteum of the posterior surface of the pubic bone at the lower border of the pubic symphysis, its fibres directed posteriorly inserting into the anococcygeal raphe and coccyx.

The pubovisceralis forms a sling around the urogenital hiatus. The puborectalis is the main part of this "U"-shaped sling and goes around the anorectum where it is attached posteriorly to the anococcygeal ligament. The puboanalis is a medially placed slip from this that runs into the anal sphincter providing striated muscle slips to the longitudinal muscle layer. Other slings have been identified: the puboprostaticus in men (or puboperineus) and pubovaginal muscle in women. The former forms a sling around the prostate to the perineal body and the latter passes along the vagina to the perineal body with attachments to the lateral vaginal walls (Sampselle and DeLancey 1998; DeLancey and Richardson 1992) (Figs. 1.9, 1.11). Both interdigitate widely. Contraction of the pubovisceralis lifts and compresses the urogenital hiatus.

1.3.2.3
Perineal Membrane (Urogenital Diaphragm)

The perineal membrane, also named the urogenital diaphragm, is a fibromuscular layer directly below the pelvic diaphragm. The diaphragm is triangular in shape and spans the anterior pelvic outlet, and is attached to the pubic bones (Fig. 1.12). The urogenital diaphragm is crossed by the urethra and vagina. In men it is a continuous sheet, whereas in women it is attached medially to lateral vaginal walls.

Classically it is described as a trilaminar structure with the deep transverse perineal muscles sandwiched between the superior and inferior fascia. However, the superior fascia is now discounted, and even the existence of the deep transverse perinei

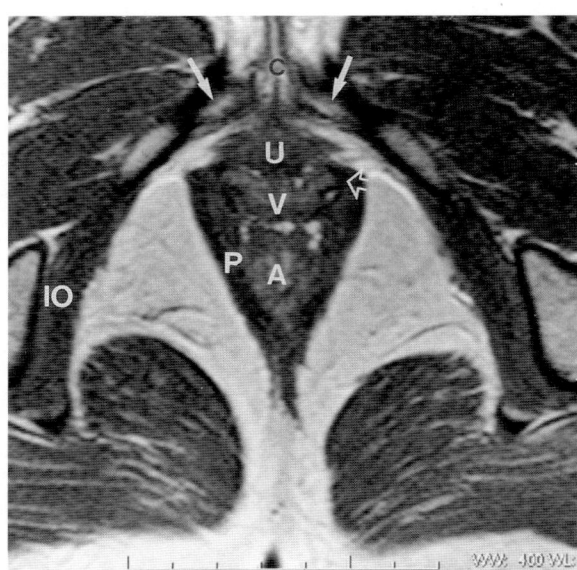

Fig. 1.11. Axial oblique T2-weighted turbo spin-echo in a woman (*U* external urethral meatus, *V* vagina, *A* anus, *P* pubovisceralis, *white arrows* ischiocavernous muscle, *IO* internal obturator muscle, *C* clitoris). Note the attachment of the vagina lateral walls to the pubovisceralis (*open arrow*)

The Anatomy of the Pelvic Floor and Sphincters

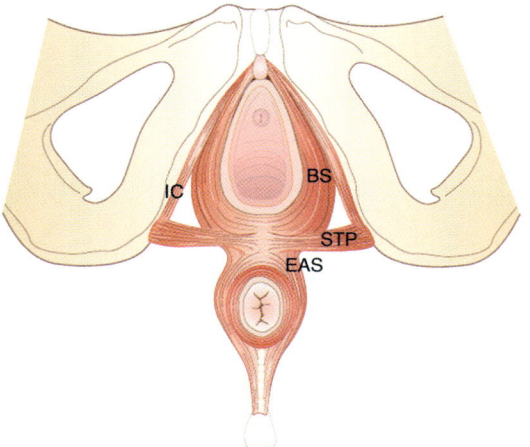

Fig. 1.12. Diagram of the perineal muscles in a female with the superficial transverse perinei (*STP*) fusing with the external anal sphincter (*EAS*) and the bulbospongiosus (*BS*) in the perineal body. The ischiocavernosus lies on the side wall of the perineal membrane

1.3.2.4
Superficial Layer (External Genital Muscles)

At the most superficial of the four layers of the pelvic floor lie the external genital muscles, derived from the cloacal sphincter, comprising the superficial transverse perinei, the bulbospongiosus and the ischiocavernosus (Fig. 1.12). The former is supportive; the other two play a role in sexual function.

In females, the bulbospongiosus courses from the clitoris along the vestibulum to the perineal body (Figs. 1.4–1.16). The ischiocavernosus originates from the clitoris, covers the crus of the clitoris that has a posterolateral course and terminates at the ischiopubic ramus (Figs. 1.14, 1.17). Both muscles compress the venous return of the clitoris (and crus of the clitoris), leading to erection of the clitoris. In males both muscles have a similar erectile function, but different anatomy. The bulbospongiosus (bulbocavernous) (Figs. 1.14–1.16, 1.18) is attached to the perineal body.

has been questioned in cadaveric and MRI studies (OELRICH 1983; DORSCHNER et al. 1999). It is likely that these are really fibres from the compressor urethrae and urethrovaginalis (Fig. 1.13) (see section 1.3.4.3 Urethral Support), which lie above the perineal membrane, or transverse fibres inserting into the vagina (OELRICH 1983) that can be identified at this level on MRI (TAN et al. 1998) (Fig. 1.9).

1.3.2.4.1
Transverse Perineal Muscles

The superficial transverse perinei span the posterior edge of the urogenital diaphragm (Figs. 1.12, 1.14, 1.15, 1.18, 1.19), inserting into the perineal body and external sphincter. In men this is into the central point of the perineum, with a plane of cleavage

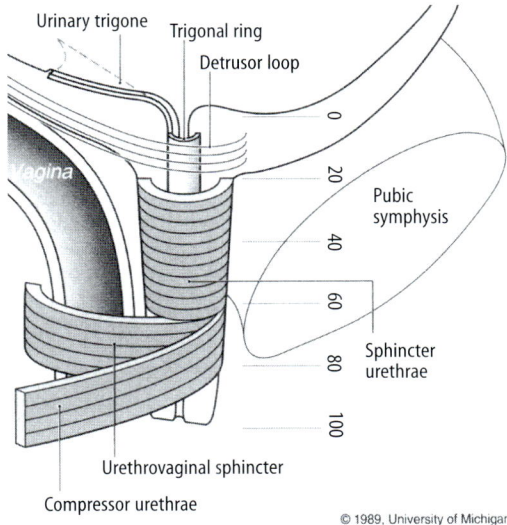

Fig. 1.13. The internal and external urethral sphincteric mechanisms and their locations. The sphincter urethrae, urethrovaginal sphincter and compressor urethrae are all parts of the striated urogenital sphincter muscle. Reprinted from CARDOZO (1997, p. 34), by permission of the publisher Churchill Livingstone

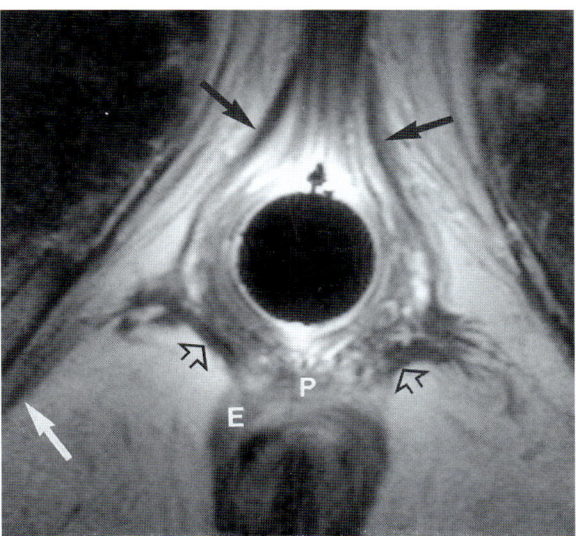

Fig. 1.14. Endovaginal axial oblique T2-weighted turbo spin-echo (*black arrows* bulbospongiosus, *open arrows* transverse perinei, *P* perineal body, *E* external anal sphincter, *white arrow* insertion of the ischiocavernous). Reprinted with permission from TAN et al. (1998)

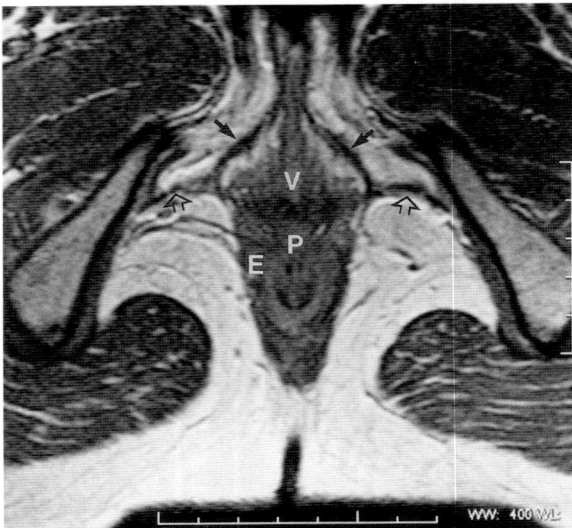

Fig. 1.15. Axial oblique T2-weighted turbo spin-echo in a woman (*E* external anal sphincter, *P* perineal body, *V* vagina, *black arrows* bulbospongiosus, *open arrows* transverse perinei)

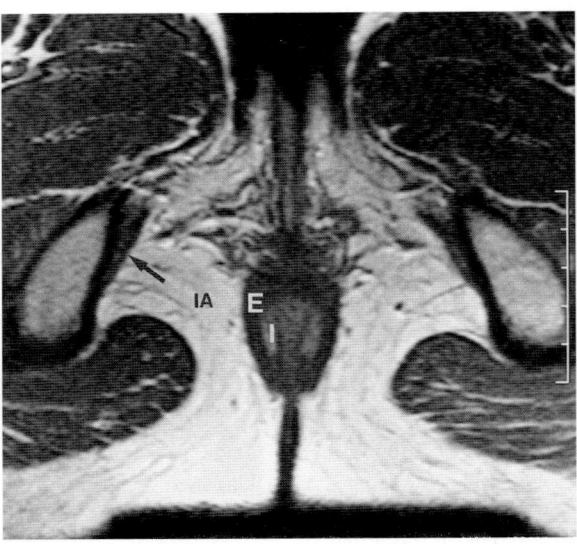

Fig. 1.17. Axial oblique T2-weighted turbo spin-echo in a woman (*E* external anal sphincter, *I* internal anal sphincter, *IA* ischioanal space, *arrow* ischiocavernosus insertion)

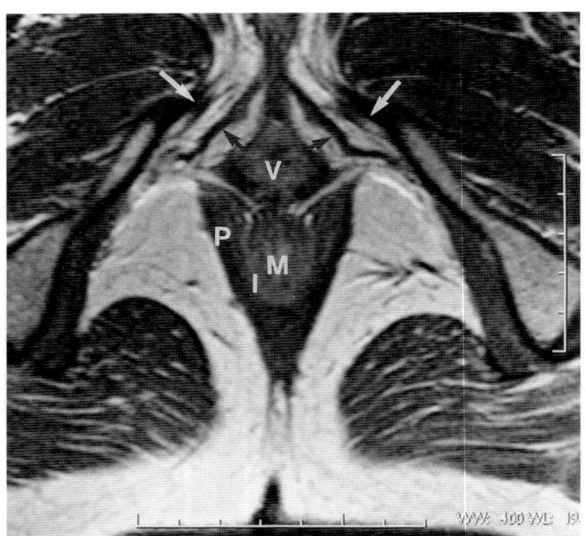

Fig. 1.16. Axial oblique T2-weighted turbo spin-echo in a woman (*I* internal anal sphincter, *M* mucosa/submucosa, *P* pubovisceralis, *V* vagina, *black arrows* bulbospongiosus, *white arrows* ischiocavernous)

between this and the external sphincter. There is no such plane in women as the fibres decussate directly with the external sphincter (Fig. 1.20).

The transverse perinei are variable in presence and often less well developed in women.

1.3.3
Bladder

The bladder is the reservoir for urine and crucial for proper lower urinary tract function. It lies posterior to the pubic bones, and is separated from the pubic bones by the retropubic space (space of Retzius), containing areolar tissue, veins and supportive ligaments. The wall has three layers: an inner mucous membrane, a smooth muscle layer – the detrusor – and an outer adventitial layer in part covered by peritoneum. The lax, distensible mucosal membrane of the bladder comprises transitional epithelium supported by a layer of loose fibroelastic connective tissue, the lamina propria. No real muscularis mucosae is present. At the trigone of the bladder the mucosa is adherent to the underlying muscle layer. Laterally at the trigone the ureteric orifices are present, with the ureteric folds. The internal urethral orifice is at the apex of the trigone, posteriorly bordered by the uvula in men (elevation caused by the median prostate lobe). During distension the trigone remains relatively fixed as the dome of the bladder rises into the abdomen.

1.3.3.1
Detrusor

The detrusor is the muscular wall of the bladder. The smooth muscle bundles are arranged in whorls and

The Anatomy of the Pelvic Floor and Sphincters

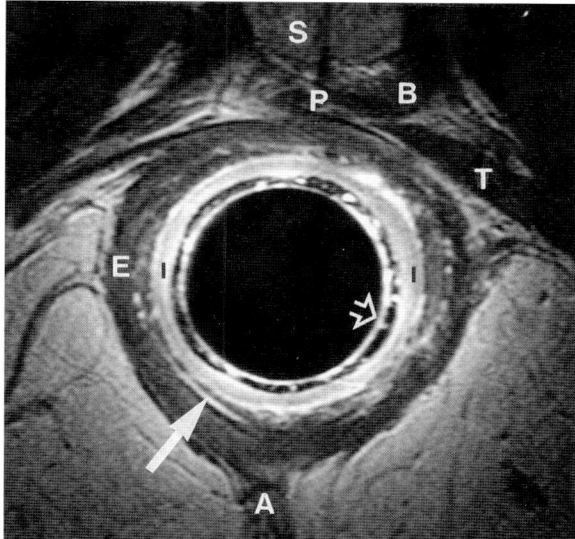

Fig. 1.18. Endoanal axial oblique T2-weighted turbo spin-echo orthogonal to the axis of the anal canal in a male volunteer (inferior to Fig. 1.30). The mucosa/submucosa is relatively hyperintense (*open arrow*) with hypointense muscularis submucosae ani. The internal anal sphincter (*I*) is relatively hyperintense and forms a ring of uniform thickness. The external sphincter (*E*) ring is relatively hypointense. In between the internal and external anal sphincter is the fat-containing hyperintense intersphincteric space with the relatively hypointense longitudinal layer (*white arrow*). The external sphincter (*E*), transverse perinei (*T*) and the bulbospongiosus (*B*) attach to the perineal body (*P*). Spongiose body of the penis (*S*). The external anal sphincter has a posterior attachment to the anococcygeal ligament (*A*)

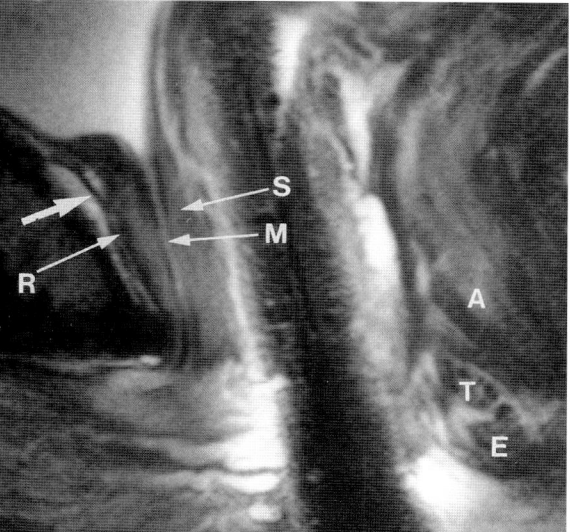

Fig. 1.20. Endovaginal sagittal oblique T2-weighted turbo spin-echo (*white arrow* pubovesicalis, *R* outer striated urethral muscle (rhabdosphincter), *S* inner smooth urethral sphincter, *M* urethral mucosa/submucosa, *A* anus). The transverse perinei (*T*) and external anal sphincter (*E*) are part of the midline perineal body. Reprinted with permission from TAN et al. (1998)

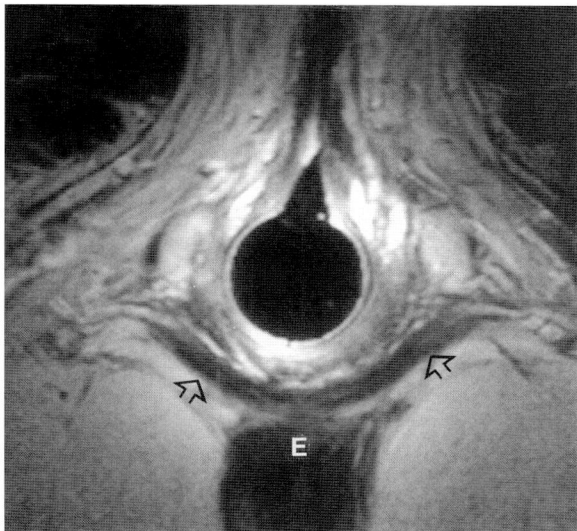

Fig. 1.19. Endovaginal axial oblique T2-weighted turbo spin-echo through the vaginal introitus. The transverse perinei (*open arrows*) course posterior to the vagina and anterior to the external anal sphincter (*E*)

spirals, with the fibres of more circular orientation in the middle layer, and more longitudinal in the inner and outer layers. Functionally the detrusor acts as a single unit. Some of the outer longitudinal fibres of the detrusor are continuous with the pubovesical muscles (ligaments), the capsule of the prostate in men and the anterior vaginal wall in women (BANNISTER et al. 1995). Some bundles, the rectovesicalis, are continuous with the rectum. At the trigone two muscular layers can be identified. The deep layer is the continuation of the detrusor muscle, while the superficial layer is composed of small-diameter bundles of smooth muscle fibres, continuous with the muscle of the intramural ureters as well as with the smooth muscle of the proximal urethra in both sexes. More recent work has shown that the superficial layer constitutes two muscular structures, a musculus interuretericus and a sphincter trigonalis or sphincter vesicae (BANNISTER et al. 1995; DORSCHNER et al. 1999). The latter surrounds the urethral orifice, is reported not to extend into the urethra and a dual role in men is hypothesized: preventing urinary incontinence and retrograde ejaculation.

1.3.3.2
Adventitia

The adventitia of the bladder is loose, except behind the trigone. At this site the bladder is anchored to the cervix uteri and anterior fornix in women. In men this part of the fascia is the upper limit of the rectovesical fascia (fascia of Denonvilliers). At the base of the bladder, condensations of areolar tissue envelop the inferior vesical artery, lymphatics, nerve supply and the vesical veins, forming the lateral ligaments or pillars of the bladder. The upper surface of the bladder is covered by peritoneum, while the rest of the bladder is surrounded by areolar tissue.

1.3.3.3
Bladder Support

The bladder is supported by several ligaments and by connections to surrounding structures. Anteriorly, the fibromuscular pubovesical muscle (ligament) is a smooth muscle extension of the detrusor muscle of the bladder to the arcus tendineus fascia pelvis and the inferior aspect of the pubic bone (DeLancey and Starr 1990). Based on a cadaver study, others have considered this structure as a ligament, anterior part of the hiatal membrane of the levator hiatus (Shafik 1999). This muscle is closely related to the pubourethral ligaments in females and puboprostatic ligaments in males. The pubovesical muscle (ligament) has been identified at MRI and may assist in opening the bladder neck during voiding (Strohbehn et al. 1996). Apart from the pubovesical muscle, other condensations of connective tissue around neurovascular structures can be found. The bladder neck position is influenced by connections between the pubovisceral (puborectal) muscle, vagina and proximal urethra. At the apex of the bladder is the median umbilical ligament, a remnant of the urachus. Posteroinferior support to the trigone in women is given by the lateral ligaments of the bladder, and attachments to the cervix uteri and to the anterior vaginal fornix. In men posteroinferior support is from the lateral ligaments and attachment to the base of the prostate. The base of the bladder rests on the pubocervical fascia, part of the endopelvic fascia, suspended between the arcus tendineus fasciae.

1.3.3.4
Neurovascular Supply

The innervation of the bladder (detrusor) is complex, involving parasympathetic and sympathetic nerve components (Chai and Steers 1997). Sympathetic fibres from the hypogastric nerves (lumbar splanchnic, or presacral nerves) reach the bladder via the pelvic plexuses. The parasympathetic nerve supply is via the nervi erigentes (S2 and S3 or S3 and S4) via the pelvic plexuses and innervates the detrusor. For the efferent sympathetic innervation there are differences in receptors. At the bladder neck and urethra α-adrenergic sympathetic innervation is predominant, leading to contraction. At the bladder dome there is predominant β-adrenergic sympathetic innervation leading to relaxation. Sympathetic stimulation from the spinal cord (T10–L2) via the hypogastric plexus with parasympathetic inhibition causes relaxation of the bladder dome and neck, with urethral contraction. In micturition the opposite mechanism, i.e. bladder contraction, relaxation of bladder neck and urethra is established by parasympathetic activity and sympathetic inhibition. The ultimate control of the lower urinary function is in the central nervous system (CNS), including regions in the sacral spinal cord (S2–S4; Onuf), pons and cerebral cortex.

1.3.4
Urethra and Urethral Support

The control of micturition depends on a complex interaction between sphincteric components of the urethra, supportive structures, and CNS coordination.

1.3.4.1
Female Urethra

The female urethra has a length of approximately 4 cm. The wall of the female urethra comprises an inner mucous membrane and an outer muscular coat. The latter consists of an inner smooth muscle coat (lissosphincter) and an outer striated muscle sphincter (rhabdosphincter) (Figs. 1.20, 1.21). This outer striated muscle is anatomically separated from the adjacent striated muscle of the pelvic diaphragm. On T2-weighted MRI the urethra is seen embedded in the adventitial coat of the anterior vaginal wall, which is attached to the arcus tendineus fascia by the endopelvic fascia. In women the urethra is attached anteriorly to the pubic bone by the pubovesical ligaments, which are bordered laterally by the pubovaginal muscle (Last 1978).

Urethral closure pressure depends on the resting tone of the smooth and striated urethral muscles, and on a process of coaptation of the vascular plexus to form a complete mucosal seal.

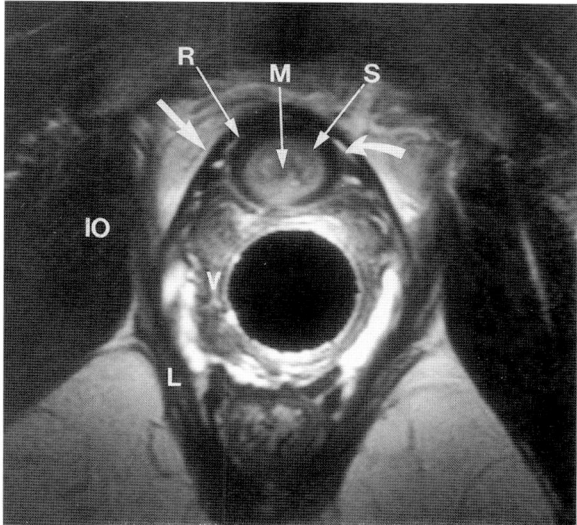

Fig. 1.21. Endovaginal axial oblique T2-weighted turbo spin-echo through the superior part of the urethra (white arrow pubovisceralis, *curved arrow* urethral supports, R outer striated urethral muscle (rhabdosphincter), S inner smooth urethral muscle, M mucosa/submucosa, V vagina, L levator ani muscle, IO internal obturator muscle). Reprinted with permission from Tan et al. (1998)

1.3.4.1.1
Urethral Mucosa

The mucosal membrane of the urethra comprises epithelium and underlying lamina propria. The lumen of the urethra at rest is crescentic and slit-like in shape in the transverse plane, with a posterior midline ridge (urethral crest, crista urethralis). The proximal epithelium of the female urethra is transitional epithelium, changing to nonkeratinizing stratified epithelium for the major portion of the urethra. At the external meatus the epithelium becomes keratinized and is continuous with the vestibular skin. The lamina propria is a supportive layer of loose tissue underlying the epithelium and consists of collagen fibrils and longitudinally and circularly orientated elastic fibres and numerous veins. The rich vascular supply of the lamina propria has a function in urethral closure by coaptation of the mucosal surfaces (mucosal seal), a mechanism influenced by oestrogen levels. Pudendal nerve branches are found in the lamina propria. Afferent pathways transmit the sensation of temperature and urine passage via the pudendal nerve.

1.3.4.1.2
Smooth Muscle Urethral Coat

The smooth muscle urethral coat is in the form of a cylinder and present along the length of the female urethra. The fibres have a predominantly oblique or longitudinal orientation, although at the outer border circularly orientated fibres are present that intermingle with the inner fibres of the external urethral sphincter. The circular orientation of these fibres and the outer striated muscle suggest a role in constricting the lumen at contraction. Strata of connective tissue have been described dividing the smooth muscles of the proximal two-thirds of the female urethra into three layers and thin fibres of the pelvic plexus course to this part of the urethra (Colleselli et al. 1998). These layers comprise a thin inner longitudinal layer, thinning out to the external meatus, a thicker transverse layer and an outer longitudinal layer. The smooth muscles have primarily a parasympathetic autonomic nerve supply originating from the pelvic plexus. The innervation and fibre orientation make a role for this muscle coat during micturition more likely than in preserving continence.

1.3.4.1.3
External Urethral Sphincter

The external urethral sphincter has circularly disposed slow-twitch fibres forming a sleeve that is thickest at the middle of the urethra (rhabdosphincter). At this level the external urethral sphincter is a continuous ring, although it is relatively thin and largely devoid of muscle fibres posteriorly (Colleselli et al. 1998) (Fig. 1.21). This is the level of maximal closure pressure. At the superior and inferior part of the urethra the external urethral sphincter is deficient posteriorly. The external sphincter slow-twitch fibres exert a constant tone upon the urethral lumen and play a role in active urethral closure at rest. During raised abdominal pressure additional closure force is provided by fast-twitch fibres. There is a close relationship with the smooth muscle urethral coat and some have indicated that smooth muscle fibres are part of the external sphincter and comprise a separate medial layer of the external sphincter (Dorschner et al. 1999). The striated sphincter muscle is closely related to the perineal membrane (urogenital diaphragm), and is separate from the adjacent striated muscle of the pubovaginal muscle. At the distal end of the rhabdosphincter, striated muscle has been identified forming two other elements: the compressor urethrae and urethrovaginal sphincter, formerly called the deep transverse perineal muscle. The anatomy of the striated urethral muscle was described in detail by OELRICH 1983 (see section 1.3.4.3 Urethral Support). Nerve fibres from the second to fourth sacral nerve supply the external urethral sphincter. Controversy exists as to which nerve fibres supply the external urethral sphincter (pudendal nerve, pelvic nerve, hypogastric nerve). Afferent nerve fibres pass through the pudendal nerve.

1.3.4.2
Male Urethra

The male urethra extends from the internal orifice (meatus) to the external urethral orifice (meatus) beyond the navicular fossa. The length is approximately 18–20 cm. In general the male urethra is considered in four parts: preprostatic, prostatic, membranous and spongiose. In this chapter on anatomy of the pelvic floor emphasis is on the former three as part of the lower urinary tract.

1.3.4.2.1
Lining of the Male Urethra

The preprostatic and proximal prostatic urethra is lined by urothelium that is continuous with the bladder lining as well as with the ducts entering this part of the urethra (e.g. ducts of the prostate). Below the ejaculatory ducts the epithelium changes into (pseudo)stratified columnar epithelium lining the membranous urethra and part of the penile urethra. The distal part of the urethra is lined with stratified squamous epithelium.

1.3.4.2.2
Preprostatic Urethra

The preprostatic urethra is approximately 1–1.5 cm in length. Superficial smooth muscle fibres surrounding the bladder neck are continuous around the preprostatic urethra and the prostatic capsule. The smooth muscle fibres surrounding the preprostatic urethra form bundles including connective tissue with elastic fibres. These bundles have been identified as an internal sphincter at the bladder neck, the musculus sphincter trigonalis or musculus sphincter vesicae (BANNISTER et al. 1995; GILPIN and GOSLING 1983). The rich sympathetic adrenergic supply of this smooth muscle sphincter has been suggested as indicative of a function in preventing retrograde ejaculation.

1.3.4.2.3
Prostatic Urethra

The prostatic urethra is embedded within the prostate, emerging just anterior to the apex of the prostate. In the posterior midline the urethral crest is present, with the verumontanum. At this level the ejaculatory ducts and prostatic ducts enter. The lower part of the prostatic urethra has a layer of smooth muscle fibres and is enveloped by striated muscle fibres continuous with the external urethral sphincter of the membranous part of the urethra.

1.3.4.2.4
Membranous Urethra and Spongiose Urethra

The membranous urethra extends from the prostatic urethra to the bulb of the penis and is approximately 2 cm long. The urethra transverses the perineal membrane with a close relationship with the membrane, especially laterally and posteriorly. Under the lining of membranous urethra is fibroelastic tissue that is bordered by smooth muscle. This smooth muscle is continuous with the smooth muscle of the prostatic urethra. Outside this smooth muscle layer is a prominent circular layer of slow-twitch striated muscle fibres, the external urethral sphincter. The fibres of the external urethral sphincter are capable of prolonged contraction, resulting in muscle tone and urethral closure, important for continence. A study using dissection of cadavers and MRI in volunteers has indicated the presence of an outer striated muscle and inner smooth muscle part of the rhabdosphincter, introducing the terms musculus sphincter urethrae transversostriatus and musculus sphincter urethrae glaber (DORSCHNER et al. 1999). The innervation of the external urethral sphincter is from S2 to S4. The spongiose urethra commences below the perineal membrane and is within the spongiose body.

1.3.4.3
Urethral Support

Urethral support is complex and not fully elucidated, although importantly more insight has been gained in recent decades. In females the urethra is supported by numerous structures, including the endopelvic fascia, the anterior vagina and arcus tendineus fascia pelvis. The endopelvic fascia (also named pubocervical fascia at this location) is attached at both lateral sides to the arcus tendineus fascia pelvis (primarily attached to the levator ani muscle as well to the pubic bone) (Fig. 1.10) and superiorly continuous with the sacrouterine and cardinal ligaments. This layer of anterior vaginal wall and pubocervical fascia suspended between the tendineus arcs at both sides forms a "hammock" underlying and supporting the urethra (DELANCEY 1994b) (Figs. 1.6, 1.22). Contraction of the levator ani muscles elevates the arcus tendineus fascia pelvis and thereby the vaginal wall. This leads to compression of the urethra by the hammock of supportive tissue. Close to the midline a pair of fibromuscular ligaments – pubourethral ligaments – anchor the urethra and vagina (Fig. 1.23). These pubourethral ligaments contain smooth muscle fibres, an inferior extension of the detrusor muscle. The ligaments give support to the bladder neck and urethra (PAPA PETROS 1998), and this may be enhanced by contraction of the smooth muscle fibres in the ligaments.

Anterior to the urethra a sling-like structure can be identified (Figs. 1.4, 1.8, 1.20–1.22, 1.24). This structure courses just anterior to the urethra and has lateral attachments to the levator ani muscle (TAN et al. 1998; TUNN et al. 2001). This structure has been identified as the inferior extension of the pubovesical muscle, originating from the vesical neck (TUNN et al. 2001) and has also been named the periurethral ligament (TAN et al. 1998). The aspect of the structure resembles the configuration of the compressor urethrae (see below), but the pubovesical muscle has a higher position, namely at the superior urethra. At high resolution endovaginal MRI, urethral support structures (paraurethral ligaments) originating from the urethra and vaginal surface of the urethra seem to attach to this sling-like structure (Fig. 1.21). This structure seems to have an intimate relationship with the inferior urethral supportive structures (Figs. 1.20, 1.24).

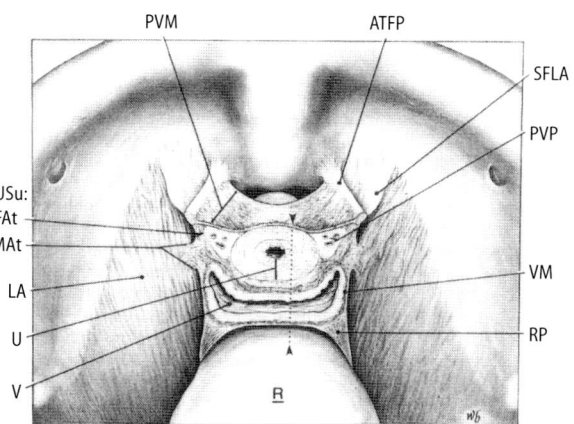

Fig. 1.22. Cross-section of the urethra (*U*), vagina (*V*), arcus tendineus fasciae pelvis (*ATFP*) and superior fascia of the levator ani muscle (*SFLA*) just below the vesical neck (drawn from cadaveric dissection). The pubovesicalis (*PVM*) lies anterior to the urethra, and anterior and superior to the paraurethral vascular plexus (*PVP*). The urethral supports (*USu*) attach the vagina and vaginal surface of the urethra to the levator ani (*LA*) muscles (*MAt* muscular attachment) and to the superior fascia of the levator ani muscle (*FAt* fascial attachment) (*R* rectum, *RP* rectal pillar, *VM* vaginal wall muscularis). Reprinted from CARDOZO (1997, p. 36), by permission of the publisher Churchill Livingstone

The urethra is in females at the level of the pelvic diaphragm bordered by the most medial part of the pubococcygeus muscle (i.e. pubovaginal muscle), which inserts posteroinferiorly into the perineal body. The pubococcygeus (pubovaginal) muscle is not directly attached to the urethra, but with contraction the proximity and orientation results in a closing force on the urethral lumen. In males, the medial part of the pubococcygeus muscle (puboperineales) has

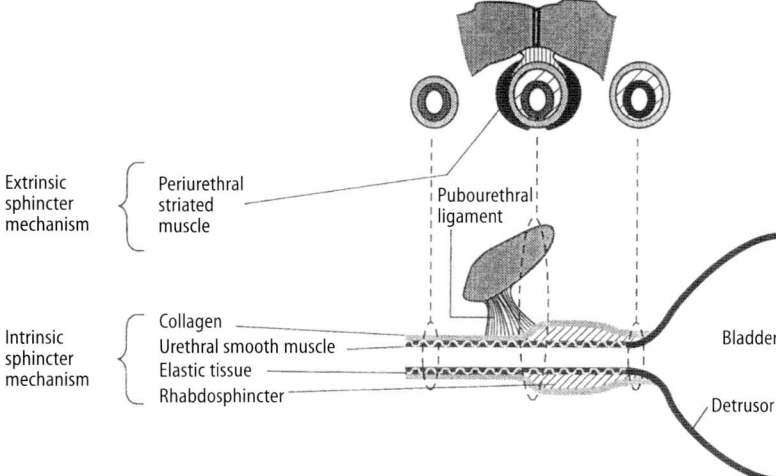

Fig. 1.23. Schematic representation of the urethra sphincter. Reprinted from CARDOZO (1997, p. 35), by permission of the publisher Churchill Livingstone

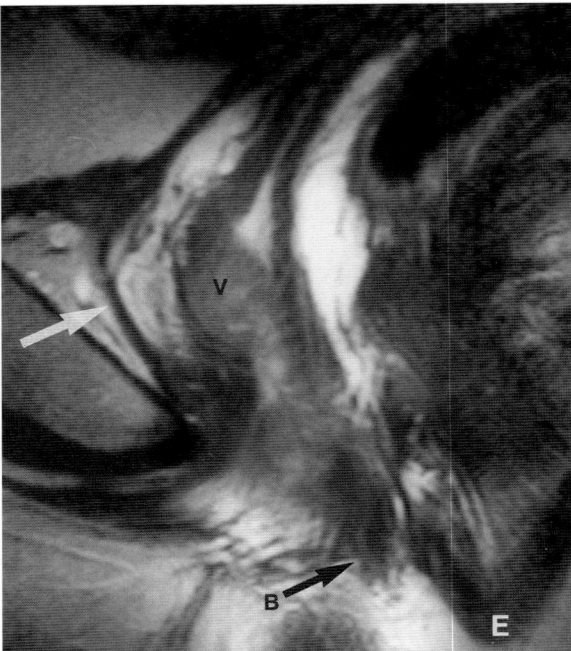

Fig. 1.24. Endovaginal parasagittal oblique T2-weighted turbo spin-echo parallel to the vaginal axis (*white arrow* pubovesicalis, *V* vagina). The bulbospongiosus (*B*) and external anal sphincter (*E*) course to the midline perineal body. Reprinted with permission from TAN et al. (1998)

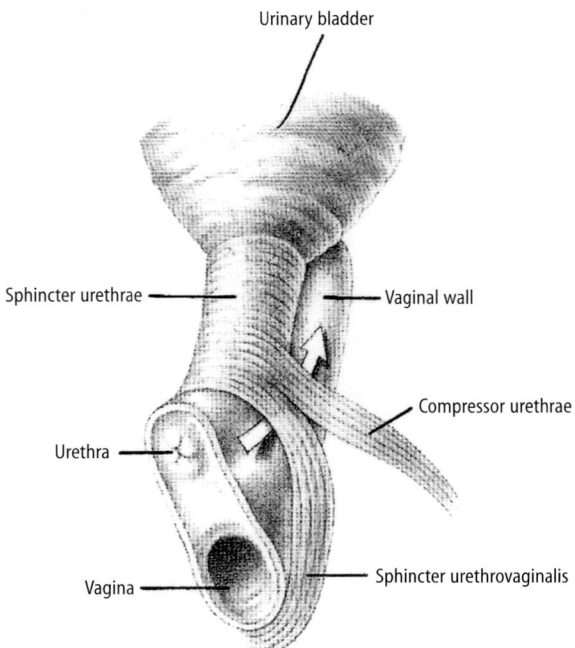

Fig. 1.25. Urethrovaginal sphincter, compressor urethrae and urethral sphincter (sphincter urethrae). Reprinted from BANNISTER et al. (1995, p. 834), by permission of Churchill Livingstone

a close relationship but no direct attachments to the urethra. Contraction of this muscle has an occlusive effect on the urethra to a certain extent and is considered important in the quick stop of micturition (MYERS et al. 2000).

At the inferior half of the urethra, striated muscle has been identified forming two elements: compressor urethrae and urethrovaginal sphincter, formerly considered part of the deep transverse perineal muscle (OELRICH 1983) (Fig. 1.25). The slow-twitch fibres compressor urethrae arises with a small tendon from the ischiopubic rami, forming a broad arching muscular sheet with the contralateral counterpart. The most anterior part is in the midline ventral to the urethra. It has been described as being below the sphincter urethrae and has been reported to be approximately 6 mm wide (OELRICH 1983). The superior edge lies within the urogenital hiatus of the pelvic diaphragm and is continuous with the lower fibres of the anterior rhabdosphincter. The compressor urethrae compresses the urethra. As it is orientated at an angle of 130° to the urethra, it can pull the external meatus inferiorly (OELRICH 1983). This, in combination with bladder elevation by other pelvic floor structures (levator ani) will elongate the urethra. Visualization of the compressor urethrae at MRI is not fully elucidated. A sling-like structure can be identified, although this has a relatively superior position and also has been identified as the pubovesical muscle (TUNN et al. 2001) (Figs. 1.4, 1.8, 1.21). Other striated muscle fibres encircle the vagina, forming the urethrovaginal sphincter (Fig. 1.25). The urethrovaginal sphincter can be identified as a low signal intensity fibrous structure at MRI (TAN et al. 1998) (Fig. 1.26). This structure is a thin flat muscle up to 5 mm wide that blends anteriorly with the compressor urethrae. Posterior fibres may extend to the perineal body. Both the compressor urethrae and the urethrovaginal sphincter are variable in form and presence. The distal part of the urethra is closely related to the bulbospongiose muscles. MRI studies have confirmed the close anterior relationship of the urethrovaginal sphincter and the compressor urethrae presenting a more or less anterior sheet (TAN et al. 1998) (Figs. 1.20, 1.24).

1.3.5 Uterus and Vagina

The uterus is a midline visceral organ, pear-shaped and mainly horizontal in orientation. The upper two-

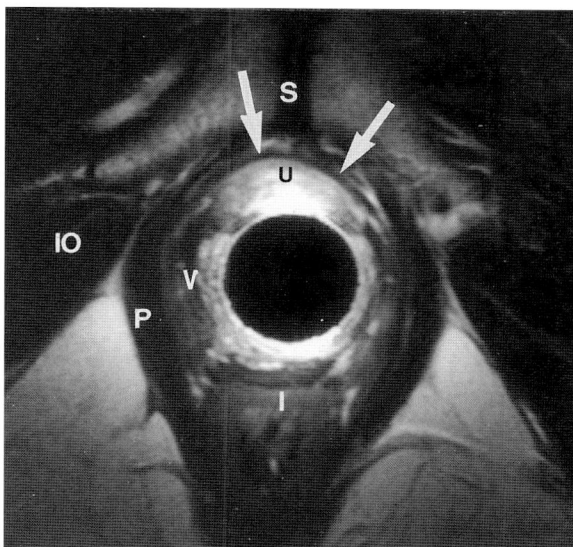

Fig. 1.26. Endovaginal axial oblique T2-weighted turbo spin-echo (*S* pubic symphysis, *white arrows* urethrovaginal sphincter, *U* external urethral meatus, *V* vaginal wall, *P* pubovisceralis, *I* internal anal sphincter, *IO* internal obturator). Reprinted with permission from TAN et al. (1998)

taining anteversion of the uterus. The endopelvic fascia covering the parametrium is continuous with the endopelvic fascia supporting the paracolpium and has been indicated as level I vaginal support (DELANCEY 1993) (Figs. 1.6, 1.22).

The second level of support is at the uterine cervix and primarily concerns the uterosacral and cardinal ligaments. The uterosacral ligaments are attached to the posterolateral aspect of the cervix, form the lateral margins of the pouch of Douglas and insert fan-like at the presacral fascia at the level of the second to fourth sacral foramen. The cardinal ligament arises from the area of the greater sciatic foramen and courses to the uterine cervix. Both the cardinal and sacrouterine ligaments surround the cervix forming a pericervical ring and have attachments to the bladder base. The ligaments also envelop the superior part of the vagina. Both ligaments have a vertical orientation, suspending the cervix and upper vagina and act as a single unit (DELANCEY 1994a). The cardinal ligaments comprise perivascular connective tissue and the sacrouterine ligaments are predominantly smooth muscle and connective tissue (DELANCEY and RICHARDSON 1992).

One level inferiorly, support is given by several structures. The cardinal and sacrouterine ligaments have downward extensions forming the pubocervical fascia and rectovaginal fascia, both with attachment to the pelvic side wall (DELANCEY 1988; DELANCEY 1994a). These fasciae (all part of the endopelvic fascia) act as a single unit, just as the sacrouterine and cardinal ligaments. The fasciae give lateral support and have been indicated as level II support (DELANCEY 1993). The anteromedial part of the vagina is suspended by the pubocervical fascia. This fascia is embedded with smooth muscles fibres and is attached to the arcus tendineus fascia pelvis. The attachment of the anterior vaginal wall to the tendineus arcs at both sides forms a supportive "hammock" of vaginal tissue and endopelvic fascia underneath the urethra (Fig. 1.22). The rectovaginal fascia of the rectovaginal septum supports the posterior part of the vagina. This septum is a sheet of fibromuscular tissue with an abundant venous supply. The rectovaginal fascia is suspended by attachments to the cardinal and sacrouterine ligaments and is laterally attached to the superior fascia of the pelvic diaphragm (DELANCEY and RICHARDSON 1992). The rectovaginal fascia has attachments to the perineal body. The vagina also has lateral support from the medial part of the levator ani (level III support), just caudal to the arcus tendineus fasciae pelvis (Figs. 1.9, 1.11), and from the perineal membrane (DELANCEY and STARR 1990; DELANCEY 1993, 1994a). This sup-

thirds constitutes the body and the lower one-third the uterine cervix. In general, the cervix is tilted forward from the coronal plane (anteversion), while the body is slightly flexed on the cervix (anteflexion). The uterus is above the pelvic diaphragm.

The vagina transverses the pelvic floor in a sagittal oblique plane, parallel to the pelvic inlet. The vagina is a fibromuscular sheath extending from the uterine cervix to the vestibule. The unstretched length is approximately 7.5 cm anteriorly and 8.5 cm posteriorly. The vagina is lined by stratified squamous epithelium. The mucous coat is corrugated by transverse elevations, the vaginal rugae. The walls are collapsed with the lumen flattened in the anteroposterior plane (H-shape) in the lower third, while the vestibular entrance is a sagittal cleft. The smooth muscle coat primarily has a longitudinal and oblique orientation.

1.3.5.1
Uterus and Vaginal Support

Support to the uterus and vagina artificially can be divided into several levels. The endopelvic fascia covering the parametrium (broad ligament) is the most superior, first layer of pelvic support. The parametrium enveloped by endopelvic fascia gives lateral support. At the anterior side of the parametrium the round ligament gives accessory support in main-port has been described as attachment and has also been identified as a separate part of the levator ani: the pubovaginal muscle. The perineal body and its attachments give inferior support.

1.3.6 Perineum and Ischioanal Fossa

The perineum is the region below the pelvic diaphragm extending to the perineal skin. The region is bordered from anterior to posterior by the pubic arch, the inferior pubic ramus, ischial tuberosity, ischial ramus, sacrotuberous ligament and the coccyx. Often the term perineum is used in a more restrictive manner, indicating the region of the perineal body and overlying skin.

1.3.6.1 Perineal Body

The perineal body (also named the central perineal tendon) is a pyramidal fibromuscular node located at the midline between the urogenital region and the anal sphincter. At this centre numerous striated muscles and fascia converge and interlace: the longitudinal muscle of the anorectum, the pubovaginal (puboprostaticus) part of the pubococcygeus muscle, the perineal membrane, the superficial transverse perineal muscle, the bulbospongiosus and the external anal sphincter (Figs. 1.14, 1.15, 1.18, 1.20). In men, this structure is more like a central point and may be named the central perineal tendon. In women the insertion is larger, and the imbrication of the muscle fibres is more pronounced; therefore, it is often described as the perineal body. The involvement of numerous muscles with their attachments to several parts of the pelvic ring (for example, the anal sphincter is connected to the coccyx by the anococcygeal ligament) gives the perineal body an important function in the complex interaction of the pelvic floor muscles.

1.3.6.2 Ischioanal Fossae

The fat-containing space lying below the levator ani between the pelvic side wall and the anus (Figs. 1.17, 1.27) is properly termed the ischioanal fossa. The ischioanal fossa is a wedge-shaped region, extending from the perineal skin to the under-surface of the pelvic diaphragm. The base of the fossa is at the perineum and the apex is superior. The lateral margin

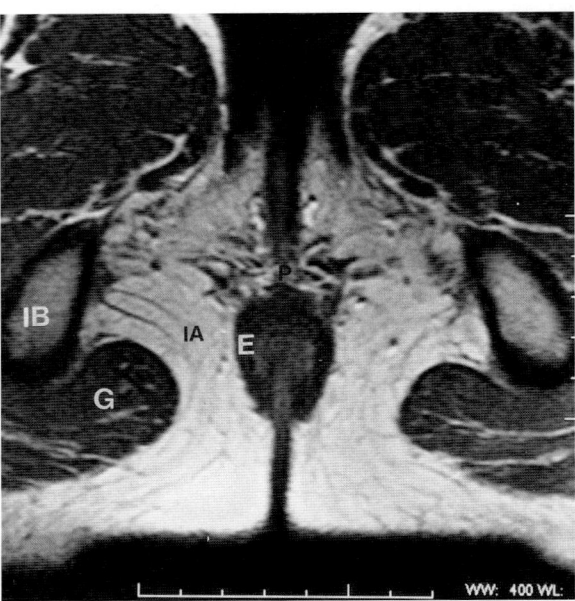

Fig. 1.27. Axial oblique T2-weighted turbo spin-echo through the lower edge of the anal sphincter in a woman (*E* external anal sphincter, *P* perineum, *IA* ischioanal space, *IB* ischial bone, *G* gluteal musculature)

is the internal obturator fascia and posteriorly the fossa is bordered by the gluteus fascia. The anterior margin is the perineal membrane, with a recess at each side extending anteriorly. The ischioanal fossa is lined by the deep perineal fascia. This fascia is attached to the ischiopubic rami, the posterior margin of the perineal membrane and the perineal body. The pudendal canal with the pudendal nerve and vessels lies at the lateral wall of the ischioanal fossa.

1.3.6.3 Perianal Connective Tissue

The superficial perineal fascia envelops a pad of fat tissue filling a large part of the ischioanal space. A network of fibroelastic connective tissue fibres traverses the perianal fat. This arises from the connective tissue within the longitudinal layer (conjoined longitudinal coat) (Haas and Fox 1977) (Fig. 1.28), and permeates through the sphincters, interlacing with each other as well as with the perimysium and endomysium to the pelvic side wall to connect with the caudal levator fascia and to the perianal skin, thus anchoring the anus within the pelvic cavity.

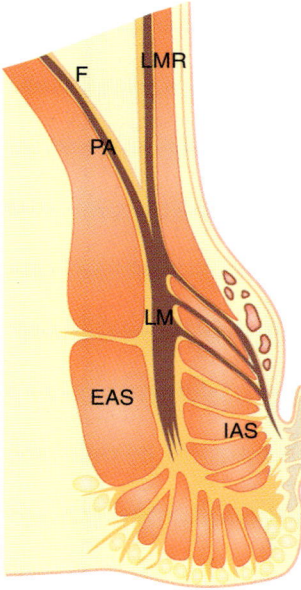

Fig. 1.28. Diagram of the anal sphincter in coronal section showing the contributions of the longitudinal muscle of the rectum (*LMR*), fascia (*F*) and puboanalis (*PA*) to form the longitudinal muscle (*LM*) running between the external anal sphincter (*EAS*) and the internal anal sphincter (*IAS*)

1.3.7
Rectum

The rectum commences where the taeniae coli fuse to form a continuous longitudinal muscular coat. The intraperitoneal rectum is related anteriorly in women to the upper vagina and uterus, and in men to the seminal vesicles with the pouch of Douglas in between. Anterior to the extraperitoneal rectum are the posterior vaginal wall and rectovaginal septum in women and the prostate and seminal vesicles in men. The ampullary portion of the rectum rests on the pelvic diaphragm. At this level the tube turns backward and downward at about a 90° angle at the anorectal junction. The inferior rectum has no mesentery but is enveloped in fat bordered by the mesorectal fascia. The length of the rectum is approximately 12 cm. The rectum has three lateral curves, the rectal valves of Houston, often two on the left and one on the right.

1.3.7.1
Rectal Wall

The epithelium of the upper rectum is continuous with the colon. The lining comprises columnar cells, goblet (mucous) cells and microfold cells overlying lymphoid follicles. Within the mucosa are distension-sensitive nerve endings, while in the muscular wall nerve endings are more sensitive to the intensity of distension (Hobday et al. 2001). The lining is supported by the lamina propria, composed of connective tissue. Below this layer are the muscularis mucosae (with longitudinal and circular layers) and submucosa.

The muscularis propria of the rectum comprises an outer longitudinal layer and an inner circular layer. This layer is uniform except for some thickening of the longitudinal layer anteriorly and posteriorly (anterior and posterior bands). The inner circular layer thickens at the anorectal junction, forming the internal sphincter. The longitudinal layer continues as the longitudinal layer of the anal sphincter. Some anterior fibres of the longitudinal layer run into the perineal body as the musculus rectourethralis (Bannister et al. 1995).

1.3.7.2
Rectal Support

The rectum is supported by several condensations of the rectal fascia (ligaments) and by the pelvic floor. The rectum is surrounded by fat and the mesorectal fascia. It is fixed to the sacrum posteriorly by the presacral fascia (fascia of Waldeyer). Lateral condensations of the endopelvic fascia, as also present at the bladder and vagina, give lateral support: the lateral rectal ligaments (or pillars). The lateral ligaments course from the posterolateral pelvic wall at the level of the third sacral vertebra to the rectum. The ligaments have a divergent spiral course, being posterior at the rectosigmoid junction and anterolateral at the lower third of the rectum (Muntean 1999). Within these ligaments run nerves and the middle rectal vessels. The lateral ligaments divide the loose connective tissue-containing pelvirectal space in an anterior and posterior region. In men, the posterior layer of the rectovesical fascia is continuous with the prostatic fascia and the peritoneum of the rectovesical pouch (prostatoperitoneal membrane, Denonvilliers' fascia) giving some anterior support (Muntean 1999). In women the rectovaginal fascia gives anterior support.

1.3.7.3
Neurovascular Supply of the Rectum

The arterial supply of the rectal mucosal membrane is by the superior rectal branch of the inferior mesenteric artery (hindgut artery), with arterial supply also to the superior anal sphincter. The muscularis propria also receives branches of the middle rectal artery, coursing through the lateral rectal ligament. Small branches of the median sacral artery are also part of the arterial supply of the posterior rectum and anorectal junction (LAST 1978; BANNISTER et al. 1995). Venous return follows the arterial supply, although there is an extensive anastomosis between the venous tributaries. Lymphatic drainage follows the arterial sources of supply. The superior rectal vessels are enveloped in a sheet, the fascia of Waldeyer. There are above the level of the pelvic floor at both sides of the rectum condensations of areolar tissue, the lateral ligament (pillar). These condensations include the middle rectal artery and branches of the pelvic plexuses.

The nerve supply of the rectum is by the autonomic system. Sympathetic supply is by branches of the superior hypogastric plexus and by fibres accompanying the inferior mesenteric and superior rectal arteries from the coeliac plexus. Parasympathetic (motor) supply is from S2–S4 to the inferior hypogastric plexuses by the nervi erigentes. These fibres give sensory supply (crude sensation and pain) and have a role in discriminating between flatus and faeces.

1.3.8
Anal Sphincter

The anal sphincter envelops the anal canal, and is tilted anteriorly in the sagittal plane with the cranial part forward. The canal is 4–6 cm (average 5 cm) in length (ROCIU et al. 2000; BEETS-TAN et al. 2001).

The anal sphincter is composed of several cylindrical layers (Fig. 1.18). The innermost layer is the subepithelium that seals off the anal canal (anal cushions) (GIBBONS et al. 1986). The next layer is the cylindrical smooth muscle of the internal sphincter, often separated from the longitudinal layer by a thin fat-containing layer that represents the surgical intersphincteric space. The outermost layer is the striated muscle of the external sphincter. The cranial part of the external sphincter is fused with the puborectalis (Fig. 1.29). The sphincter is surrounded by the ischioanal fossae. The anococcygeal ligament lies posteriorly in the midline and attaches the external sphincter to the coccyx (Figs. 1.18, 1.30). The anococcygeal raphe is superior to this ligament.

1.3.8.1
Lining of the Anal Canal

The lining of the anal canal varies according to embryological origin. There is variation in the relative contribution between the various linings in individuals and a transitional zone is present (FENGER 1988).

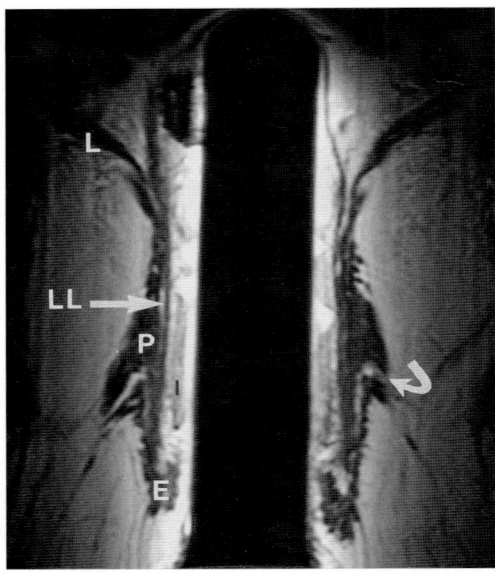

Fig. 1.29. Endoanal coronal oblique T2-weighted turbo spin-echo at the midanal canal in a 45-year old man (posterior to Fig. 1.33) (*I* internal sphincter with some internal haemorrhoids at the upper half of the sphincter, *LL* longitudinal layer in the intersphincteric space, *E* external sphincter, *P* pubovisceralis (puborectalis), *L* levator ani (iliococcygeus) muscle). Note the close relationship of the deep part of the external sphincter and the puborectalis (*curved arrow*)

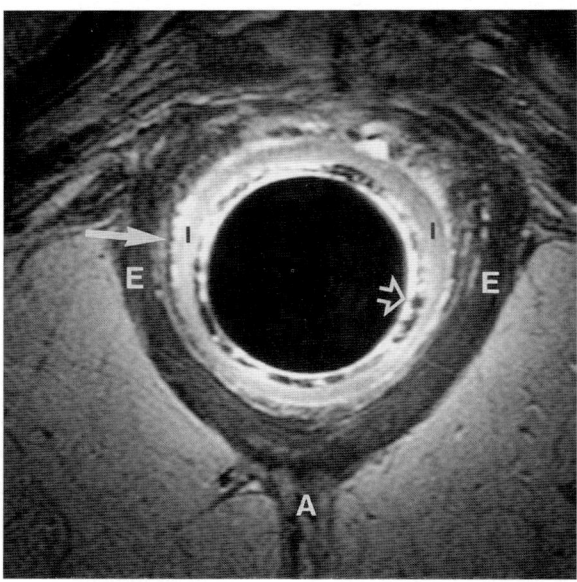

Fig. 1.30. Endoanal axial oblique T2-weighted turbo spin-echo in a male volunteer (superior to Fig. 1.18) (*open arrow* mucosa/submucosa with hypointense submucosal muscularis ani, *I* internal anal sphincter, *white arrow* intersphincteric space with the relatively hypointense longitudinal muscle, *E* external sphincter, *A* anococcygeal ligament). The external anal sphincter shortest longitudinal dimension is anterior, and at this level, the ring is incomplete anteriorly (see also Fig. 1.33)

The upper part of the anus is lined by mucosa that is colonic in type. The uppermost part still has muscularis mucosae so that there is a true submucosa present, but there is no muscularis in most of the canal, so that "subepithelium" is used. The mucosa is arranged into six to ten vertical folds, called the anal columns, which are separated by grooves (WOODBURNE 1983). A small crescentic mucous fold, the anal valves, join the caudal ends of each column. The submucosal anal glands open just above the valves. The valves are situated at the dentate line, which may represent the junction of the endoderm and ectoderm (anal membrane), although this is disputed.

The anal cushions are three specialized vascular engorgements of the submucosa that act as seals for the anal canal. The lining directly below the anal columns is smooth hairless skin of the about 1 cm wide transitional zone, the dentate line. The dentate line separates the neurovascular supply of the upper and lower part of the anus; above is autonomic, below is somatic. There is a portosystemic venous connection at this level. The lining is nonkeratinized cuboidal epithelium and this region is richly supplied with sensory nerve endings (both free and organized nerve endings), important in the continence mechanism (FENGER 1988). The lowest part of the anal canal is lined by keratinized stratified squamous epithelium with underlying subcutis with sweet and sebaceous glands similar to and continuous with the perianal dermis.

The muscularis submucosae ani is derived from the longitudinal muscle and forms a thin band of smooth muscle in the subepithelial layer. Fibres are orientated downwards towards the dentate line and are not seen in the lower canal.

1.3.8.2
Internal Sphincter

The internal sphincter is the continuation of the circular layer of the muscularis propria of the rectum. This layer increases in thickness below the anorectal junction to form the circular internal sphincter. The internal sphincter is approximately 2.8 mm thick on endoluminal imaging (ROCIU et al. 2000) (Figs. 1.18, 1.29, 1.30). The inferior border of the internal sphincter is approximately 1 cm above the inferior edge of the sphincter complex (i.e. inferior edge of the external sphincter). On MRI with a T2-weighted sequence the internal sphincter appears as a relatively hypertense circular structure with a homogeneous, uniform architecture (Fig. 1.18).

1.3.8.3
Intersphincteric Space

The intersphincteric space, is the plane of surgical dissection between the sphincters. This is presumed to be the thin sheet of fat containing loose areolar tissue seen as a bright line on T2-weighted MRI (Figs. 1.18, 1.29). It lies either between the internal sphincter and the longitudinal layer, or between this layer and the external sphincter, or both. The width of this space varies considerably.

1.3.8.4
Longitudinal Layer

In the last decade several studies have increased our understanding of the complex anatomy of the longitudinal layer (LUNNISS and PHILLIPS 1992). The longitudinal layer (conjoint longitudinal layer, or longitudinal muscle) is the continuation of the smooth muscle longitudinal layer of the rectum, with striated muscles from the levator ani, particularly the puboanalis (LUNNISS and PHILLIPS 1992), and a large fibroelastic element derived from the endopelvic fascia.

The layer is 2.5 mm thick (ROCIU et al. 2000). Cranially it is predominantly muscular, and fibroelastic caudally. The fibroelastic tissue forms a network throughout the sphincter, and passes through the subcutaneous external sphincter as bundles or fibres to insert into the perianal skin. Some fibres running into the lower canal have been considered to form the corrugator cutis ani, though this is disputed, as is even the existence of any such muscle (LUNNISS and PHILLIPS 1992; BANNISTER et al. 1995). On T2-weighted MRI the longitudinal muscle layer is seen as a relatively hypointense layer within the hyperintense intersphincteric space (Figs. 1.18, 1.29, 1.30), with its termination into multiple bundles in the lower sphincter visible on MRI.

1.3.8.5
External Anal Sphincter

The external sphincter envelops the intersphincteric space and represents the inferior outer aspect of the anal sphincter. The external sphincter is approximately 2.7 cm high, while it is shorter anteriorly in women, approximately 1.5 cm (ROCIU et al. 2000). The lateral part of the external sphincter is approximately 2.7 cm high. The external sphincter has a thickness of 4 mm on endoluminal imaging. The external sphincter extends approximately 1 cm beyond the internal sphincter (Figs. 1.29, 1.31–1.33). The muscle is a stri-

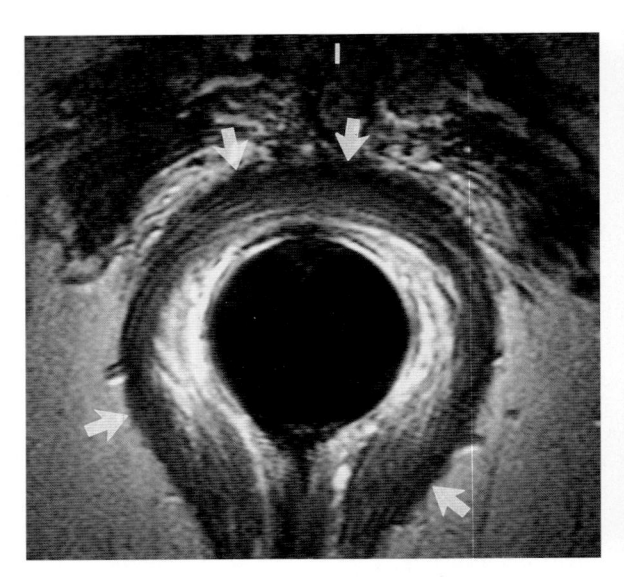

Fig. 1.31. Endoanal axial oblique T2-weighted turbo spin-echo in a woman through the lower aspect of the external sphincter (*arrows*) with a complete anterior ring (*I* vaginal introitus)

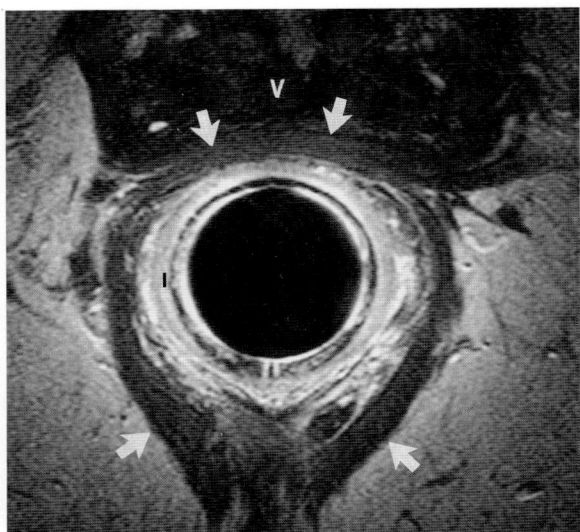

Fig. 1.32. Endoanal axial oblique T2-weighted turbo spin-echo through the lower edge of the internal sphincter (*I*) in a woman at a higher level than Fig. 1.31 (*arrows* external sphincter, *V* vagina)

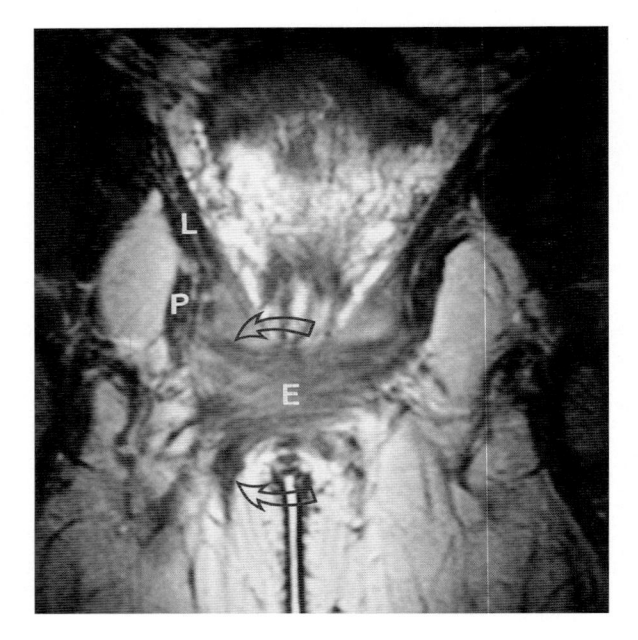

Fig. 1.33. Endoanal coronal oblique T2-weighted turbo spin-echo anterior to Fig. 1.29, through the anterior part of the external anal sphincter. Note that the external sphincter is shorter anteriorly (*E*) than laterally (*curved arrows*) (*P* pubovisceralis, *L* levator ani)

ated muscle under voluntary control and comprises predominantly slow-twitch muscle fibres, capable of prolonged contraction. There is with increasing age a shift towards more type II (rapid) fibres (LIERSE et al. 1993). The action of the external sphincter is voluntary closure and reflex closure of the anal canal and it contributes to the sphincter tonus to some extent.

The concept of the anatomy of the external sphincter with respect to the pubovisceral (puborectal/puboanal) muscle has changed over time (MILLIGAN and MORGAN 1934; GOLIGHER 1967; OH and KARK 1972). Some consider the external sphincter to constitute the complete or largest part of the outer cylinder of the anal sphincter. The pubovisceral (puborectal/puboanal) muscle is described as being present at the level of the anorectal junction or most superior part of the anal sphincter. These concepts are based on findings at dissection and at surgery. Imaging studies, especially endoluminal MRI, have supported the concept that the pubovisceral (puborectal) muscle comprises approximately the upper outer half of the anal sphincter (HUSSAIN et al. 1995; ROCIU et al. 2000) (Figs. 1.29, 1.34). The pubovisceral muscle forms a sling around the upper half. Because of the sling-form no striated muscle is present anteriorly at this level. The pubovisceral (puboanal) muscle can be separated from the external sphincter muscle on imaging (MRI, endosonography) and cadaver studies (HUSSAIN et al. 1995; ROCIU et al. 2000; FUCINI et al. 1999) (Fig. 1.29).

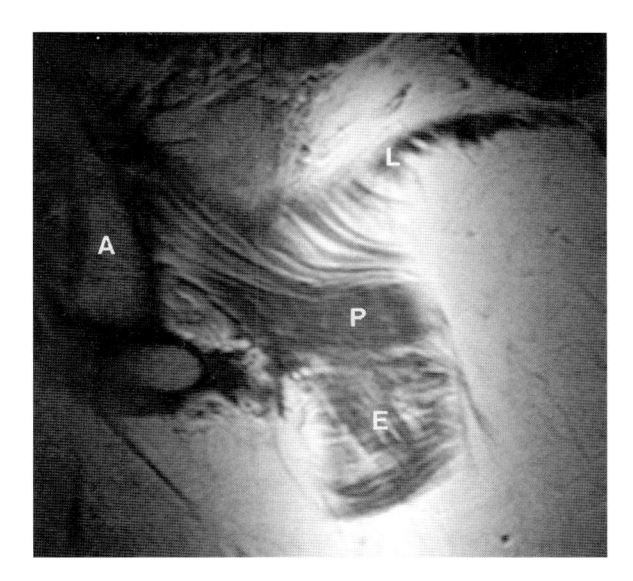

Fig. 1.34. Endoanal parasagittal oblique T2-weighted turbo spin-echo in a male volunteer. Note the difference in orientation of the external sphincter (E) and pubovisceralis (P) (A anterior, L levator ani)

In the literature the external sphincter is often described as subdivided in the coronal plane: the subcutaneous, superficial and deep part. However, this concept is not supported by all studies and also single-layer and bilayer concepts have been described as well as a triple-loop concept (BANNISTER et al. 1995; GOLIGHER 1967; OH and KARK 1972; SHAFIK 1975; GARAVOGLIA et al. 1993; BOGDUK 1996). MRI studies have identified different aspects of the external sphincter at certain levels, which to some extent supports a multilayer anatomy (ROCIU et al. 2000). Clefts between parts of the external sphincter can be identified at MRI in some individuals, although often only several bundles (also more than three) can be identified without clear clefts. The external sphincter has posterior fibres continuous with the anococcygeal ligament. Some of the anterior fibres decussate into the superficial transverse perineal muscle and perineal body. The deep part of the external sphincter is intimately related to the puborectal muscle (Fig. 1.29).

1.3.8.6
Pubovisceral (Puborectal) Muscle

The pubovisceral part of the levator ani comprises the puborectalis, and pubococcygeus. The pubovisceral (puborectal) muscle is approximately 2.8 cm high and 5.6 mm thick when measured on endoanal MRI (ROCIU et al. 2000) (Fig. 1.29). The sling-like puborectalis has a somewhat tilted transverse orientation with the open ends attached to the pubic bone (see section 1.3.2.2 Pelvic Diaphragm) (Fig. 1.35). The puborectalis displays some resting tone, but contracts rapidly in response to any sudden increase in intraabdominal pressure to prevent incontinence. The urogenital hiatus with urethra, vagina and anus and supportive structures is bordered and supported by the puborectalis (see section 1.3.2.2 Pelvic Diaphragm).

1.3.8.7
Anal Sphincter Support

The anal sphincter has numerous attachments. For anterior support the perineal body and its attachments are important, as well as other supportive structures in the anovaginal septum in females and the Denonvilliers' fascia in males. Lateral support is given by the levator ani muscle (pubovisceral muscle) and superficial transverse perineal muscle. Posterior support is given by the attachment of the anococcygeal ligament to the coccyx and superiorly by the continuity with the rectum. The fibroelastic network surrounding and involving the anal sphincter gives more general support.

1.3.8.8
Anal Sphincter Anatomy Variance and Ageing

Normal variants of anal sphincter anatomy have been identified, such as differing relationships between the superficial transverse perineal muscle and the exter-

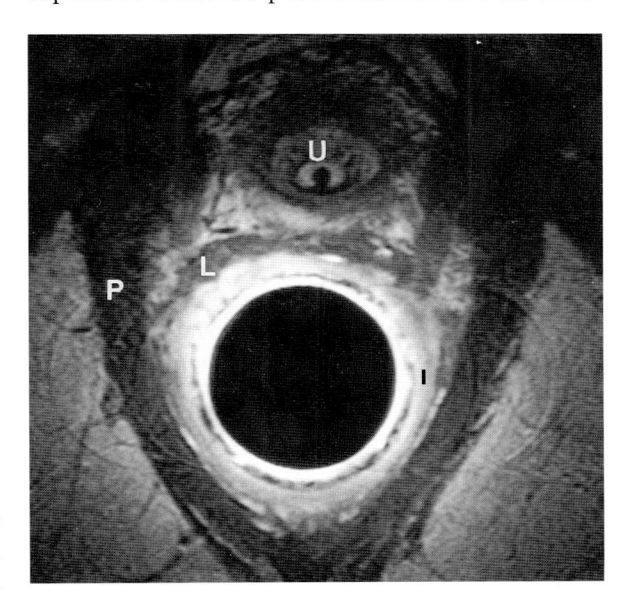

Fig. 1.35. Endoanal axial oblique T2-weighted turbo spin-echo in a male volunteer (superior to Fig. 1.30) (P pubovisceralis, L longitudinal layer, I internal sphincter, U urethra)

nal sphincter (HAAS and FOX 1977). The inferior edge of the external sphincter may have a closed circular configuration or may be open anteriorly and posteriorly. After trauma (e.g. obstetric), the anal sphincter anatomy may be disturbed without clinical symptoms. These findings may possibly be related to late-onset incontinence.

Sex-related differences include a significantly shorter external sphincter in women than in men, especially anteriorly. The central perineal tendon in men is a central muscular insertion point; in women, it represents an area where muscle fibres imbricate. The external sphincter has a more horizontal orientation in women. In women, the longitudinal muscle terminates just cranial to the external sphincter, whereas in men it extends to the caudal part of the external sphincter. The superficial transverse perineal muscle is close to the external sphincter, and their relationship in the craniocaudal direction is different between the sexes. In women, the superficial transverse perineal muscle is directly superior to the external sphincter, often with some overlap (Fig. 1.20). In men, the superficial perineal muscle is directly anterior to the external sphincter. The central perineal tendon is an insertion common to all the striated muscles, which anchors the anal sphincter to the surrounding structures (superficial transverse perineal muscle, bulbospongiosus muscle, urogenital diaphragm). In men, this structure is more like a central point, whereas in women this insertion is larger, and the imbrication of the muscle fibres is more pronounced; therefore, it is often described as the perineal body.

Age-related variations included a significant decrease in the thickness of the longitudinal muscle and an increase in the thickness of the internal sphincter in both sexes (ROCIU et al. 2000). A decrease in the thickness of the external sphincter in men with age has been demonstrated. In females this is also most likely in normal ageing, however when coinciding with external sphincter defects this may lead to incontinence. No significant age-related differences in the lengths of the anal canal, external sphincter, and puborectalis are found.

1.3.8.9
Neurovascular Supply of the Anal Sphincter

The arterial, venous, lymphatic and nerve supply of the superior two-thirds of the anus (hindgut origin) is different from the inferior one-third (proctoderm origin) (MOORE and PERSAUD 1998). The arterial supply of the superior two-thirds is mainly by the inferior rectal artery, a branch of the inferior mesenteric artery (hindgut artery). Small branches of the median sacral artery also are part of the arterial supply of the posterior anorectal junction (BANNISTER et al. 1995; LAST 1978). Venous drainage is by the superior rectal vein, draining to the inferior mesenteric artery. For the inferior one-third of the anus, arterial supply is by inferior rectal branches of the internal pudendal artery and venous drainage by the inferior rectal vein, a tributary of the internal pudendal vein draining into the internal iliac vein. The submucosa of the anal canal is a junction of the portal and systemic venous systems. Longitudinal veins, cross-connecting at the anal valves are connected to the veins of the transitional zone (dentate or pectineal line) and cutis and to radicles crossing the anal sphincters forming the inferior and middle rectal veins draining to the internal iliac vein and inferior caval vein. Ascending mucosal veins will drain into the superior rectal vein and portal system.

The lymphatics of the (cloacal) anus primarily follow the supplying and draining vessels, especially the superior rectal vessels to the inferior mesenteric nodes. Lymphatic drainage of the lowest (proctoderm) part of the anal sphincter is to the superficial inguinal nodes.

The autonomic nerve supply of the internal sphincter is by sympathetic fibres along the superior rectal artery via the inferior pelvic plexus and parasympathetic (inhibitory) fibres through the inferior pelvic plexus and splanchnic nerves (S2–S4). For the function of the internal sphincter, the enteric plexus and associated autonomic and visceral sensory nerves are involved. Afferent impulses (distension) pass through the parasympathetic nerves and pain impulses through sympathetic and parasympathetic nerves (BANNISTER et al. 1995). The external sphincter has nerve supply by the inferior rectal branch of the pudendal nerve (S2, S3) and the perineal branch of the fourth sacral nerve (S4). The puborectalis is supplied by the inferior rectal branch and from the perineal ramus of the fourth sacral nerve. For both external sphincter and puborectalis, regulation is partly reflex (e.g. sudden increase in abdominal pressure) and partly voluntary through the visceral and somatic afferent and somatic efferent nerves. Important for proper function of the anal sphincter is the rich supply of sensory endings at the dentate line and proprioceptive fibres. Motor control and sensory input are processed at several levels of the central nervous system. Nerve supply to the superior two-thirds of the anal lining is by the autonomic nervous system, for the lower part by the inferior rectal nerve.

1.3.9
Nerve Supply of the Pelvic Floor

In this section the main nerve supply of the pelvic floor is described. The specific nerve supply for parts of the pelvic floor has been described in the sections describing these structures. The nerve supply to the pelvic floor and related organs is by branches of the sacral plexus – the pudendal nerve, the perineal branch of S4 and the parasympathetic nervi erigentes – and the sympathetic supply by the hypogastric nerve. Higher regulating levels of the central nervous system (e.g. pontine micturition centre, cerebral cortex) are crucial for proper function of the pelvic floor.

1.3.9.1
Somatic Nerve Supply

The pudendal nerve supplies the majority of the somatic innervation of the pelvic floor region. The pudendal nerve courses through the greater sciatic foramen, travelling dorsal to the ischial spine to the pudendal canal at the lateral side of the ischiorectal fossa (Colleselli et al. 1998). At the level of the pelvic floor the inferior rectal nerve, perineal nerves and the dorsal nerve of the clitoris branch off the pudendal nerve in females. From the terminal branch of the pudendal nerve multiple thin branches run to the external urethral sphincter, entering at the lateral aspect (Colleselli et al. 1998). Other somatic nerves give additional supply. For example, the perineal branch of S4 runs forward on the coccygeus muscle and passes through the pelvic diaphragm between the coccygeus and iliococcygeus muscle. This nerves supplies the perianal skin and gives off branches to the external anal sphincter.

1.3.9.2
Autonomic Nerve Supply

The autonomic nerve supply of the pelvic floor is by the pelvic plexus (inferior hypogastric plexus), receiving sympathetic nerves from the hypogastric nerves and parasympathetic nerves from the pelvic splanchnic nerves. This pelvic plexus is a coarse, flat meshwork, enlarged in places by ganglia. The pelvic plexus is on the pelvic sidewall and within the parietal pelvic fascia. The visceral branches form, together with the arterial and venous supply, neurovascular bundles. These bundles coursing medially having fibrous tissue condensations, forming "ligaments", such as the lateral ligaments of the bladder, cervix and rectum.

The pelvic parasympathetic supply (nervi erigentes) arises from S2–S4. These nerves pass anteriorly towards the pelvic plexus and are distributed along with the sympathetic supply. These fibres travel to the pelvic organs through a sagittal orientated vessel nerve plate between rectum and pelvic wall. Some thin fibres run alongside the lateral vaginal wall to the bladder neck and proximal urethra (Colleselli et al. 1998).

The sympathetic nerves arising from T10–T12 course through the sympathetic chain and preaortic plexus (superior hypogastric plexus) to the hypogastric nerve. The hypogastric nerve gives off somatic branches (lower limb and perineum) to the sacral nerves and visceral branches to the pelvic plexus.

Acknowledgements. Mirjam Evers van Bavel, Astrid Kooren van der Vuurst and Marga Nuberg Post are acknowledged for their secretarial help.

References

Arey LB (1966) Developmental anatomy, 7th edn. Saunders, Philadelphia
Bannister LH, Berry MM, Collins P, Dyson M, Dussek JE, Ferguson MWJ (1995) Gray's anatomy, 38th edn. Churchill Livingstone, New York
Beets-Tan RGH, Morren GL, Beets G, et al (2001) Measurement of anal sphincter muscles: endoanal US, endoanal MR imaging, or phased array MR imaging? A study with healthy volunteers. Radiology 220:81–89
Bogduk N (1996) Issues in anatomy: the external anal sphincter revisited. Aust N Z J Surg 66:626–629
Cardozo L (ed) (1997) Urogynecology. Churchill Livingstone, Edinburgh
Chai TC, Steers WD (1997) Neurophysiology of micturition and continence in women. Int Urogynecol J Pelvic Floor Dysfunct 8:85–97
Colleselli K, Stenszl A, Eder R, Strasser H, Poisel S, Bartsch G (1998) The female urethral sphincter: a morphological and topographical study. J Urol 160:49–54
De Caro R, Aragona F, Herms A, Guidolin D, Brizzi E, Pagano F (1998) Morphometric analysis of the fibroadipose tissue of the female pelvis. J Urol 160:707–713
DeLancey JOL (1988) Structural aspects of the extrinsic continence mechanism. Obstet Gynecol 72:296–301
DeLancey JOL (1993) Anatomy and biomechanics of genital prolapse. Clin Obstet Gynecol 36:897–909
DeLancey JOL (1994a) Functional anatomy of the female pelvis. In: Kursh ED, McGuire EJ (eds) Female urology, 1st edn. Lippincott, Philadelphia
DeLancey JOL (1994b) Structural support of the urethra as it relates to stress urinary incontinence: the hammock hypothesis. Am J Obstet Gynecol 170:1713–1723
DeLancey JOL, Richardson AC (1992) Anatomy of genital support. In: Benson JT (ed) Female pelvic floor disorders: investigation and management, 1st edn. Norton Medical Books, New York

DeLancey JOL, Starr RA (1990) Histology of the connection between the vagina and levator ani muscles. Implications for urinary tract function. J Reprod Med 35:765–771

Dorschner W, Biesold M, Schmidt F, Stolzenburg JU (1999) The dispute about the external sphincter and the urogenital diaphragm. J Urol 162:1942–1945

Fenger C (1988) Histology of the anal canal. Am J Surg Pathol 12:41–55

Fucini C, Elbetti C, Messerini L (1999) Anatomic plane of separation between external anal sphincter and puborectalis muscle. Clinical implications. Dis Colon Rectum 42:374–379

Garavoglia M, Borghi F, Levi AC (1993) Arrangement of the anal striated musculature. Dis Colon Rectum 36:10–15

Gibbons CP, Trowbridge EA, Bannister JJ, Read NW (1986) Anal cushions. Lancet 8486:886–887

Gilpin SA, Gosling JA (1983) Smooth muscle in the wall of the developing human urinary bladder and urethra. J Anat 137:503–512

Goligher J (1967) Surgery of the anus, rectum and colon, 2nd edn. Baillière Tindall, London

Haas PA, Fox TA (1977) The importance of the perianal connective tissue in the surgical anatomy and function of the anus. Dis Colon Rectum 20:303–313

Hamilton WJ, Mossman HW (1972) Hamilton, Boyd and Mossman's human embryology, 4th edn. Williams and Wilkins, Baltimore

Hobday DI, Aziz Q, Thacker N, Hollander I, Jackson A, Thompson DG (2001) A study of the cortical processing of anorectal sensation using functional MRI. Brain 124:361–368

Hussain SM, Stoker J, Laméris JS (1995) Anal sphincter complex: endoanal MR imaging of normal anatomy. Radiology 197:671–677

Lansman HH, Robertson EG (1992) Evolution of the pelvic floor. In: Benson JT (ed) Female pelvic floor disorders: investigation and management, 1st edn. Norton Medical Books, New York

Last RJ (1978) Anatomy. Regional and applied, 6th edn. Churchill Livingstone, Edinburgh

Li L, Li Z, Huo HS, Wang HZ, Wang LY (1992) Sensory nerve endings in the puborectalis and anal region of the fetus and newborn. Dis Colon Rectum 35:552–559

Lierse W, Holschneider AM, Steinfeld J (1993) The relative proportions of type I and type II muscle fibres in the external sphincter ani muscle at different ages and stages of development – observations on the development of continence. Eur J Pediatr Surg 3:28–32

Lunniss PJ, Phillips RKS (1992) Anatomy and function of the anal longitudinal muscle. Br J Surg 79:882–884

Mauroy B, Goullet E, Stefaniak X, Bonnal JL, Amara N (2000) Tendinous arch of the pelvic fascia application to the technique of paravaginal colposuspension. Surg Radiol Anat 22:73–79

Milligan ETC, Morgan CN (1934) Surgical anatomy of the anal canal. Lancet 2:1150–1156

Moore K, Persaud TVN (1998) The developing human: clinically oriented embryology, 6th edn. Saunders, Philadelphia

Muntean V (1999) The surgical anatomy of the fasciae and the fascial spaces related to the rectum. Surg Radiol Anat 21:319–324

Myers RP, Cahill DR, Kay PA, et al (2000) Puboperineales: muscular boundaries of the male urogenital hiatus in 3D from magnetic resonance imaging. J Urol 164:1412–1415

Nievelstein RAJ, van der Werff JFA, Verbeek FJ, et al (1998) Normal and abnormal development of the anorectum in human embryos. Teratology 57:70–78

Norton PA (1993) Pelvic floor disorders: the role of fascia and ligaments. Clin Obstet Gynecol 36:926–938

Oelrich TM (1983) The striated urogenital muscle in the female. Anat Rec 205:223–232

Oh C, Kark AE (1972) Anatomy of the external anal sphincter. Br J Surg 1972:717–723

Papa Petros PE (1998) The pubourethral ligaments. An anatomical and histological study in the live patient. Int Urogynecol 9:154–157

Rociu E, Stoker J, Eijkemans MJC, Laméris JS (2000) Normal anal sphincter anatomy and age- and sex-related variations at high spatial resolution endoanal MR imaging. Radiology 217:395–401

Sampselle CM, DeLancey JO (1998) Anatomy of female continence. J Wound Ostomy Continence Nurs 25:63–74

Shafik A (1976) A new concept of the anatomy of the anal sphincter mechanism and the physiology of defecation. III. The longitudinal muscle: anatomy and role in anal sphincter mechanism. Invest Urol 13:271–277

Shafik A (1999) Levator ani muscle: new physioanatomical aspects and role in the micturition mechanism. World J Urol 17:266–273

Strohbehn K, Ellis J, Strohbehn JA, DeLancey JOL (1996) Magnetic resonance imaging of the levator ani with anatomic correlation. Obstet Gynecol 87:277–285

Strohbehn K (1998) Normal pelvic floor anatomy. Obstet Gynecol Clin North Am 25:683–705

Tan IL, Stoker J, Zwamborn AW, Entius KAC, Calame JJ, Laméris JS (1998) Female pelvic floor. Endovaginal MR imaging of normal anatomy. Radiology 206:777–783

Tobias PV, Arnold M (1981) Man's anatomy, 3rd edn. Witwatersrand University Press, Johannesburg

Tunn R, DeLancey JOL, Quint EE (2001) Visibility of pelvic organ support system structures in magnetic resonance images without an endovaginal coil. Am J Obstet Gynecol 184:1156–1163

Van der Werff JFA, Nievelstein RAJ, Brands E, et al (2000) Normal development of the male anterior urethra. Teratology 61:172–183

van Ophoven A, Roth S (1997) The anatomy and embryological origins of the fascia of Denonvilliers: a medico-historical debate. J Urol 157:3–9

Woodburne RT (1983) Essentials of human anatomy, 7th edn. Oxford University Press, New York

2 Functional Anatomy of the Pelvic Floor

J. O. L. DeLancey

CONTENTS

2.1 Introduction 27
2.2 Support of the Pelvic Organs 27
2.2.1 Endopelvic Fascia 28
2.2.2 Uterovaginal Support 29
2.2.3 Apical Prolapse; Uterus or Vaginal Apex 30
2.2.4 Anterior Wall Support and Urethra 30
2.2.5 Posterior Support 31
2.2.6 Levator Ani Muscles 34
2.2.7 Pelvic Floor Muscles and Endopelvic Fascia Interactions 35
2.2.8 Perineal Membrane and External Genital Muscles 35
2.3 Functional Anatomy of the Lower Urinary Tract 35
2.3.1 Bladder 37
2.3.2 Urethra 37
References 38

2.1 Introduction

Pelvic organ prolapse and urinary incontinence are debilitating problems that prevent one in nine women from enjoying a full and active life (Olsen et al. 1997). They arise due to injuries and deterioration of the muscles, nerves and connective tissue that support and control normal pelvic organ function. Although it is clear that incontinence and prolapse increase with age (Olsen et al. 1997), there is no hour during a woman's life when these structures are more vulnerable than during the time a woman delivers a child. Vaginal birth confers a 4- to 11-fold increase in risk of developing pelvic organ prolapse (Mant et al. 1997).

This chapter addresses the functional anatomy of the pelvic floor in women. The anal sphincter and intestinal tract are discussed in Section 4 of this book. This chapter focuses specifically on how the pelvic organs are held in their normal positions and how pelvic visceral function affects urinary continence and prolapse of the vagina and uterus. The basic anatomy of the female pelvic floor is covered in Chapter 1, but short reviews of pertinent material are provided here to assist in orientation before describing the functional aspects of those anatomical structures.

2.2 Support of the Pelvic Organs

The pelvic organs, when removed from the body, exist only as a limp and formless mass. Their shape and position in living women is determined by their attachments to the pubic bones through the muscles and connective tissue of the pelvis. The actions of their sphincters and muscles require connection to the peripheral and central nervous systems. The structures of the pelvic organ supports are important to understanding pelvic floor dysfunction. In this chapter the term pelvic floor is used broadly to include all the structures supporting the abdominal and pelvic cavity rather than the restricted use of this term to refer to the levator ani group of muscles.

The pelvic floor consists of several components lying between the pelvic peritoneum and the vulvar skin. These are (from above downward) the peritoneum, pelvic viscera and endopelvic fascia, levator ani muscles, perineal membrane and external genital muscles. The eventual support for all of these structures comes from their connection to the bony pelvis and its attached muscles. The viscera are often thought of as being supported by the pelvic floor, but are actually a part of it. The viscera play an important role in forming the pelvic floor through their connections to the pelvis by such structures such as the cardinal and uterosacral ligaments.

The phenomenon of prolapse can be understood by analogy (Fig. 2.1). Bonney (1934) pointed out that

---

J. O. L. DeLancey, MD
Norman F. Miller Professor of Gynecology, Department of Obstetrics and Gynecology, L 4000 Women's Hospital, 1500 E. Medical Center Drive, Ann Arbor, MI 48109-0276, USA

the vagina is in the same relationship to the abdominal cavity as the in-turned finger of a surgical glove is to the rest of the glove. If the pressure in the glove is increased, it forces the finger to protrude downwards in the same way that increases in abdominal pressure force the vagina to prolapse. Figure 2.2 demonstrates this phenomenon and the strategies the body uses to prevent prolapse. Figure 2.2a and Fig. 2.2b provide a schematic illustration of this phenomenon of prolapse. In Fig. 2.2c, the lower end of the vagina is held closed by the pelvic floor muscles preventing prolapse by constriction. Figure 2.2d shows suspension of the vagina to the pelvic walls. Figure 2.2e demonstrates that spatial relationships are important. This is a flap valve closure where the suspending fibers hold the vagina in a position against the supporting walls of the pelvis so that increases in pressure force the vagina against the wall, thereby pinning it in place. Vaginal support is a combination of constriction, suspension and structural geometry.

Because the supportive tissues attach the pelvic organs to the pelvic walls, the female pelvis can naturally be divided into anterior and posterior compartments (Fig. 2.3). The levator ani muscles form the bottom of the pelvis. The organs are attached to the levator ani muscles when they pass through the urogenital hiatus and are supported by these connections.

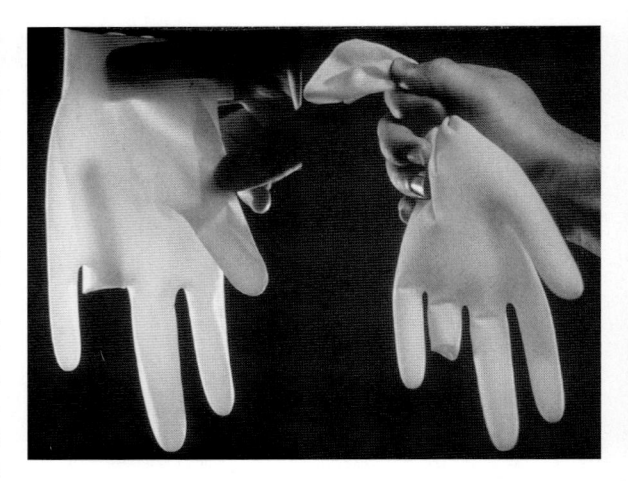

Fig. 2.1. Bonney's analogy of the eversion of an inturned surgical glove finger by increasing pressure in the glove simulating prolapse of the vagina (DeLancey 2002, with permission)

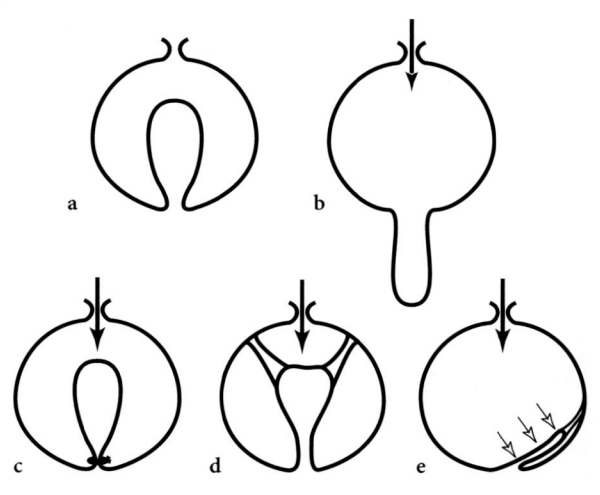

Fig. 2.2a–e. Diagrammatic display of vaginal support strategies. **a** Invaginated area in a surrounding compartment; **b** what happens when the pressure (*arrow*) is increased; **c** muscle action where closing the bottom of the vagina prevents its descent; **d** ligament suspension; **e** flap valve closure where a tethering suspension holds the vagina in such a position where it is pressed against the wall and pinned in place (DeLancey 2002, with permission)

2.2.1
Endopelvic Fascia

On each side of the pelvis the endopelvic fascia attaches the cervix and vagina to the pelvic wall (Fig. 2.4). This fascia forms a continuous sheet-like mesentery – extending from the uterine artery at its cephalic margin to the point at which the vagina fuses with the levator ani muscles below. The part that attaches to the uterus is called the parametrium and that which attaches to the vagina, the paracolpium (DeLancey 1992).

The vagina is attached laterally to the pelvic walls forming a single divider in the middle of the pelvis that determines the nature of prolapse. Cystoceles and rectoceles occur from the front or the back. There are no "laterocles". The division of clinical problems into cystoceles, rectoceles and apical prolapse reflects the nature of these lateral connections. Therefore, there are three types of movement that occur in patients with pelvic organ prolapse: (1) the cervix or vaginal apex can move downward between the anterior and posterior supports; (2) the anterior vaginal wall can protrude through the introitus; and (3) the posterior wall can protrude through the introitus. These different types of support loss arise because of the location of the genital tract's connection to the pelvic sidewall. The location of connective tissue damage determines whether a woman has a cystocele, rectocele, or vaginal vault prolapse, and understanding the different characters of this support helps understand the different types of prolapse that can occur.

Functional Anatomy of the Pelvic Floor

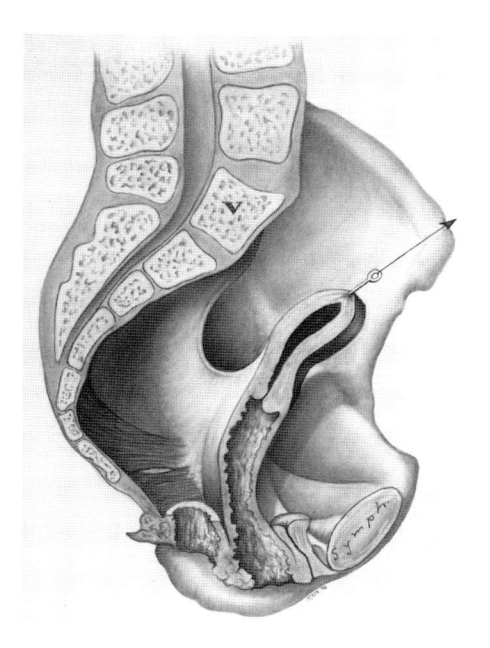

Fig. 2.3. Compartments of the pelvis. The vagina, connected laterally to the pelvic walls, divides the pelvis into an anterior and posterior compartment (DeLancey 1998, with permission; based on Sears 1933)

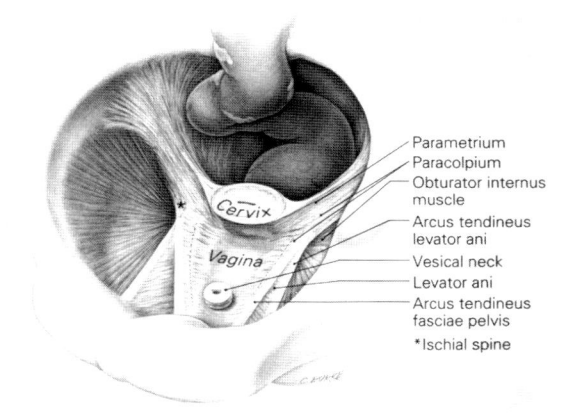

Fig. 2.4. Attachments of the cervix and vagina to the pelvic walls demonstrating different regions of support with the uterus in situ. Note that the uterine corpus and the bladder have been removed (DeLancey 2002, with permission)

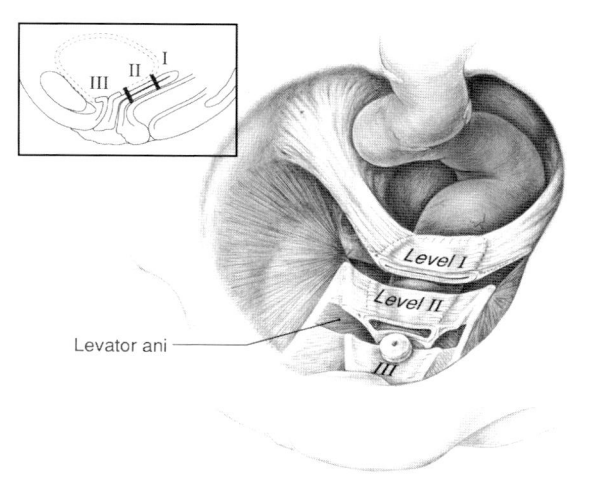

Fig. 2.5. Levels of vaginal support after hysterectomy. *Level I* (suspension) and *level II* (attachment). In *level I* the paracolpium suspends the vagina from the lateral pelvic walls. Fibers of *level I* extend both vertically and also posteriorly towards the sacrum. In *level II* the vagina is attached to the arcus tendineus fasciae pelvis and the superior fascia of levator ani (DeLancey 1992, with permission)

2.2.2
Uterovaginal Support

The attachments of the cervix and uterus to the pelvic walls are comprised of the cardinal and uterosacral ligaments (Campbell 1950; Range and Woodburne 1964), tissues that can be referred to together as the parametrium (Fig. 2.4). This tissue continues downward over the upper vagina to attach it to the pelvic walls and is called the paracolpium here (DeLancey 1992). These tissues provide support for the vaginal apex following hysterectomy (Fig. 2.5). This paracolpium has two portions. The upper portion (level I) consists of a relatively long sheet of tissue that suspends the vagina by attaching it to the pelvic wall whether or not the cervix is present. In the mid-portion of the vagina, the paracolpium attaches the vagina laterally and more directly to the pelvic walls (level II). This attachment stretches the vagina transversely between the bladder and rectum and has functional significance. The structural layer that supports the bladder ("pubocervical fascia") is composed of the anterior vaginal wall and its attachment through the endopelvic fascia to the pelvic wall (Fig. 2.6). It is not a separate layer from the vagina as sometimes inferred, but is a combination of the anterior vaginal wall and its attachments to the pelvic wall.

Similarly, the posterior vaginal wall and endopelvic fascia (rectovaginal fascia) forms the restraining layer that prevents the rectum from protruding forward, blocking formation of a rectocele. In the distal vagina (level III) the vaginal wall is directly attached to surrounding structures without any intervening paracolpium. Anteriorly it fuses with the urethra, posteriorly with the perineal body, and laterally with the levator ani muscles.

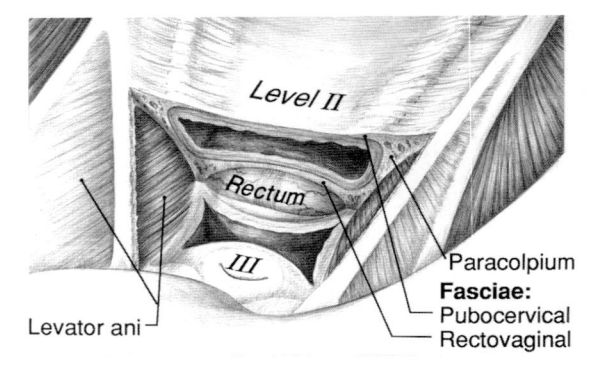

Fig. 2.6. Close-up of the lower margin of *level II* after a wedge of vagina has been removed (*inset*). Note how the anterior vaginal wall, through its connections to the arcus tendineus fascia pelvis, forms a supportive layer clinically referred to as the pubocervical fascia (DeLancey 1992, with permission)

2.2.3
Apical Prolapse; Uterus or Vaginal Apex

One common type of pelvic organ prolapse involves descent of the uterus or the vaginal apex in women that have previously undergone a hysterectomy (Fig. 2.7). The nature of uterine support can be understood when the uterine cervix is pulled downward with a tenaculum during a D&C or pushed downward during a laparoscopy. After a certain amount of descent within the elastic range of the fascia, the parametria become tight and arrest further cervical descent. Similarly, downward descent of the vaginal apex after hysterectomy is resisted by the paracolpia. The fact that these ligaments do not limit the downward movement of the uterus in normal healthy women is attested to by the observation that the cervix may be drawn down to the level of the hymen with little difficulty (Bartscht and DeLancey 1988). The same can be said of the vaginal apex after hysterectomy.

Damage to the upper suspensory fibers of the paracolpium causes uterine or vaginal vault prolapse (Fig. 2.8) and damage to the level II and III supports of the vagina, resulting in cystocele and rectocele. These defects occur in varying combinations and this variation is responsible for the diversity of clinical problems encountered within the overall spectrum of pelvic organ prolapse.

2.2.4
Anterior Wall Support and Urethra

The position and mobility of the anterior vaginal wall, bladder and urethra are important to urinary continence and cystocele (Ala-Ketola 1973). Fluoroscopic examination has shown that the upper urethra and vesical neck are normally mobile structures while the distal urethra remains fixed in position (Muellner 1951; Westby et al. 1982). Both the pelvic floor muscles and the pelvic fasciae therefore, determine the support and fixation of the urethra, and the activity of the muscles has significant impact on urethral support (Miller et. al. 2001).

The anterior vaginal wall and urethra are intimately connected. Failure of this supportive system results in downward descent of the anterior vaginal wall. Their support depends not on attachments of the urethra itself to adjacent structures, but upon the connection of the vagina and periurethral tissues to the muscles and fascia of the pelvic wall (Fig. 2.9). On either side of

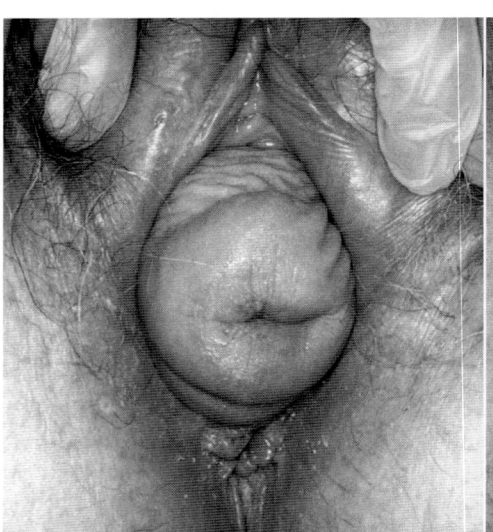

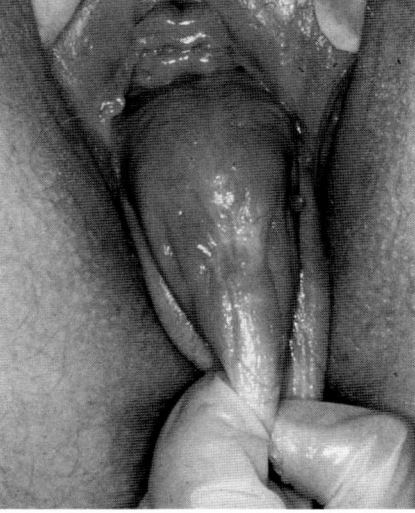

Fig. 2.7. Uterine prolapse (*left*) showing the cervix protruding from the vaginal opening and vaginal prolapse (*right*) where the puckered scar from where the cervix used to be and upper vagina are prolapsed (DeLancey 2002, with permission)

the pelvis, the arcus tendineus fasciae pelvis is found as a band of connective tissue attached at one end to the lower sixth of the pubic bone, 1 cm from the midline, and at the other end to the ischial spine. The anterior portion of this band lies on the inner surface of the levator ani muscle that arises some 3 cm above the arcus tendineus fasciae pelvis.

The layer of tissue that provides urethral support has two lateral attachments; a fascial attachment and a muscular attachment (Fig. 2.9) (DeLancey 1994). The fascial attachment of the urethral supports connects the periurethral tissues and anterior vaginal wall to the arcus tendineus fasciae pelvis and has been called the paravaginal fascial attachments by Richardson et al. (1981). They observed that it is a lateral detachment of the connections of the pubocervical fascia from the pelvic wall that is associated with stress incontinence and cystourethrocele (Fig. 2.10). The muscular attachment connects these same periurethral tissues to the medial border of the levator ani muscle. These attachments allow the levator ani muscle's normal resting tone to maintain the position of the vesical neck, supported by the fascial attachments. When the muscle relaxes at the onset of micturition, it allows the vesical neck to rotate downward to the limit of the elasticity of the fascial attachments, and then contraction at the end of micturition allows it to resume its normal position.

Loss of anterior vaginal support results in what gynecologists call a cystocele or anterior wall prolapse (Fig. 2.11). This can occur either because of lateral detachment of the anterior vaginal wall at the pelvic side wall, referred to as a displacement cystocele, or as a central failure of the wall ("pubocervical fascia") itself that results in a distension cystocele.

The urethral support mechanism influences stress incontinence, not by determining how high or how low the urethra is, but by how it is supported. In examining anatomic specimens, simulated increases in abdominal pressure reveal that the urethra lies in a position where it can be compressed against the supporting hammock by rises in abdominal pressure (Fig. 2.12) (DeLancey 1994). In this hypothesis, it is the stiffness of this supporting layer under the urethra rather than the height of the urethra that would influence stress continence. In an individual with a firm supportive layer the urethra would be compressed between abdominal pressure and pelvic fascia in much the same way that you can stop the flow of water through a garden hose by stepping on it and compressing it against an underlying sidewalk. If, however, the layer under the urethra becomes unstable and does not provide a firm backstop for abdominal pressure to compress the urethra against, the opposing force that causes closure is lost and the occlusive action diminished. This latter situation is similar to trying to stop the flow of water through a garden hose by stepping on it while it lays on soft soil.

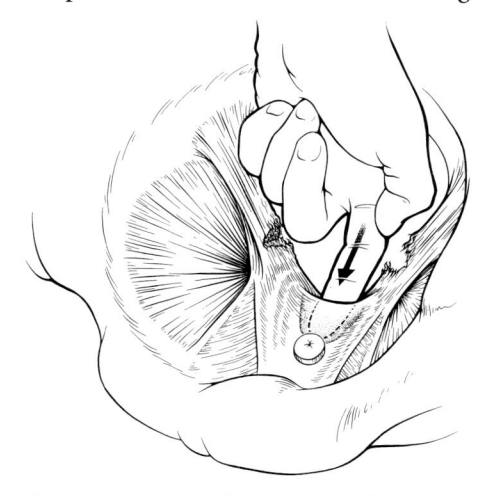

Fig. 2.8. Damage to the suspensory ligaments that can lead to eversion of the vaginal apex when subjected to downward force (DeLancey 2002, with permission)

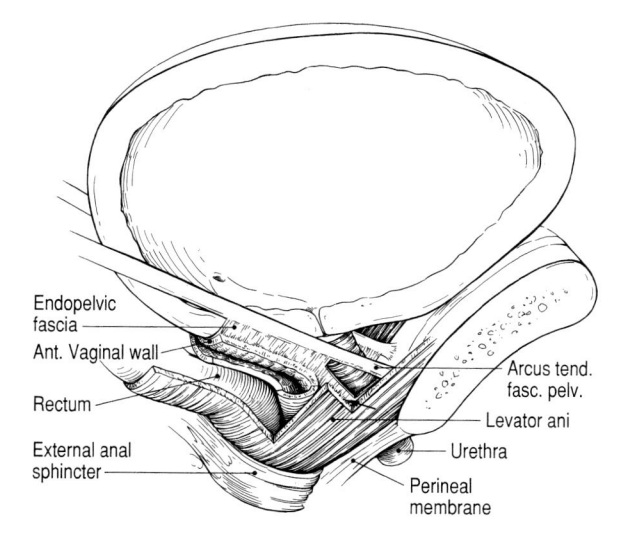

Fig. 2.9. Lateral view of the pelvic floor structures related to urethral support seen from the side in the standing position, cut just lateral to the midline. Note that windows have been cut in the levator ani muscles, vagina, and endopelvic fascia so that the urethra and anterior vaginal walls can be seen (DeLancey 2002, with permission; redrawn after DeLancey 1994)

2.2.5
Posterior Support

The posterior vaginal wall is supported by connections between the vagina, the bony pelvis and the

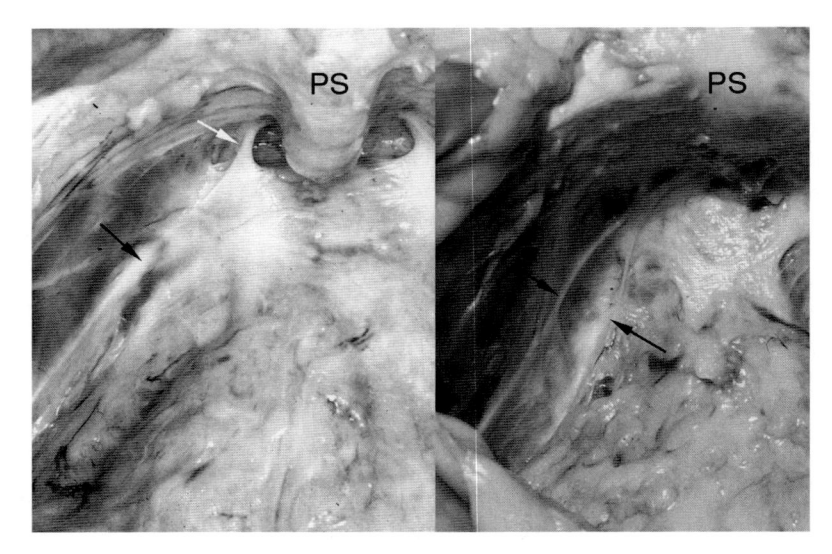

Fig. 2.10. *Left panel* shows normal attachment of the arcus tendineus fascia pelvis to the pubic bone (*white arrow*) showing the arcus tendineus fascia pelvis (*black arrow*). *Right panel* shows a paravaginal defect where the pubocervical fascia has separated from the arcus tendineus (*black arrows* mark the sides of the split) (*PS* pubic symphysis) (DeLancey 2002, with permission)

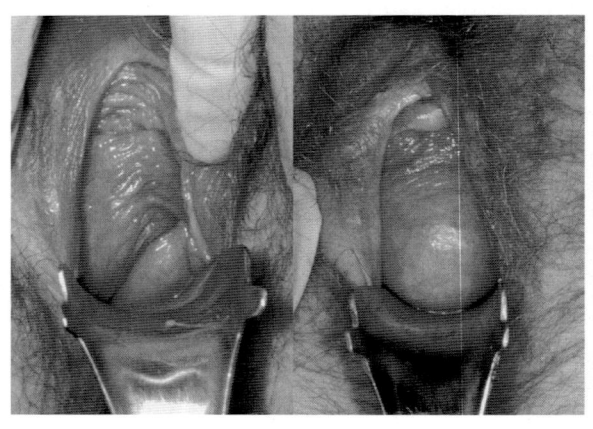

Fig. 2.11. *Left* Displacement cystocele where the intact anterior vaginal wall has prolapsed downward due to paravaginal defect. Note that the right side of the patient's vagina and cervix has descended more than the left because of a larger defect on this side. *Right* Distension cystocele where the anterior vaginal wall fascia has failed and the bladder is distending the mucosa (DeLancey 2002, with permission)

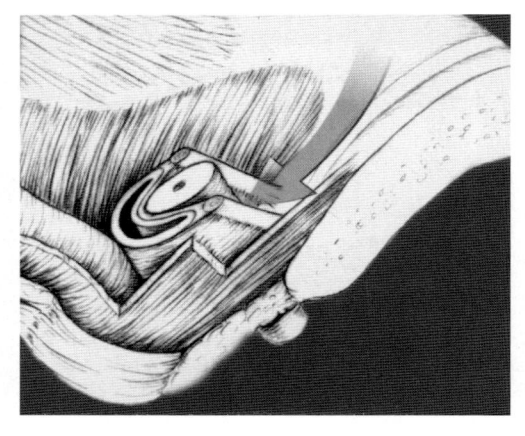

Fig. 2.12. Lateral view of pelvic floor with the urethra, vagina and fascial tissues transected at the level of the vesical neck drawn indicating compression of the urethra by downward force (*arrow*) against the supportive tissues indicating the influence of abdominal pressure on the urethra (DeLancey 1994, with permission)

levator ani muscles (DeLancey 1999). The lower one-third of the vagina is fused with the perineal body (Fig. 2.13). This structure is the attachment between the perineal membranes on either side. This connection prevents downward descent of the rectum in this region. If the fibers that connect one side with the other rupture, then the bowel can protrude downward. (Fig. 2.14)

The mid-posterior vaginal wall is connected to the inside of the levator ani muscles by sheets of endopelvic fascia (Fig. 2.15). These connections prevent the ventral movement of the vagina during increases in abdominal pressure. These paired sheets are sometimes called the rectal pillars. In the upper one-third of the vagina, the vaginal wall is connected laterally by the paracolpium and in this region there is a single attachment for the vagina and there is not a separate system for the anterior and posterior vaginal walls. This is essentially the same support provided by level I.

When abdominal pressure forces the posterior vaginal wall downward towards the introitus, these attachments between the posterior vaginal wall and the levator muscles prevent this downward movement. The uppermost area of the posterior wall is suspended and descent of this area is most closely associated with the clinical problem of enterocele and vaginal vault prolapse. The lateral connections in the mid-vagina hold this portion of the vaginal wall

Functional Anatomy of the Pelvic Floor

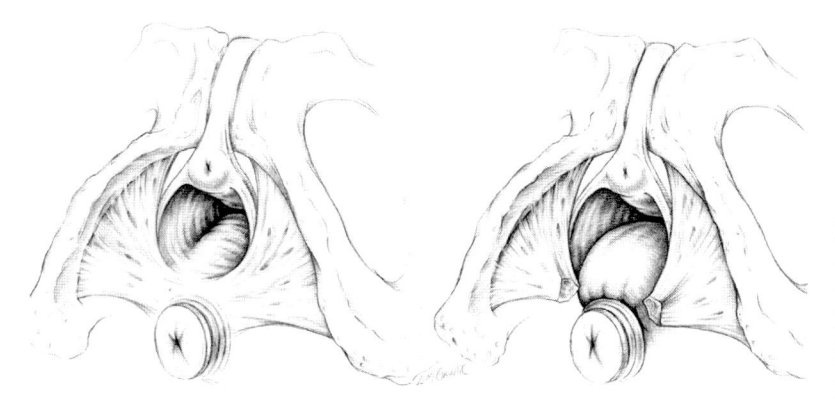

Fig. 2.13. The perineal membrane spans the arch between the ischiopubic rami with each side attached to the other through their connection in the perineal body. Note that separation of the fibers in this area leaves the rectum unsupported and results in a low rectocele (DeLancey 1999, with permission)

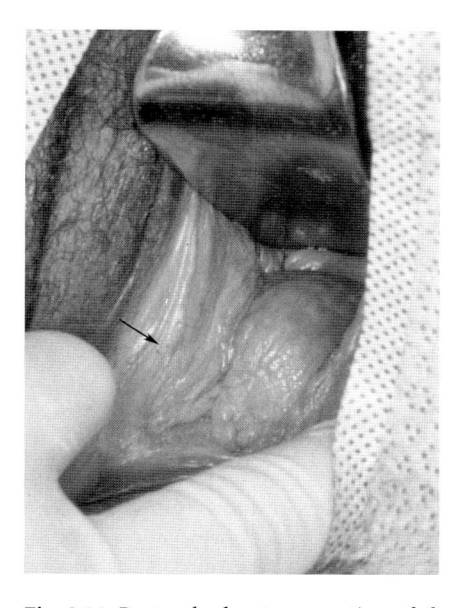

Fig. 2.14. Rectocele due to separation of the perineal body. Note the end of the hymenal ring that lies laterally on the side of the vagina, no longer united with its companion on the other side (DeLancey, with permission)

in place and prevent a mid-vaginal rectocele from occurring (Fig. 2.16). The multiple connections of the perineal body to the levator muscles and the pelvic sidewalls prevent a low rectocele from descending downward through the opening of the vagina (the urogenital hiatus and the levator ani muscles). These defects in the support at the level of the perineal body most frequently occur during vaginal delivery and are the most common type of posterior vaginal wall support problem.

The attachment of the levator ani muscles into the perineal body is important and damage to this part of the levator ani muscle during birth is one of the unrepairable aspects of pelvic floor dysfunction. Recent magnetic resonance imaging has vividly depicted these defects and will add greatly to our understanding of pelvic organ prolapse etiology. It is the author's personal belief that this muscular damage is one of the important factors that results in recurrence. An individual with muscles that do not function properly has a problem that is not surgically correctable. A more complete understanding of the biomechanics

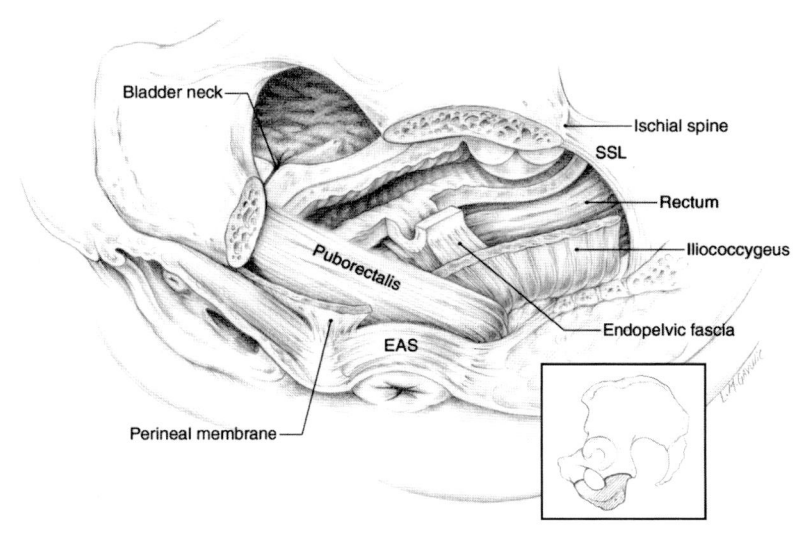

Fig. 2.15. Lateral view of the pelvis showing the relationships of the puborectalis, iliococcygeus and pelvic floor structures after removal of the ischium below the spine and sacrospinous ligament (*SSL*) (*EAS* external anal sphincter). The bladder and vagina have been cut in the midline yet the rectum left intact. Note how the endopelvic fascial "pillars" hold the vaginal wall dorsally preventing its downward protrusion (DeLancey 1999, with permission)

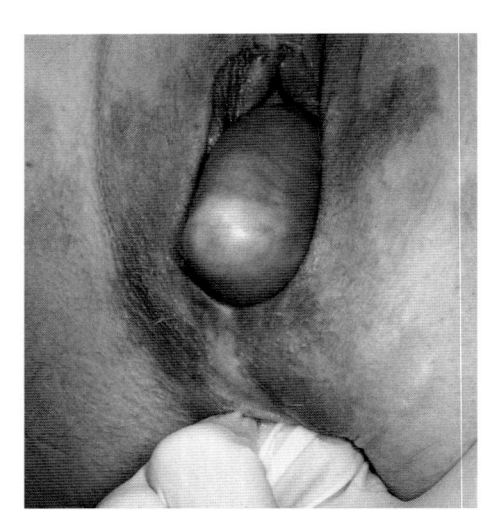

Fig. 2.16. Mid-vaginal rectocele that protrudes through the introitus despite a normally supported perineal body (DeLancey, with permission)

of this region will be needed for us to fully appreciate the importance of this injury.

2.2.6
Levator Ani Muscles

The levator ani muscles play a critical role in supporting the pelvic organs (Halban and Tandler 1907, summarized in Porges and Porges 1960; Berglas and Rubin 1953). Not only has evidence of this been seen in magnetic resonance scans (Kirschner-Hermanns et al. 1993; Tunn et al. 1998) but histological evidence of muscle damage has been found as well (Koelbl et al. 1989) and tied to operative failure (Hanzal et al. 1993). Any connective tissue within the body may be stretched by subjecting it to a constant force. Skin expanders used in plastic surgery stretch the dense and resistant dermis to extraordinary degrees and flexibility exercises practiced by dancers and athletes elongate leg ligaments with as little as 10 min of stretching a day. Both of these observations underscore the malleable nature of connective tissue when subjected to force over time. If the ligaments and fasciae within the pelvis were subjected to the continuous stress imposed on the pelvic floor by the great force of abdominal pressure, they would stretch. This stretching does not occur because the constant tonic activity of the pelvic floor muscles (Parks et al. 1962) closes the pelvic floor and carries the weight of the abdominal and pelvic organs, preventing constant strain on the ligaments.

Below the fascial layer is the levator ani group of muscles (Lawson 1974). (Fig. 2.17). They have a connective tissue covering on both superior and inferior surfaces called the superior and inferior fasciae of the levator ani. When these muscles and their fasciae are considered together, the combined structure is called the pelvic diaphragm.

The opening within the levator ani muscle through which the urethra and vagina pass (and through which prolapse occurs), is called the urogenital hiatus of the levator ani. The rectum also passes through this opening, but because the levator ani muscles attach directly to the anus it is not included in the name of the hiatus. The hiatus, therefore, is bounded ventrally (anteriorly) by the pubic bones, laterally by the levator ani muscles and dorsally (posteriorly) by the perineal body and external anal sphincter. The normal baseline activity of the levator ani muscle keeps the urogenital hiatus closed (Taverner 1959). It squeezes the vagina, urethra and rectum closed by compressing them against the pubic bone and lifts the floor and organs in a cephalic direction.

There are two basic regions of the levator ani muscle. One, the iliococcygeal portion, forms a relatively flat, horizontal shelf that spans the pelvic opening from one pelvic sidewall to the other. The second portion of the pubovisceral muscle is a sling of muscle that arises from the pubic bone on either side forming a sling around and behind the pelvic organs and also attaches to the walls of the pelvic organs. This includes what is generally referred to as the pubococcygeus and the puborectalis portions. This medial portion has constant activity and is responsible for holding the pelvic floor closed by constricting the urogenital hiatus in the levator ani muscles.

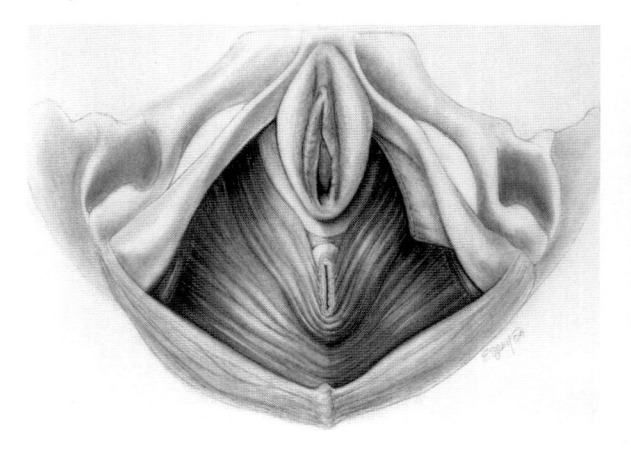

Fig. 2.17. Levator ani muscles seen from below. The cut edge of the perineal membrane ("urogenital diaphragm") can be seen on the left of the specimen (DeLancey, with permission)

The constant activity of the levator ani muscle is similar to other postural muscles. This continuous contraction is similar to the continuous activity of the external anal sphincter muscle and closes the lumen of the vagina in a way similar to the way in which the anal sphincter closes the anus. This constant action eliminates any opening within the pelvic floor through which prolapse could occur and forms a relatively horizontal shelf on which the pelvic organs are supported (Nichols et al. 1970).

2.2.7
Pelvic Floor Muscles and Endopelvic Fascia Interactions

The interaction between the pelvic floor muscles and the supportive ligaments is critical to pelvic organ support. As long as the levator ani muscles function properly the pelvic floor is closed and the ligaments and fasciae are under no tension. The fasciae simply act to stabilize the organs in their position above the levator ani muscles. When the pelvic floor muscles relax or are damaged, the pelvic floor opens and the vagina lies between the high abdominal pressure and low atmospheric pressure. In this situation it must be held in place by the ligaments. Although the ligaments can sustain these loads for short periods of time, if the pelvic floor muscles do not close the pelvic floor then the connective tissue must carry this load for long periods of time and will eventually fail to hold the vagina in place.

This support of the uterus has been likened to a ship in its berth floating on the water attached by ropes on either side to a dock (Paramore 1918). The ship is analogous to the uterus, the ropes to the ligaments, and the water to the supportive layer formed by the pelvic floor muscles. The ropes function to hold the ship (uterus) in the center of its berth as it rests on the water (pelvic floor muscles). If, however, the water level were to fall far enough that the ropes would be required to hold the ship without the supporting water, the ropes would all break. The analogous situation in the pelvic floor involves the pelvic floor muscles supporting the uterus and vagina that are stabilized in position by the ligaments and fasciae. Once the pelvic floor musculature becomes damaged and no longer holds the organs in place, the connective tissue fails.

2.2.8
Perineal Membrane and External Genital Muscles

In the anterior pelvis, below the levator ani muscles, is a dense triangularly shaped membrane called the perineal membrane (urogenital diaphragm). It lies at the level of the hymenal ring, and attaches the urethra, vagina, and perineal body to the ischiopubic rami (Fig. 2.18). Associated with the upper surface of the perineal membrane are the compressor urethrae and urethrovaginal sphincter muscles.

The term perineal membrane replaces the old term urogenital diaphragm, reflecting more accurate recent anatomical information (Oelrich 1983). Previous concepts of the urogenital diaphragm show two fascial layers, with a transversely oriented muscle in between (the deep transverse perineal muscle). Observations based on serial histology and gross dissection, however, reveal a single connective tissue membrane, with muscle lying immediately above. The correct anatomy explains the observation that pressures during a cough are greatest in the distal urethra (Hilton and Stanton 1983; Constantinou 1985) where the compressor urethra and urethrovaginal sphincter can compress the lumen closed in anticipation of a cough (DeLancey 1986, 1988).

2.3
Functional Anatomy of the Lower Urinary Tract

The inseparable link between structure and function found in living organisms is one of the common themes found in biology. The anatomy and clini-

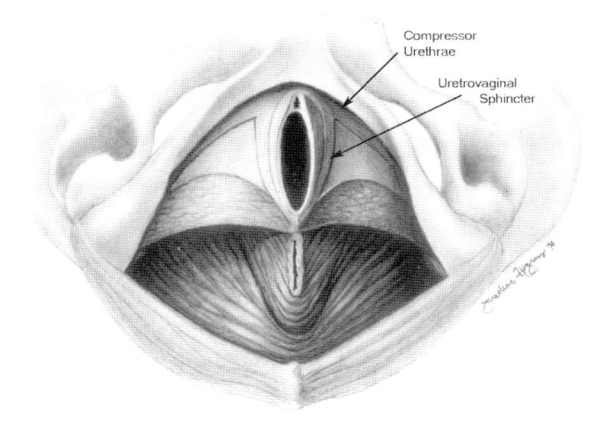

Fig. 2.18. Position of the perineal membrane and its associated components of the striated urogenital sphincter, the compressor urethra and the urethrovaginal sphincter (DeLancey, with permission)

cal behavior of the lower urinary tract exemplify this immutable link. The following descriptions are intended to offer a brief overview of some clinically relevant aspects of lower urinary tract structure that help us understand the normal and abnormal behavior of this system. The lower urinary tract can he divided into the bladder and urethra (Figs. 2.19, 2.20). At the junction of these two continuous, yet discrete structures, lies the vesical neck. This hybrid structure represents that part of the lower urinary tract where the urethral lumen traverses the bladder wall before becoming surrounded by the urethral wall. It contains portions of the bladder muscle, and also elements that continue into the urethra. The vesical neck is considered separately because of its functional differentiation from the bladder, and the urethra.

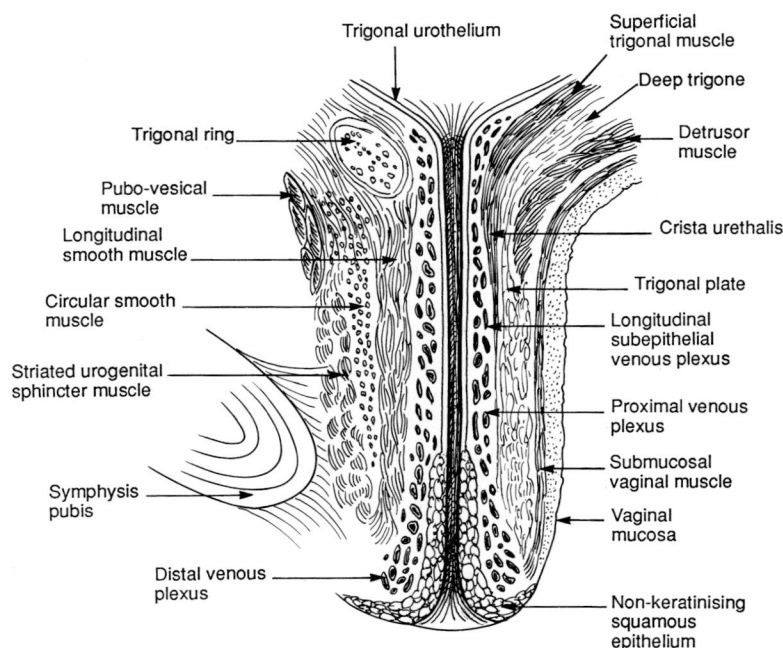

Fig. 2.19. Cross-section of the mid-urethra modified from HUISMAN (1983). From STROHBEHN and DeLANCEY (1997) (Saunders, with permission)

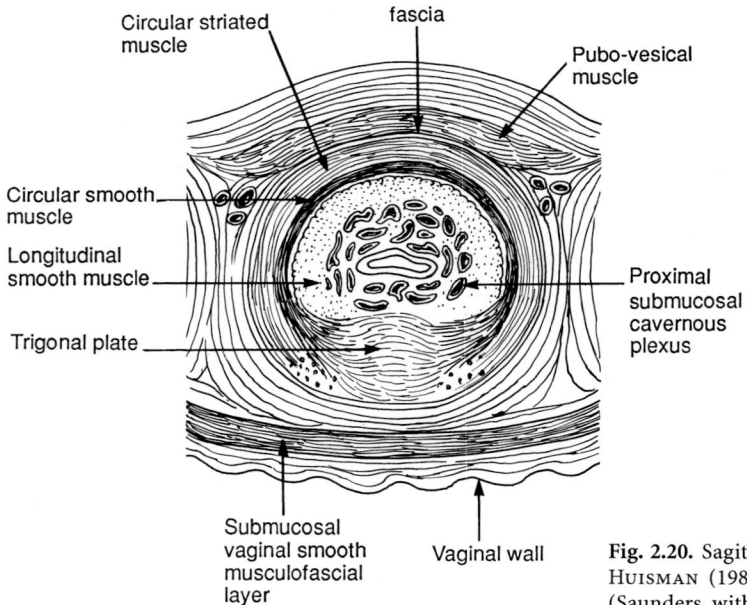

Fig. 2.20. Sagittal section of the mid-urethra modified from HUISMAN (1983). From STROHBEHN and DeLANCEY (1997) (Saunders, with permission)

2.3.1
Bladder

The bladder is a bag-like structure composed of smooth muscle. It relaxes to receive incoming urine so that increasing volumes can be stored with no appreciable increase in intravesical pressure. At a certain point, determined by multiple physiological and psychological factors, cerebral inhibition of the detrusor muscles' relaxation is released and a reflex voiding contraction initiated. The complex interactions between environmental, societal, personal, and physiological factors that determines this storage and periodic release are the subject of active clinical investigation in the field of urinary incontinence as it relates to the clinical problem of detrusor instability. From a structural standpoint, however, this has not been a particularly active area of investigation other than some studies noting the relationship between bladder wall thickness and voiding dysfunction. Bladder diverticula which can extend between fascicles of the interlacing detrusor muscles do have clinical importance and are easily documented either radiographically or cystoscopically.

2.3.1.1
Vesical Neck

The term "vesical neck" is both a regional and a functional one as previously discussed. It does not refer to a single anatomical entity. It denotes that area at the base of the bladder where the urethral lumen passes through the thickened musculature of the bladder base. Therefore, it is sometimes considered as part of the bladder musculature, but also contains the urethral lumen studied during urethral pressure profilometry. It is a region where the detrusor musculature, including the detrusor loop, surrounds the trigonal ring and the urethral meatus (GIL VERNET 1968).

The vesical neck has come to be considered separately from the bladder and urethra because it has unique functional characteristics. Specifically, sympathetic denervation or damage of this area results in its remaining open at rest (McGUIRE 1986) and when this happens in association with stress incontinence, simple urethral suspension is often ineffective in curing the problem (McGUIRE 1981).

2.3.2
Urethra

The urethra holds urine in the bladder and is therefore an important structure that helps determine urinary continence. It is a complex tubular viscus extending below the bladder. In its upper third it is clearly separable from the adjacent vagina, but its lower portion is fused with the wall of the latter structure. Embedded within its substance are a number of elements that are important to lower urinary tract dysfunction (HUISMAN 1983).

2.3.2.1
Striated Urogenital Sphincter

The striated urogenital sphincter muscle encircles the urethra in its mid portion. Distally under the arch of the pubic bone, these fibers diverge to insert into the walls of the vagina and the perineal membrane (compressor urethrae and urethrovaginal sphincter) (Fig. 2.18). This muscle is responsible for increasing intraurethral pressure during times of need and also contributes about a third of the resting tone of the urethra. Its composition primarily of slow-twitch fatigue-resistant muscle fibers belies its constant activity.

2.3.2.2
Urethral Smooth Muscle

There are two layers of the urethral smooth muscle, an outer circular layer and an inner longitudinal layer. The circular fibers contribute to urethral constriction and smooth muscle blockade reduces resting urethral closure pressure by about a third. The function of the longitudinal muscle is not entirely understood. There is considerably more longitudinal muscle than circular muscle and the reasons for this are yet to be determined.

2.3.2.3
Submucosal Vasculature

There is a remarkably prominent submucosal vasculature which is far more extensive than one would expect for such a small organ. This is probably responsible in part for the hermetic seal that maintains mucosal closure. Occlusion of arterial flow into this area decreases resting urethral closure pressure and so these vessels are felt to participate in closure function.

2.3.2.4
Glands

A series of glands are found in the submucosa primarily along the dorsal (vaginal) surface of the urethra (HUFFMAN 1948). They are most concentrated in the lower and middle thirds, and vary in number. The location of urethral diverticula, which are derived from cystic dilation of these glands, follows this distribution being most common distally, and usually originating along the dorsal surface of the urethra. In addition, their origin within the submucosa indicates that the fascia of the urethra must be stretched and attenuated over their surface, and indicates the need for its approximation after diverticular excision.

References

Ala-Ketola L (1973) Roentgen diagnosis of female stress urinary incontinence. Roentgenological and clinical study. Acta Obstet Gynecol Scand Suppl 23:1–59

Bartscht KD, DeLancey JOL (1988) A technique to study cervical descent. Obstet Gynecol 72:940–943

Berglas B, Rubin IC (1953) Study of the supportive structures of the uterus by levator myography. Surg Gynecol Obstet 97:677–692

Bonney V (1934) The principles that should underlie all operations for prolapse. J Obstet Gynaecol Br Emp 41:669–683

Campbell RM (1950) The anatomy and histology of the sacrouterine ligaments. Am J Obstet Gynecol 59:1–12

Constantinou CE (1985) Resting and stress urethral pressures as a clinical guide to the mechanism of continence in the female patient. Urol Clin North Am 12:247–258

DeLancey JOL (1986) Correlative study of paraurethral anatomy. Obstet Gynecol 68:91–97

DeLancey JOL (1988) Structural aspects of the extrinsic continence mechanism. Obstet Gynecol 72:296–301

DeLancey JOL (1992) Anatomic aspects of vaginal eversion after hysterectomy. Am J Obstet Gynecol 166:1717–1728

DeLancey JOL (1994) Structural support of the urethra as it relates to stress urinary incontinence: the hammock hypothesis. Am J Obstet Gynecol 170:1713–1720

DeLancey JOL (1999) Structural anatomy of the posterior compartment as it relates to rectocele. Am J Obstet Gynecol 180:815–823

Gil Vernet S (1968) Morphology and function of the vesicoprostato-urethral musculature. Edizioni Canova, Treviso

Halban J, Tandler J (1907) Anatomie und Aetiologie der Genitalprolapse beim Weibe. Braumuller, Vienna

Hanzal F, Berger F, Koelbl H (1993) Levator ani muscle morphology and recurrent genuine stress incontinence. Obstet Gynecol 81:426–429

Hilton P, Stanton SL (1983) Urethral pressure measurement by microtransducer: the results in symptom-free women and in those with genuine stress incontinence. Br J Obstet Gynaecol 90:919–933

Huffman J (1948) Detailed anatomy of the paraurethral ducts in the adult human female. Am J Obstet Gynecol 55:86–101

Huisman AB (1983) Aspects on the anatomy of the female urethra with special relation to urinary continence. Contrib Gynecol Obstet 10:1–31

Kirschner-Hermanns R, Wein B, Niehaus S, Schaefer W, Jakse G (1993) The contribution of magnetic resonance imaging of the pelvic floor to the understanding of urinary incontinence. Br J Urol 72:715–718

Koebl H, Strassegger H, Riss PA, Gruber H (1989) Morphologic and functional aspects of pelvic floor muscles in patients with pelvic relaxation and genuine stress incontinence. Obstet Gynecol 74:789–795

Lawson JO (1974) Pelvic anatomy. I. Pelvic floor muscles. Ann R Coll Surg Engl 54:244–252

Mant J, Painter R, Vessey M (1997) Epidemiology of genital prolapse: observations from the Oxford Family Planning Association study. Br J Obstet Gynaecol 104:579–585

McGuire EJ (1981) Urodynamic findings in patients after failure of stress incontinence operations. Prog Clin Biol Res 78:351–360

McGuire EJ (1986) The innervation and function of the lower urinary tract. J Neurosurg 65:278–285

Miller JM, Perucchini D, Carchidi LT, DeLancey JOL, Ashton-Miller J (2001) A pelvic floor muscle contraction during a cough decreases vesical neck mobility. Obstet Gynecol 97:255–260

Muellner SR (1951) Physiology of micturition. J Urol 65:805–810

Nichols DH, Milley PS, Randall CI (1970) Significance of restoration of normal vaginal depth and axis. Obstet Gynecol 36:251–256

Oelrich TM (1983) The striated urogenital sphincter muscle in the female. Anat Rec 205:223–232

Olsen AL, Smith VJ, Bergstrom JO, Coiling JC, Clark AL (1997) Epidemiology of surgically managed pelvic organ prolapse and urinary incontinence. Obstet Gynecol 89:501–506

Paramore RH (1918) The uterus as a floating organ. In: The statics of the female pelvic viscera. Lewis, London, pp 12–15

Parks AG, Porter NH, Melzak J (1962) Experimental study of the reflex mechanism controlling muscles of the pelvic floor. Dis Colon Rectum 5:407–414

Porges RF, Porges JC (1960) After office hours: the anatomy and etiology of genital prolapse in women (translated by J Halban and J Tandler). Obstet Gynecol 15:790–796

Range RL, Woodburne RT (1964) The gross and microscopic anatomy of the transverse cervical ligaments. Am J Obstet Gynecol 90:460–467

Richardson AC, Edmonds PB, Williams NL (1981) Treatment of stress urinary incontinence due to paravaginal fascial defect. Obstet Gynecol 57:357–362

Sears PS (1933) The fascia surrounding the vagina, its origin and arrangement. Am J Obstet Gynecol 25:484–492

Strohbehn K, DeLancey JOL (1997) The anatomy of stress incontinence. Oper Tech Gynecol Surg 2:5–16

Taverner D (1959) An electromyographic study of the normal function of the external anal sphincter and pelvic diaphragm. Dis Colon Rectum 2:153–160

Tunn R, Paris S, Fischer W, Hamm B, Kuchinke J (1998) Static magnetic resonance imaging of the pelvic floor muscle morphology in women with stress urinary incontinence and pelvic prolapse. Neurourol Urodyn 17:579–589

Westby M, Astumussen M, Ulmsten U (1982) Location of maximum intraurethral pressure related to urogenital diaphragm in the female subject as studied by simultaneous urethrocystometry and voiding urethrocystography. Am J Obstet Gynecol 144:408–412

3 Innervation and Denervation of the Pelvic Floor

J. T. Benson

CONTENTS

3.1 Innervation of the Pelvic Floor 39
3.1.1 Somatic Motor System 40
3.1.2 Autonomic System 41
3.1.3 Sensory System 42
3.2 Denervation of the Pelvic Floor 42
3.2.1 Motor Neuropathy 42
3.2.2 Sensory Neuropathy 43
References 44

3.1 Innervation of the Pelvic Floor

Problems with abnormal nerve function are an important cause of pelvic floor dysfunction. A knowledge of the role that nerve injury plays in these disorders will help explain visible abnormalities seen in imaging studies and is important for overall understanding of pelvic floor disorders.

The pelvic floor has complexity surpassing other muscular body areas. In addition to the considerable task of supporting the pelvic contents in the upright *Homo sapiens*, it also interacts intimately with the functions of the pelvic organs. Urinary and fecal storage, and elimination, reproductive and sexual functions are all complex processes relating to pelvic floor muscles and sphincters. This is a relationship that involves the entire nervous system, with reflex interactions at local, spinal, and supraspinal levels for "quasiautomatic" functions, and cortical levels for conscious control. The reflex mechanisms involve somatic motor, autonomic and sensory nerves.

The major innervation of the pelvic floor is via the sacral peripheral nerves. Their anatomical disposition makes them particularly vulnerable at certain points: the nerve roots in the cauda equina, in part of their course in the pelvic plexus, and the extrapelvic course of the sacral nerves forming the pudendal nerve.

The cauda equina (Fig. 3.1) is formed by the lumbosacral nerve roots descending from their origin in the spinal cord to their respective vertebral exits. Such descent is caused by the spinal cord growing disproportionately to the vertebral column so that in the adult, the cord ends at about the first lumbar vertebra. Nerve roots, such as those of the cauda equina, do not have the firm protection of a perineurium (Fig. 3.2) surrounding the nerve fascicles, and are therefore even more subject to trauma. After the nerve roots meet and form the nerve at the sacral exit foramina, they split into posterior rami, innervating episacral cartilaginous and ligamentous structures, and anterior rami.

J. T. Benson, MD
Clinical Professor, Obstetrics and Gynecology, Director, Female Pelvic Medicine and Reconstructive Surgery, Indiana University, Diplomate American Board of Electrodiagnostic Medicine, 1633 North Capitol Avenue, Suite 436, Indianapolis, IN 46202-1227, USA

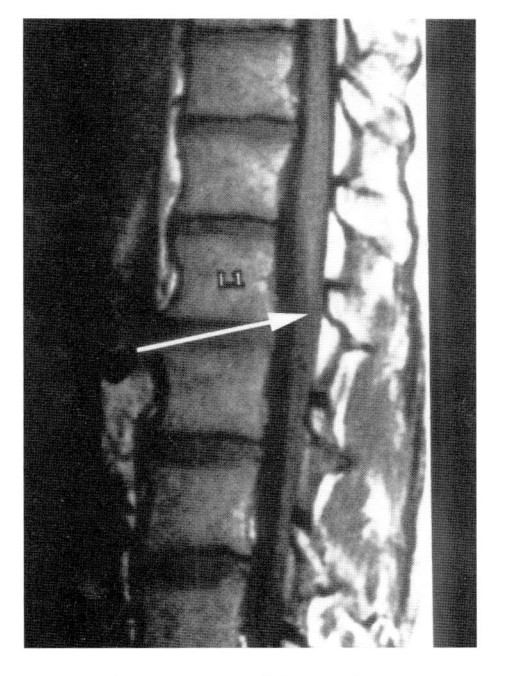

Fig. 3.1. The nerve roots of the sacral nerves traverse the cauda equina from vertebral level L1 to the sacral foramina

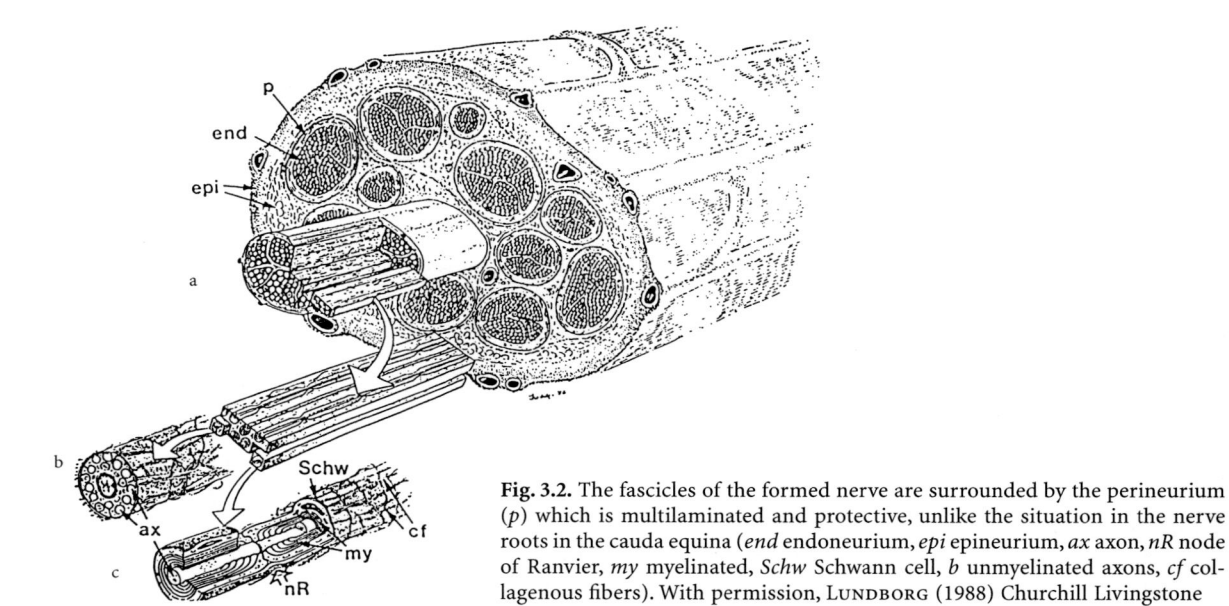

Fig. 3.2. The fascicles of the formed nerve are surrounded by the perineurium (*p*) which is multilaminated and protective, unlike the situation in the nerve roots in the cauda equina (*end* endoneurium, *epi* epineurium, *ax* axon, *nR* node of Ranvier, *my* myelinated, *Schw* Schwann cell, *b* unmyelinated axons, *cf* collagenous fibers). With permission, LUNDBORG (1988) Churchill Livingstone

The anterior rami course around and through overlying muscle, forming the lowermost components of the lumbosacral plexus. Branches of the lumbosacral plexus meet with small visceral nerves and form the pelvic plexus. The pelvic plexus overlies and invests the pelvic muscular floor, thus supplying pelvic floor muscles from a "superior" aspect, and surrounds and supplies the pelvic viscera. This plexus is subject to trauma from obstetric delivery and pelvic surgery (Fig. 3.3).

The pudendal nerve is formed in the lower division of the lumbosacral plexus. It leaves the pelvis through the greater sciatic foramen, wraps around the ischial spine, and is firmly invested in obturator fascia (Alcock's canal). It then courses back into the pelvis through the lesser sciatic foramen to provide muscular innervation to the superficial muscles of the pelvic floor from an "inferior" aspect. The area of fascial investment of the nerve in Alcock's canal locks it in place, subjecting it to stretch injury when the pelvic floor descends.

3.1.1 Somatic Motor System

The somatic motor nerves supply skeletal muscle have their nerve cell bodies in the anterior gray matter of the spinal cord (anterior horn cells), and a single axon from each cell goes to the effector organ (muscle). Such somatic motor nerves supply the skeletal muscle of most of the pelvic floor, e.g. the

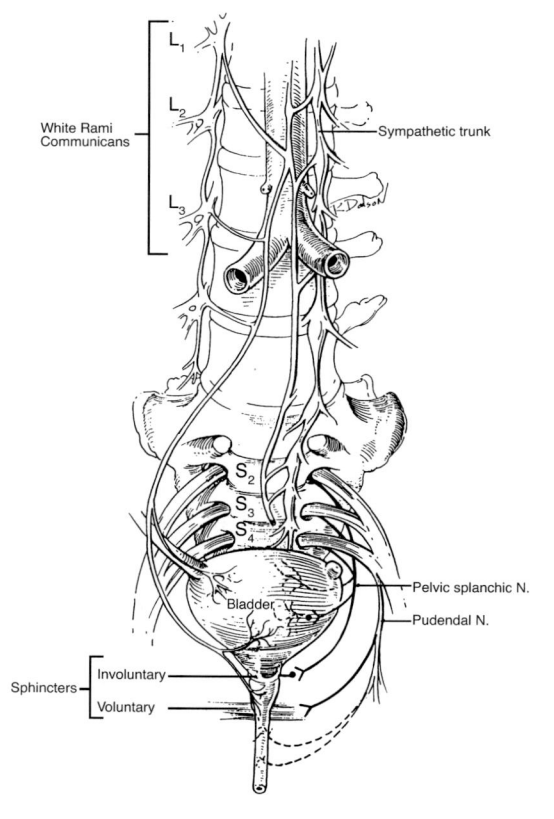

Fig. 3.3. The pelvic plexus has somatic supply via sacral nerves, visceral parasympathetic supply with preganglionic pelvic splanchnic nerves, and sympathetic supply with sympathetic postganglionic nerves and visceral afferents. The pudendal nerve bypasses the pelvic plexus to supply superficial pelvic muscles and urethral and anal sphincters

levator ani muscle mass. However, the group of cell bodies in the spinal cord that give rise to the motor axons supplying the pelvic floor sphincters, chiefly via the pudendal nerve, are different. These anterior horn cells are collectively called "Onuf's nucleus." They are somewhat smaller than other anterior horn cells. Unlike other motoneurons, these sacral motoneurons have reciprocal inhibitory interactions with sacral parasympathetic neurons and receive input not only from somatic upper motoneuron pathways but also from the hypothalamus and other autonomic regions. They are also frequently less involved in disease processes affecting other anterior horn cells (e.g., amyotrophic lateral sclerosis or polio). Both norepinephrine and serotonin mechanisms, usually present with sympathetic activity, are active with the pudendal motoneurons.

Alpha one adrenoceptor antagonists reduce striated urethral sphincter tone acting via inhibition of sacral pudendal motoneurons, which have noradrenergic nerve terminals and alpha adrenoceptors (THIND 1995) 5-Hydroxytryptamine (5-HT, serotonin) systems also are active at the pudendal motoneurons with evidence that 5-HT receptor agonists facilitate pudendal reflexes (DAUNSER and THOR 1996). Hence, the sacral motoneurons have distinct properties resembling autonomic motoneurons, unlike other somatic motoneurons. Thus, the innervation of the pelvic floor sphincters is unlike either the innervation of a typical skeletal or a typical smooth muscle elsewhere in the body, being "intermediate" in type between somatic and autonomic innervation.

3.1.2
Autonomic System

The autonomic or visceral motor nervous system controls the activity of the bladder, anorectal, and other pelvic smooth muscles. It exerts influences that are more continuous and generalized than those of the somatic system. The visceral motor system, unlike the somatic, is a two-neuron pathway with at least one synapse in the autonomic ganglia. It is separated morphologically and functionally into sympathetic ("thoracolumbar") and parasympathetic ("craniosacral") divisions. The preganglionic autonomic neurons occupy the visceral motor column of the cord (intermediolateral cell column), with sympathetic ones from T1 to L3 segments of the spinal cord and pelvic parasympathetic neurons from S2 to S4 segments. These neurons originate from the basal plate of the neural groove and use acetylcholine as the principle neurotransmitter. They also synthesize nitric oxide and some release enkephalin or neurotensin. Their axons leave the cord as small myelinated fibers and synapse with autonomic ganglion neurons.

The autonomic ganglion neurons affect transmission of preganglionic inputs into postganglionic neurons and use acetylcholine with fast excitation (nicotinic receptors), slower excitation (muscarinic receptors), and late slow response mediated by neuropeptides (e.g., substance P). The postganglionic axons are unmyelinated and release acetylcholine (parasympathetic) or norepinephrine (sympathetic) and neuropeptides and ATP (purine) cotransmitters. Sympathetic postganglionic receptors are alpha and beta adrenergic. Postganglionic parasympathetic receptors are chiefly muscarinic.

Pelvic preganglionic sympathetic axons from L1 to L3 exit via ventral roots to enter either the paravertebral or the prevertebral sympathetic systems (Fig. 3.4). The paravertebral preganglionic sympathetic axons pass by white rami communicants (white because they are myelinated) of the corre-

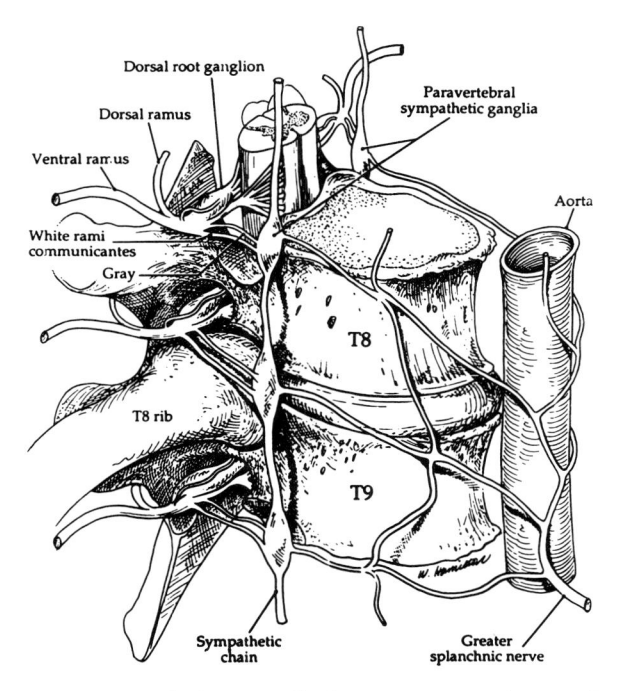

Fig. 3.4. Sympathetic preganglionic nerves traverse the ventral root, and the white rami communicantes; some synapse in the paravertebral sympathetic chain and post ganglionic neurons go via the gray rami communicantes to the somatic peripheral nerves. Others pass through the paravertebral chain to travel with the vessels in the prevertebral areas. Some visceral sensory nerves traverse the prevertebral system and pass via the white rami communicantes to their cell body in the dorsal root ganglia

sponding spinal nerve to reach the paravertebral chain. At this level, some run rostrally and caudally, synapsing with postganglionic axons, which return to peripheral nerves via gray (unmyelinated) rami communicants. These then travel with the nerves, such as the pudendal and pelvic somatic nerves. The axons of the prevertebral sympathetic preganglionic neurons pass through the paravertebral chain without synapsing to follow prevertebral vessels. These lumbar splanchnic nerves synapse on inferior mesenteric (presacral) ganglia and provide postganglionic sympathetic input to hypogastric and pelvic plexuses to innervate pelvic and perineal organs and glands.

Preganglionic parasympathetic fibers arise from S2 to S4 spinal cord segments, exit via ventral roots, and join the pelvic plexus by direct branches (nervi erigentes) to synapse at the ganglia. The ganglia are located within the visceral walls, so postganglionic fibers are very short.

3.1.3
Sensory System

The sensory, or afferent system is comprised of sensory nerves from the skin (cutaneous afferents), the muscles (somatic afferents), the viscera (visceral afferents), and other autonomic structures, e.g., the vessels and glands. Sensory nerves have their nerve cell bodies outside the spinal cord proper, in the dorsal root ganglion. Embryologically, the dorsal root ganglion neurons, like autonomic ganglion neurons and adrenal medullaris cells, arise from the neural crest, whereas the spinal cord and cell bodies located within it arise from a separate location, the basal plate of the neural groove. This partly explains certain disease processes and growth factors with an affinity for secretory and autonomic nerves.

The axon of the dorsal root ganglion neurons is a "split" axon (like a "T") with the distal process receiving the action potentials from the periphery, and the central process conveying the potentials to the spinal cord. The majority of the pelvic floor afferents traverse the pelvic plexus and the sacral nerves. Some follow prevertebral (and possibly paravertebral) sympathetic pathways, traversing the white rami communicantes to reach the dorsal root ganglia (Fig. 3.4). The elaborate system of reflex neural organization of the pelvic floor and the pelvic viscera to accomplish bowel, bladder, reproductive, sexual, and supportive functional missions begins with the afferent messages of the pelvic sensory nerves.

3.2
Denervation of the Pelvic Floor

Denervation of the pelvic floor is associated not only with muscular weakness that underlies pelvic organ prolapse, but is of paramount importance in functional disturbance of pelvic organs. Bladder and rectal storage, elimination, reproductive and sexual activities are all dependent on neuronal reflex activity, and may be affected by denervating processes.

3.2.1
Motor Neuropathy

Denervation of motor nerves has differing effects when the target organ is smooth muscle, as with autonomic denervation, or skeletal muscle, as with somatic denervation. Smooth muscle cells that are denervated maintain the property of automatism, the ability to sustain rhythmic contractions in the absence of innervation. Intramural conduction is also maintained following denervation. Such conduction between smooth muscle cells may occur electrically (ionic transfer) with gap junctions as in the heart and blood vessels, or mechanically with intramural connections as in the gut and bladder. In addition, most autonomic effectors develop denervation supersensitivity in response to postganglionic denervation. Such supersensitivity is the exaggerated response to the specific neurotransmitter, and involves several mechanisms, including upregulation of postjunctional receptors and reduced reuptake of the neurotransmitter.

The main consequence of skeletal muscle denervation is paralysis and atrophy, with the muscle fiber shrinking to less than 5% of its previous size unless it becomes reinnervated. Reinnervation is usual unless nerve damage was so severe that all the axons were destroyed and axon regrowth becomes impossible. Reinnervation is identified either by electrodiagnosis, or by biopsy to recognize muscle fiber type "grouping".

The muscle fibers belong to motor units. A motor unit is one anterior horn cell, its axon, and all the muscle fibers innervated by the branches of that axon. Muscle fibers are classified into generally three classes or functional groups. The slow-twitch, nonfatiguing, oxygen-using, red-colored (secondary to cytochrome oxidase and increased blood) muscle fibers with increased mitochondria are type I. Type II fibers are faster twitch, more anaerobically energized, thus higher in glycogen content and ATPase, and are generally recruited at stronger effort. The type II fibers are subclassified into two groups depending on the level of oxygen versus glycogen metabolism. Each motor unit is composed of a distinct class of muscle fiber, and the fibers are interspersed in the muscle to give a "checkerboard" type of appearance on histological study. When denervation of one axon occurs, the neighboring axon will sprout branches to innervate the adjacent muscle fibers which have lost neural supply. These reinnervated muscle fibers will assume the characteristics of the fibers of the reinnervating motor unit, and there will be a resultant grouping of muscle fiber type, replacing the checker-board configuration of muscle that has not undergone denervation.

Somatic motor neuromuscular damage may occur at any point from the anterior horn cell to the root (radiculopathy), plexus (plexopathy), peripheral nerve (neuropathy), neuromuscular junction, or muscle fibers. Anterior horn cell diseases typically do not involve Onuf's nucleus, reflecting the unique properties of these neurons. Lumbosacral radiculopathies commonly involve bladder and bowel dysfunction. In fact, bladder and bowel involvement is a clinical marker to separate radiculopathy from anterior horn cell disease. Ankylosing spondylitis, ependymomas, lipomas, dermoid cysts, transverse myelitis, arteriovenous malformations, and congenital meningomyelocele with cord tethering may all produce conus medullaris lesions. It is a fairly common complication of abdominal aortic aneurysm surgery secondary to prolonged aortic clamping. Cauda equina lesions are very common. Central disc protrusion can affect the bladder and bowel nerve roots, and many clinicians consider bladder and bowel involvement to be a chief indication for surgical treatment of disc protrusion. Cauda equina lesions are seen with congenital caudal aplasia (from diabetic mothers) and congenital and acquired spinal stenosis (pseudoclaudication syndrome). Ankylosing spondylitis, schwannomas, primary and metastatic malignancies, lymphomas, meningiomas, neurofibromas, chordomas, AIDS, and cytomegalovirus infection are other causes of cauda equina disease. Damage may also occur with distal aortic occlusive disease. Cauda equina lesions secondary to arachnoiditis are seen in episodic fashion, suggesting contamination of epidural agents. Arachnoiditis is also seen with injections of alcohol, phenol, or with very high dosages of intrathecal penicillin therapy. Diabetic lumbosacral radiculopathies most commonly involve the L3–L4 roots and are bilateral in half of all cases.

Lumbosacral plexus lesions are most commonly associated with malignancies (cervical, rectal, lymphoma), radiation damage, or hematomas. Pelvic plexus lesions may occur with these processes as well, but are more commonly seen with obstetric injury. Mechanical compressive nerve damage of a permanent nature has been shown to occur with a pressure of 80 mm Hg for 8 h. Because the forces during the second stage of labor normally reach a maximum pressure of 240 mm Hg (REMPEN and KRAUS 1991), it is not surprising to see nerve lesions. The pelvic plexus contains somatic motor nerves to the pelvic floor striated muscle, preganglionic parasympathetic nerves and postganglionic sympathetic nerves to smooth muscle and viscera, and somatic and visceral sensory nerves. Pathological processes in the plexus areas may have many resulting dysfunctions.

Mononeuropathies occur frequently in pelvic nerves secondary to injury that may be mechanical, thermal, electrical, radiation-induced, vascular, granulomatous, or from primary or metastatic neoplastic lesions. The leading cause of pelvic mononeuropathy is the mechanical effect (compression and stretching) of labor and delivery. Stretch has been shown to cause nerve demyelination if the nerve is stretched by 15% of its length (LUNDBORG 1988). The pudendal nerve is stretched by 15% with descent of the pelvic floor by only 1.35 cm. This amount of descent occurs commonly with exaggerated Valsalva action such as occurs with labor and delivery and with constipation disorders. Pelvic floor prolapse, which may well have neuropathy as a precipitating factor, may in itself add to continued stretch effects on pudendal (and other) nerves, creating a continuing cycle of chronic nerve damage.

3.2.2
Sensory Neuropathy

Peripheral nerves, when injured, have a capacity for repair, whereas nerves within the central nervous system have much less. Hence, the distal process of a sensory nerve may regenerate after injury, but if the proximal branch of the sensory nerve is damaged, it is capable of regeneration up to its junction with the central nervous system only.

Sensory effects are possible with involvement of the central nervous system conducting the impulses to the cerebral cortex, involvement of the proximal axon of the sensory ganglion cell, such as with radiculopathy, involvement of the nerve cell (neuronopathy), or involvement of the distal axon by plexopathy or neuropathy. Hence, all of the conditions affecting somatic motor axons beyond the central nervous system may also affect somatic the sensory system. Certain processes, however, have a predilection for predominantly sensory neuronal and axonal involvement.

Understanding pelvic floor neuropathy has led to improvements in therapy for pelvic floor disorders. Manipulation of sacral neurons via affecting neurotransmitter reuptake, application of sensory stimulants or suppressants to influence spinal and supraspinal reflex responses, restricting or increasing nerve growth factors to influence development of "pathological" reflexes, and electrical stimulation of sacral nerves to affect both bladder storage and emptying reflexes are a few of the avenues of therapy in research trials and in clinical practice today. The ever-increasing number of patients in our society suffering from pelvic floor disorders may look forward to improvement in their care fostered by increasing understanding of the significant role of neuropathic processes.

References

Daunser H, Thor K (1996) Spinal 5-HT2 receptor-mediated facilitation of pudendal nerve reflexes in the anaesthetized cat. Br J Pharmacol 118:150–154

Lundborg G (1988) Nerve injury and repair. Churchill Livingstone, New York, p 54

Rempen A, Kraus M (1991) Measurement of head compression during labor: preliminary results. J Perinat Med 19:115–120

Thind P (1995) The significance of smooth and striated muscles in the sphincter function of the urethra in healthy women. Neurourol Urodyn 14:585–618

4 Imaging Techniques (Technique and Normal Parameters)

S. Halligan, F. M. Kelvin, H. K. Pannu, C. I. Bartram, E. Rociu. J. Stoker, K. Strohbehn, A. V. Emmanuel

4.1 Evacuation Proctography

S. Halligan

CONTENTS

4.1.1 Introduction 45
4.1.2 Technique 45
4.1.3 Normal Findings 46
4.1.3.1 Pre-evacuation 47
4.1.3.2 Evacuation 48
4.1.3.3 Post-evaluation 48
4.1.4 Alternative Approaches 49
4.1.5 Summary 49
        References 49

4.1.1 Introduction

Evacuation proctography is a simple radiological technique that images rectal voiding of a barium paste enema. Evacuating proctography serves two main purposes: it images rectal configuration throughout all phases of rectal evacuation and also provides an assessment of whether voiding is normal or difficult (which usually means prolonged). Thus it provides both morphological and functional information.

Radiological studies of rectal evacuation have been performed for over 50 years (Wallden 1953) but it was the description in 1984 of a relatively simple technique along with parameters for interpretation that was the impetus for more general acceptance (Mahieu et al. 1984). Evacuation proctography is now widely disseminated, even though it remains predominantly confined to specialist centres. Although requested most by coloproctological surgeons, proctography is also useful to both urogynaecologists and gastroenterologists. Difficult rectal evacuation is by far the most common reason for referral. The examination is frequently termed defaecography and other terms are also occasionally used; videoproctography, cinedaefecography, dynamic rectal examination. Whatever the terminology, it should be remembered that the findings are based on voluntary rectal evacuation and not physiological defaecation. The latter is accompanied by colonic contraction and complex anorectal reflexes, many of which may be normally absent during the proctography. Because of this, terminology that implies physiological defaecation is probably best avoided.

4.1.2 Technique

There are possibly as many different techniques practised as there are practitioners (Finlay 1988). Opinions differ as to the type of contrast used, its consistency, the volume instilled, imaging modality, manoeuvres taken, and the images acquired. Furthermore, the basic technique may be modified so that other pelvic organs are imaged at the same sitting, the ultimate expression of which is dynamic cystoproctography (see Section 4.2). The purpose of this Section is to describe the basic proctographic technique, which the author feels should be as rapid and simple as possible.

Assessment of evacuation rate and completeness is an essential part of the examination, possibly the most important part (Halligan et al. 1995a). Because of this, the author prefers the rectum to be emptied before proctography, simply achieved in most subjects by inserting two glycerine suppositories and asking the patient to visit the lavatory after having retained these for approximately 20 minutes. Alternatively, an enema may be administered in the department. The same volume of contrast (120 ml for example) is then used in all patients so that meaningful comparison of rectal evacuation can be made with established normal values derived from normal subjects (Kamm et al. 1989). Furthermore, a consistent standardized technique means that follow-up studies are comparable when clinically necessary, and comparisons between patients is possible for research. Alternatively, some investigators

S. Halligan, MD, MRCP, FRCR
Intestinal Imaging Centre, Level 4V, St. Mark's Hospital, Watford Road, Northwick Park, Harrow, Middlesex, HA1 3UJ, UK

omit rectal emptying and instil contrast until an urge to evacuate is elicited. It has been suggested that this approach is more physiological but, for the reasons described above, the entire examination is unphysiological whatever the technique used. Furthermore, an empty rectum is more acceptable to staff for obvious reasons. It is also possible that stool may inhibit some findings such as intussusception.

It is generally accepted that contrast consistency should be approximately the same as faeces. Mahieu used a barium suspension mixed with potato starch. Others have used methylcellulose, and commercial preparations specifically designed for the purpose are now easily available. However, there is good evidence that the consistency of the contrast used is largely irrelevant (IKENBERRY et al. 1996), which is in accord with physiological studies of constipated patients that suggest evacuation is disordered regardless of the consistency of rectal content. Interestingly, large stools are actually easier to pass than small ones (BANNISTER et al. 1987).

The paste is administered with the patient in the left-lateral position on the fluoroscopy table. A simple approach is to fill two bladder syringes (which have a wide-tipped nozzle) with 60 ml of contrast each and then to syringe the contrast directly into the rectum after lubricating the syringe tip. If the paste is very viscous, then a caulking gun can be used instead of simple hand injection. The syringe is withdrawn towards the end of injection in order to mark the anal canal and verge.

The patient then steps off the table whilst it is brought upright and a commode placed on the footrest. Commercial commodes are available, although it is a simple job to build one. The commode should be comfortable and the seat should be relatively radiolucent; Perspex or wood is commonly used. The commode also needs to be able to support a disposable plastic bag for the patient to evacuate into and must also incorporate some filtration underneath the seat to balance radiographic exposure and prevent screen flare; our commode uses 4-mm of copper plate (Fig. 4.1.1), whilst others have used water-filled rubber rings or a Perspex sheet. Some commodes incorporate a radiographic ruler for precise measurements when felt clinically necessary. Although the more sensitive seated position is preferable, proctography can be performed in the left-lateral position if a commode is unavailable or if the patient is incontinent (POON et al. 1991), but it should be borne in mind that static values for pelvic floor position are higher (JORGE et al. 1994). It may be helpful to shield the patient behind a portable screen, especially if the radiographic unit is remotely controlled, so that some privacy is afforded and embarrassment potentially avoided.

It is essential to obtain continuous or rapid recording of rectal evacuation, either by spot filming, cineradiography or videofluoroscopy. Although spot filming provides the best spatial resolution, the facility to replay the entire examination at any speed is an invaluable feature of video; this is also possible with some digital systems, which also convey the lowest dose. Radiation dose has been a major and persistent concern, not least because many patients are young women in their childbearing years. However, because high spatial resolution is not a prerequisite for proctography, low-dose digital algorithms and added filtration may be applied without any diagnostic loss (HARE et al. 2001). Intermittent imaging should also be employed to reduce dose in patients whose evacuation is prolonged; there is no benefit to having multiple, identical images of an atonic rectum!

4.1.3
Normal Findings

Based on the findings in 56 asymptomatic patients, Mahieu et al. defined five criteria for a normal examination: increased anorectal angulation, obliteration of the puborectal muscle impression, wide anal canal

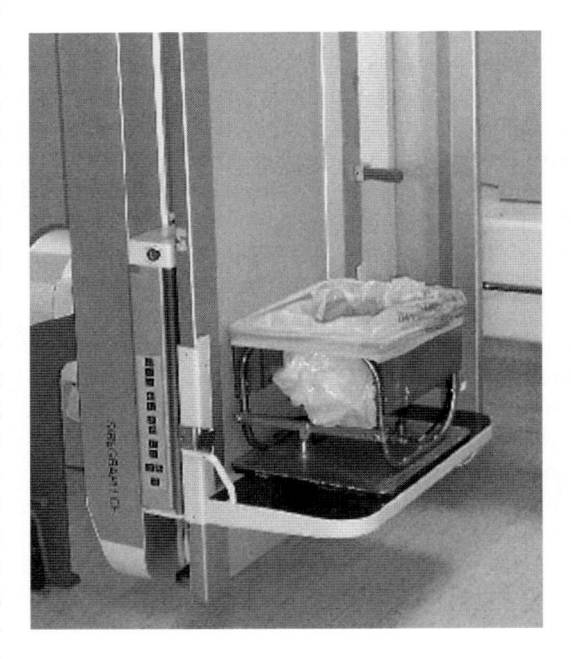

Fig. 4.1.1. The proctography commode placed on the footrest of the upright fluoroscopy table. Note the copper sheet immediately below the seat to balance radiographic contrast

opening, total evacuation of contrast, and normal pelvic floor resistance (MAHIEU et al. 1984). Several subsequent studies of asymptomatic volunteers have revealed a wide range of normal values, including some overlap with pathology, but the general consensus of what is normal is broadly in agreement with Mahieu's original description. There have been several studies of asymptomatic volunteers following Mahieu's description, with varying degrees of selection bias, sometimes unavoidable because of perceived problems with radiation dose. Others have defined normality retrospectively on the basis of a "normal" proctogram, which is scientifically unsatisfactory. Probably the best study is that by SHORVON and coworkers (1989), who examined 47 asymptomatic volunteers, most of whom were under 30 years old. Any proctographic examination can be considered in three stages; pre-evacuation, evacuation and post-evacuation.

4.1.3.1
Pre-evacuation

The patient should be initially imaged in the lateral position, which provides most information about anorectal configuration and pelvic floor position, and from which it is easiest to assess the degree of rectal emptying; a single lateral image at rest will suffice (Fig. 4.1.2a). The funnelled junction between the rectal ampulla and anal canal, the anorectal junction, is easy to appreciate at rest and for practical purposes defines the level of the posterior pelvic floor. The pubococcygeal line, a line drawn between the inferior border of the symphysis pubis and the sacrococcygeal junction, is generally believed to indicate the normal position of the pelvic floor. However, these bony landmarks may be difficult to identify with a limited field of view and the inferior surface of the ischial tuberosities are often used instead. An even simpler approach is to use the top of the commode seat as a rough and ready estimate of pelvic floor position. The anorectal junction should be at or just above this plane (0.4 cm above this level in women and 1.6 cm in men) (SHORVON et al. 1989). The canal should also be tightly closed without any contrast leakage.

The anorectal angle (ARA) is the angle subtended between the anal canal axis and the posterior distal rectal wall. An alternative measurement uses the central rectal axis rather than the posterior rectal wall. The ARA is formed in part by the puborectalis muscle, which slings behind the anorectal junction, and is thought to be important in maintaining continence because of the resultant acute angle between the rectal and anal axis; the "flap-valve" theory of anal continence (BARTOLO et al. 1986). Indeed, incontinent patients often have an obtuse ARA and postanal repair, used to treat incontinence, aims to restore the ARA in these patients. However, although considerable attention has been devoted to this measurement, there is little evidence that it is worthwhile. Most

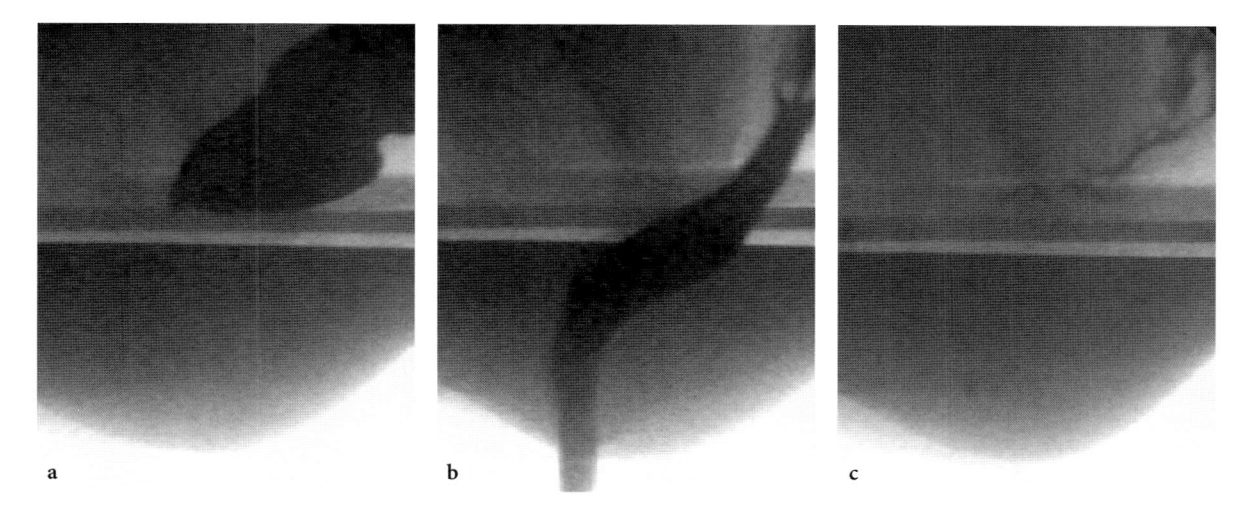

Fig. 4.1.2a–c. Normal evacuating proctogram. Asymptomatic volunteer. **a** Pre-evacuation phase. Resting rectal position and configuration is normal. The anal canal is tightly closed and the anorectal junction is approximately at the level of the seat top. **b** Evacuation phase. The anorectal junction has descended, the anal canal has opened widely, and the anorectal angle has become more obtuse. The rectum empties smoothly and completely within 30 s. **c** Post-evacuation phase. The rectum is empty, the anal canal closed, and the anorectal junction has returned to its pre-evacuation position

investigators have abandoned it, not least because the normal range of values is very wide and there is considerable overlap with symptomatic patients (SHORVON et al. 1989). Nevertheless, as a broad guide the ARA should be approximately 90° at rest.

Before formal evacuation, many investigators advocate additional manoeuvres: "squeeze" views to evaluate the strength of voluntary pelvic floor musculature; "cough" views to stress the continence mechanism; "strain" views to assess pelvic floor descent. Although these seem sensible, in reality there is little evidence that they discriminate enough between patients to be clinically useful and it is likely they merely add procedural complexity. It is interesting to note that the ARA may paradoxically increase during strain manoeuvres in up to 30% of normal subjects, reflecting pelvic floor contraction secondary to a desire to remain continent (KELVIN et al. 1994).

Lastly, when centering the pre-evacuation image it is important to allow for pelvic floor descent during subsequent evacuation. This may be considerable and can result in the rectum being displaced out of the radiographic field of view.

4.1.3.2
Evacuation

After an initial lateral resting view has been obtained, the patient is asked to evacuate their rectum as rapidly and completely as possible. Evacuation should be initiated quickly after the appropriate command since delay is positively associated with pelvic incoordination and indicates functional disorder (HALLIGAN et al. 1995a). Embarrassment may also cause delay. The anorectal junction should descend in response to raised intraabdominal pressure; failure to descend represents inadequate effort and may also be a sign of functional disorder (HALLIGAN et al. 1995b). Once initiated, evacuation should be rapid and complete; asymptomatic individuals are able to void the majority of a 120-ml contrast enema within 30 seconds (KAMM et al. 1989). Prolonged evacuation is usually abnormal and is occasionally associated with repetitive jerky pelvic floor movements. Pelvic floor descent (represented by inferior movement of the anorectal junction) should be no more than approximately 3.0 cm. The puborectal impression should flatten and the ARA become more obtuse. The anal canal should shorten and widen to allow evacuation (Fig. 4.1.2b). Generally, the rectal ampulla should empty smoothly and symmetrically, rather like a toothpaste tube, although a wide variety of configurations are possible (SHORVON et al. 1989). Patients who need to use digital manoeuvres to aid rectal emptying, such as applying vaginal or posterior perineal pressure, should be instructed to do so, so that their effect may be evaluated.

4.1.3.3
Post-evacuation

The examination generally finishes once evacuation is complete, or when it is clear that little or no evacuation is likely. After evacuation the anal canal closes and the anorectal junction should ascend, returning to its pre-evacuation resting position (Fig. 4.1.2c). The ARA should also return to its pre-evacuation configuration. The rectum should be empty or nearly so. Occasionally, when the evacuation phase has raised the possibility of intussusception predominantly within the coronal plane (the rectal valves of Houston are best seen in this plane, for example), it may be worthwhile examining the patient in the frontal position, which is also the best position to evaluate perineal hernias. The commode is simply turned around on the footrest and the subject asked to strain during fluoroscopy; there is usually enough residual barium to render the fold configuration visible (MCGEE and BARTRAM 1993). After the examination the patient should visit the lavatory in order to void any residual barium and to clean him or herself. The bag can then be simply lifted from the commode and disposed of. The entire room time for the examination should be approximately 5 minutes. Evacuation proctography can be a rapid and simple technique, requiring much less effort from staff and patient than a barium enema, for example.

The radiological report should comment on rectal configuration at rest, the degree of pelvic floor descent during evacuation, the degree and rapidity of evacuation, and the presence of any associated structural abnormality. In day-to-day practice, a formal measurement of various angles and distances is not required; an understanding of what is broadly normal and abnormal will suffice and will come with experience.

Extension of this basic technique is discussed in Chapter 4.2. but, as a routine, the author administers 100 ml oral barium suspension (100% weight/volume) diluted with 200 ml water to which 10 ml Gastrografin has been added. This is administered 30 min before proctography in order to facilitate diagnosis of enterocoeles. Alternatively, contrast gel may be injected to the vaginal apex using a syringe; enterocoeles are then revealed by significant rectovaginal separation. However, tampons should not be used because of their propensity to splint the vagina and thus inhibiting enterocoele formation (ARCHER et al. 1992).

4.1.4 Alternative Approaches

It is worth noting that evacuation proctography can be performed using scintigraphic methods (HUTCHINSON et al. 1993). Although spatial resolution is poor, impairing diagnosis of intussusception, for example, the technique provides very accurate assessments of the rate and degree of rectal emptying, and radiation dose may be less than with some conventional systems. Recognizing that the ability to evacuate is more important than the rectal configuration adopted to do so, some authors have employed a radio-opaque rectal balloon instead of contrast (PRESTON et al. 1984). Such an approach will not reliably diagnose many structural abnormalities. Indeed, it has frequently been argued that the imaging component of the examination can be dispensed with altogether and a balloon (BARNES and LENNARD-JONES 1985) or fluid used instead (ALSTRUP et al. 1997). Again, these methods will miss many morphological abnormalities, the significance of which remains controversial (see Chapter 6.2). Other investigators have performed proctography following injection of intraperitoneal water-soluble contrast medium (HALLIGAN and BARTRAM 1995), but this has not found general acceptance, possibly because it has been superseded by MR imaging. In the final analysis, the level of information needed by the referring physician will largely define the radiological approach used.

4.1.5 Summary

Evacuation proctography is a simple and rapid technique with which to assess morphological and functional aspects of rectal evacuation. It is generally extremely well tolerated by patients, much more so than the barium enema, for example. The examination may be extended so that a global pelvic floor assessment is achieved, but this adds to procedural complexity and is probably best reserved for urogynaecological practice. However, addition of oral barium to diagnose enterocoeles as described is worthwhile and simple. In day-to-day practice, a formal measurement of various angles and distances is not required; an understanding of what is broadly normal and abnormal will suffice and will come with experience. Abnormal findings and their relevance are discussed in Chapter 6.2.

References

Alstrup N, Ronholt C, Chuangang F, Rasmussen O, Sorensen M, Christiansen J (1997) Viscous fluid expulsion in the evaluation of the constipated patient. Dis Colon Rectum 40:580–584

Archer BD, Somers S, Stevenson GW (1992) Contrast medium gel for marking vaginal position during defecography. Radiology 182:278–279

Bannister JJ, Davison P, Timms JM, Gibbons C, Read NW (1987) Effect of stool size and consistency on rectal evacuation. Gut 28:1246–1250

Barnes PRH, Lennard-Jones JE (1985) Balloon expulsion from the rectum in constipation of different types. Gut 26:1049–1052

Bartolo DC, Roe AM, Locke-Edmunds JC, Virjee J, Mortensen NJ (1986) Flap valve theory of anorectal continence. Br J Surg 73:1012–1014

Finlay IG (1988) Symposium: Proctography. Int J Colorectal Dis 3:67–89

Halligan S, Bartram CI (1995) Evacuation proctography combined with positive contrast peritoneography to demonstrate pelvic floor hernias. Abdom Imaging 20:442–445

Halligan S, Bartram CI, Park HY, Kamm MA (1995a) The proctographic features of anismus. Radiology 197:679–682

Halligan S, Thomas J, Bartram CI (1995b) Intrarectal pressures and balloon expulsion related to evacuation proctography. Gut 31:100–104

Hare C, Halligan S, Bartram CI, Gupta R, Walker AE, Renfrew I (2001) Dose reduction in evacuation proctography. Eur Radiol 11:432–434

Hutchinson R, Mostafa AB, Grant EA, Smith NB, Deen KI, Harding LK, Kumar D (1993) Scintigraphic defecography: quantitative and dynamic assessment of anorectal function. Dis Colon Rectum 36:1132–1138

Ikenberry S, Lappas JC, Hana MP, Rex DK (1996) Defecography in healthy subjects: comparison of three contrast media. Radiology 201:233–238

Jorge JMN, Ger GC, Gonzalez L, Wexner SD (1994) Patient position during cinedefecography. Dis Colon Rectum 37: 927–931

Kamm MA, Bartram CI, Lennard-Jones JE (1989) Rectodynamics – quantifying rectal evacuation. Int J Colorectal Dis 4:161–163

Kelvin FM, Maglinte DD, Benson JT, Brubaker LP, Smith C (1994) Dynamic cystoproctography: a technique for assessing disorders of the pelvic floor in women. AJR Am J Roentgenol 163:368–370

Mahieu P, Pringot J, Bodart P (1984) Defecography 1. Description of a new procedure and results in normal patients. Gastrointest Radiol 9:247–251

McGee SG, Bartram CI (1993) Intra-anal intussusception: diagnosis by posteroanterior stress proctography. Abdom Imaging 2:136–140

Poon FW, Lauder JC, Finlay IG (1991) Technical report: evacuating proctography – a simplified technique. Clin Radiol 44:113–116

Preston DM, Lennard-Jones JE, Thomas BM (1984) The balloon proctogram. Br J Surg 71:29–31

Shorvon PJ, McHugh S, Diamant NE, Somers S, Stevenson GW (1989) Defecography in normal volunteers: results and implications. Gut 30:1737–1749

Wallden L (1953) Roentgen examination of the deep rectogenital pouch. Acta Radiol 39:105–116

4.2 Dynamic Cystoproctography: Fluoroscopic and MRI Techniques for Evaluating Pelvic Organ Prolapse

F. M. Kelvin and H. K. Pannu

CONTENTS

4.2.1 Introduction 51
4.2.2 Fluoroscopic Dynamic Cystoproctography 51
4.2.2.1 Technique 52
4.2.2.2 Radiologic Definitions and Grading of Prolapse 53
4.2.2.3 Specific Sites of Prolapse on Fluoroscopic Examination 53
4.2.2.4 Comparison with Physical Examination 57
4.2.3 Dynamic MR Imaging of the Pelvic Floor 58
4.2.3.1 Technique 58
4.2.3.2 Evolution of Dynamic MR Imaging 58
4.2.3.3 Specific Sites of Prolapse on MR Examination 60
4.2.3.4 Criteria for Diagnosing Pelvic Organ Prolapse on MR Imaging 63
4.2.4 Comparison of MR and Fluoroscopic Techniques 65
References 66

4.2.1 Introduction

Pelvic organ prolapse is a major cause of morbidity in women. Surgical repair of sites of prolapse is often unsuccessful. The relatively high reoperation rate may, in some instances, reflect failure to recognize the full extent of prolapse preoperatively, if assessment is based predominantly on physical examination.

Physical examination is the main diagnostic test used to evaluate patients with known or suspected prolapse. However, physical landmarks may be altered in patients with recurrent prolapse after surgery. Also,

F. M. Kelvin, MD
Department of Radiology, Methodist Hospital of Indiana, Clinical Professor of Radiology, Indiana University School of Medicine, 1701 North Senate Boulevard, Indianapolis, IN 46202, USA
H. K. Pannu, MD
Assistant Professor of Radiology, The Russell H. Morgan Department of Radiology and Radiological Science, Johns Hopkins Medical Institutions, 600 North Wolfe Street, Room 100, Baltimore, MD 21287, USA

in patients with severe prolapse and complete vaginal eversion, it may be difficult on physical examination to determine with certainty the identity of all the prolapsing organs (Brubaker et al. 1993). In these situations, imaging can be helpful to confirm clinically suspected prolapse, distinguish the prolapsing organ, as well as to identify unsuspected defects in pelvic floor support (Weidner and Low 1998). Imaging can also help guide surgical repair in patients with inconclusive clinical findings (Tunn et al. 2000). Other than ultrasonography, the main imaging techniques used to assess pelvic organ prolapse are fluoroscopic dynamic cystoproctography and dynamic magnetic resonance (MR) imaging of the pelvic floor.

4.2.2 Fluoroscopic Dynamic Cystoproctography

Evacuation proctography (defecography) has traditionally been limited to the study of anorectal dysfunction. Colpocystography has been used by some radiologists and gynecologists for over 3 decades to study pelvic organ prolapse. (Bethoux et al 1965) In women, the role of evacuation proctography may be extended if the small bowel and vagina are opacified in addition to the rectum, as this facilitates the detection of an enterocele (Kelvin et al. 1992). The addition of a cystogram provides a more comprehensive radiologic method of assessing the pelvic organs. Sites of weakness involving these organs are then imaged at rest, during straining, and during and after evacuation. The term "dynamic cystoproctography" (DCP) or, more completely "dynamic cystocolpoproctography" has been attached to this procedure, as well as other terms such as colpocystodefecography (Hock et al. 1993) and four-contrast defecography (Altringer et al. 1995).

This radiographic approach was developed to serve as a complement to the physical examination for the evaluation of pelvic organ prolapse. Weakness of the pelvic floor muscles in women usually involves multiple organ systems and, therefore, a global approach to pelvic floor imaging is preferable, whether by DCP or MR imaging. The varied sites of injury or weakness lead to the development of specific anatomic defects such as rectocele, cystocele, enterocele and sigmoidocele, as well as symptoms of stress urinary incontinence and fecal incontinence.

4.2.2.1
Technique

Several items of specialized equipment are utilized during the examination. These include a radiolucent commode, video recording with slow motion play-back capability, and a thick barium paste that approximates the consistency of fecal material. Because proctography depends upon opacification of multiple pelvic organs, it is unquestionably an intrusive procedure. Irrespective of the form of proctography employed, it is crucial to explain the procedure thoroughly to the patient beforehand and to provide maximal privacy and reassurance for the patient during the procedure. Respect for the dignity of the patient in an unfamiliar environment is of paramount importance (KELVIN et al. 2000).

In most centers, DCP is performed in one phase after all the constituent pelvic organs have been opacified. There is, however, only a limited amount of space within the confines of the bony pelvis. As a result, unemptied organs may prevent recognition of other prolapsed organs which are competing for available space. This is particularly true of the bladder; an insufficiently drained cystocele often prevents descent of small bowel and may minimize a rectocele (Fig. 4.2.1). Similarly, an incompletely emptied rectocele or rectum may also hide an enterocele. In view of these common problems, a triphasic approach based upon sequential organ emptying is optimal (KELVIN et al. 2000). The following account is a brief summary of this technique.

A special radiolucent commode that can be safely attached to the fluoroscopic table for fluoroscopy in the seated upright position is required. Initially, the pelvic small bowel is opacified with oral barium. The bladder is then catheterized and approximately 50 ml of cystographic contrast material is introduced. This amount is sufficient to fill the dependent part of the bladder and reduces the amount of drainage subsequently required. Lateral films of the bladder at rest and on maximal strain are obtained (cystographic phase) and the bladder then emptied as much as possible via the catheter before the latter is removed.

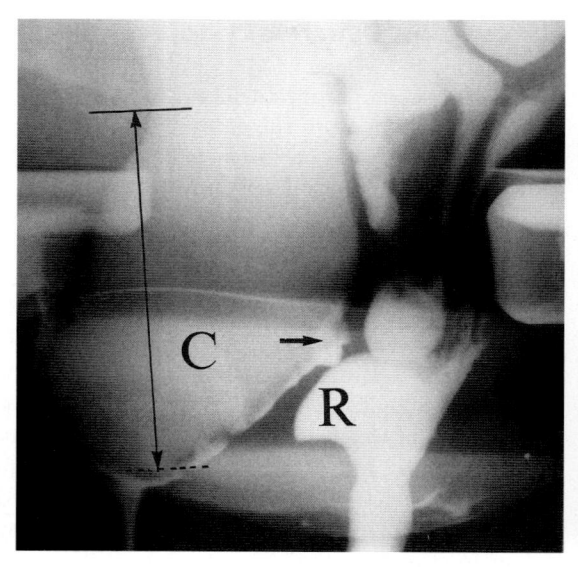

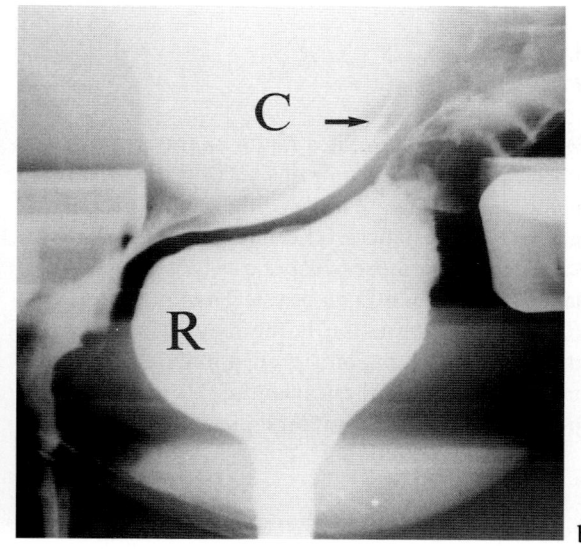

Fig. 4.2.1a, b. Cystocele minimizing size of rectocele. **a** Cystoproctogram image taken during evacuation shows a very large cystocele (*C*). The *uninterrupted line* represents the pubococcygeal line, the *dotted line* indicates the bladder base and the *arrowed line* therefore indicates the depth of the cystocele below the pubococcygeal line. There is a rectocele (*R*) but its size is minimized by pressure from the large cystocele. The *arrow* indicates the uppermost point of the vagina. **b** Six months later, following cystocele repair, urethral suspension and sacrocolpopexy, the cystoproctogram was repeated. The cystocele (*C*) is much smaller. The rectocele (*R*) is now considerably larger as it is no longer compressed by the cystocele. Note the elevation of the vaginal apex (*arrow*) as a result of sacrocolpopexy (reprinted with permission from KELVIN and MAGLINTE 1997)

After further voiding in the bathroom, the vagina is then opacified with 20 ml of a barium suspension following which a folded gauze square is inserted in the urogenital introitus to limit loss of contrast from the vagina and thereby improve vaginal opacification (Ho et al. 1999). The rectum is filled with approximately 200 ml of a high viscosity barium paste, which is introduced via a caulking gun, and lateral films of the pelvis at rest and on voluntary contraction of the pelvic floor muscles ("squeezing") are obtained. The patient is then asked to evacuate as rapidly and completely as possible and lateral films are taken during and following evacuation. The post-evacuation film is obtained with the patient straining maximally.

The patient then goes to the bathroom again to attempt further evacuation and voiding before returning for the post-toilet phase, which consists of a final lateral film on the commode with the patient again straining maximally. The entire examination is recorded on videotape for subsequent review.

A more invasive variation of proctography is to combine it with simultaneous peritoneography to directly visualize herniation of the posterior peritoneal cul-de-sac (peritoneography) (Halligan and Bartram 1995; Bremmer et al. 1997).

4.2.2.2
Radiologic Definitions and Grading of Prolapse

There are two basic considerations that are relevant to the radiologic assessment of pelvic organ prolapse. The first consideration is to determine whether prolapse of a specific organ is indeed present. If so, the degree of prolapse requires quantification, i.e. grading the extent of the prolapse is required. This grading is particularly important because minor degrees of prolapse are often asymptomatic. Unfortunately, there are no universally accepted radiologic criteria for defining prolapse of pelvic organs (Kelvin and Maglinte 2000).

Prolapse of most pelvic organs is customarily defined radiologically by reference to the pubococcygeal line, which extends from the inferior margin of the pubic symphysis to the sacrococcygeal junction. A cystocele, enterocele or sigmoidocele, and vaginal vault prolapse are defined by extension of the bladder base, small bowel or sigmoid colon, and vaginal apex respectively below this reference line (Fig. 4.2.1). An enterocele is often also defined by the extension of small bowel below the vaginal apex, but the vagina is too mobile a structure to be a reliable reference point. A radiologic grading system for prolapse of the above organs has been described: prolapse of any of these organs is graded as small if there is organ descent up to 3 cm below the pubococcygeal line, moderate if this extension measures between 3 and 6 cm, and large if descent is greater than 6 cm (Kelvin et al. 2000). These measurements are all made on the images which show maximal organ descent. The radiologic definition of a rectocele is based on different criteria (see below). Correction for magnification is made possible by the incorporation of a midline radio-opaque centimeter ruler within the commode.

Normative values for descent of the organs in the asymptomatic population are not available, and it is therefore appropriate that final determination of whether radiological findings are a cause of patient symptoms must depend on the patient's clinical status. There is considerable mobility of the pelvic organs found in normal multiparous women. A definitive-sounding radiologist's report may result in surgery, especially in the case of rectocele, when the descent of the pelvic organs is not the cause of symptoms. Therefore, open communication between the radiologist and clinician is critical to avoid surgery that will not correct a woman's problem.

4.2.2.3
Specific Sites of Prolapse on Fluoroscopic Examination

The relative prevalence of prolapsed organs at DCP in a large group of patients referred by urogynecology has been documented. A cystocele or a rectocele is present in more than 90% of such patients, and an enterocele is identified in approximately 30% (Kelvin et al. 1999). Sigmoidoceles are demonstrated in 4–5% of DCPs.

4.2.2.3.1
Rectocele

The majority of anterior rectoceles are believed to be related to vaginal delivery. Obstetric damage is thought to be responsible for weakness and even breakdown of the rectovaginal septum or fascia. Although a rectocele has often been defined radiologically as any anterior rectal bulge, such bulging is common in asymptomatic subjects (Bartram et al. 1988; Shorvon et al. 1989). An anterior rectocele, therefore, is better defined as a bulge greater than 2 cm in a symptomatic patient. The depth of the bulge is measured from a line extended upward from the anterior wall of the anal canal (Fig. 4.2.2).

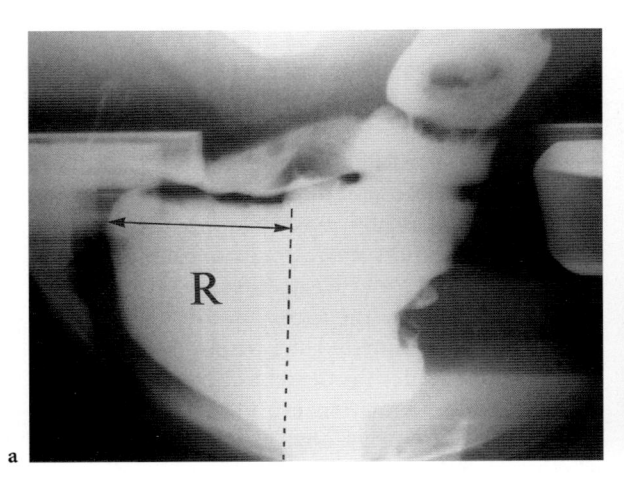

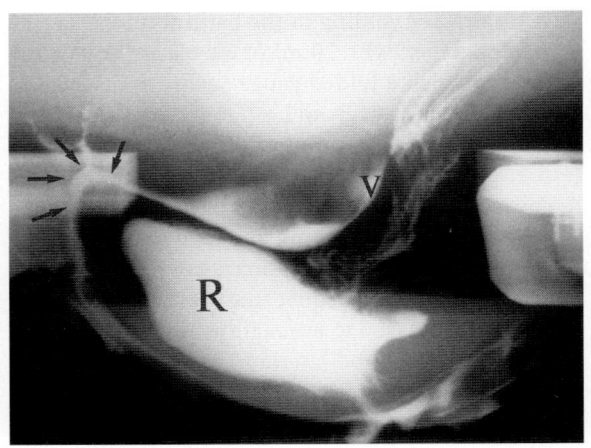

Fig. 4.2.2a, b. Large, symptomatic rectocele. Patient with rectal discomfort and sensation of incomplete emptying after bowel movement. **a** During evacuation, a large outpouching arises from the anterior aspect of the lower rectum indicating a large rectocele (*R*). The depth of the rectocele is measured by its maximal distance (*arrowed line*) from a line extended upwards from the anterior margin of the anal canal (*dotted line*). **b** Following evacuation, there is marked retention of contrast (barium trapping) within the rectocele (*R*). Note the anterior displacement of the vagina (*arrows*) by the rectal protrusion (*V* vaginal apex) (reprinted with permission from KELVIN and MAGLINTE 1997)

Proctography also determines whether barium is retained within the rectocele after evacuation (barium trapping) (Fig. 4.2.2). The likelihood of barium trapping is directly related to rectocele size (KELVIN et al. 1992). Trapping of contents is generally thought to explain the evacuation disturbance associated with a rectocele (VAN DAM et al. 1997). Recent experience has shown that barium trapping diminishes considerably if a post-toilet image is obtained (GREENBERG et al. 2001). This is presumably related to more effective evacuation in the privacy of the bathroom. Trapping is an important radiographic observation, as many surgeons are reluctant to operate on a rectocele unless it retains contrast.

If symptomatic, rectoceles usually are associated with straining and a sensation of incomplete evacuation. In some patients, impaired evacuation is probably associated with anismus rather than with the rectocele itself (JOHANSSON et al. 1992). Proctography may suggest the presence of anismus (HALLIGAN et al. 1995) and, therefore, the need for biofeedback therapy instead of surgery.

Posterior or lateral rectoceles (see Fig. 4.2.3a) may also occur (see section 4.2.3 Dynamic MR Imaging of the Pelvic Floor).

4.2.2.3.2
Enterocele

An enterocele is a mass effect produced by distending herniation of small bowel into the posterior peritoneal cul-de-sac in the rectovaginal space (Fig. 4.2.4) and/or into the vagina itself (Fig. 4.2.5). Definitive diagnosis therefore depends upon opacification of both the pelvic small bowel and the vagina. Since the normal posterior cul-de-sac extends 4 cm below the cervix, the simple presence of this space in this location should not be confused with the distension of this area by intestinal contents (KUHN and HOLLYOCK 1982) Enterocele is not uncommon after hysterectomy and cystourethropexy, as these procedures may open up the posterior cul-de-sac.

Unlike rectoceles, which are usually maximal during evacuation, enteroceles often become evident only at the end of evacuation. Repeated straining after evacuation may be essential for recognition of enteroceles (Fig. 4.2.4). In one study, almost half (43%) of the enteroceles were only seen on postevacuation or post-toilet radiographs with the patient straining maximally, thus emphasizing the importance of this maneuver (KELVIN et al. 1999). Evacuation should be as complete as possible because the unemptied rectum or rectocele may prevent descent of an enterocele (KELVIN and MAGLINTE 1997). Obtaining a post-toilet image on straining after the patient has been to the bathroom to carry out further rectal evacuation therefore offers the best proctographic opportunity to detect an enterocele (Fig. 4.2.3). Enteroceles that are intravaginal rather than extending into the rectovaginal space may compete with a cystocele (Fig. 4.2.5). If the cystocele is not sufficiently drained, the presence of a coexistent enterocele may be overlooked or minimized.

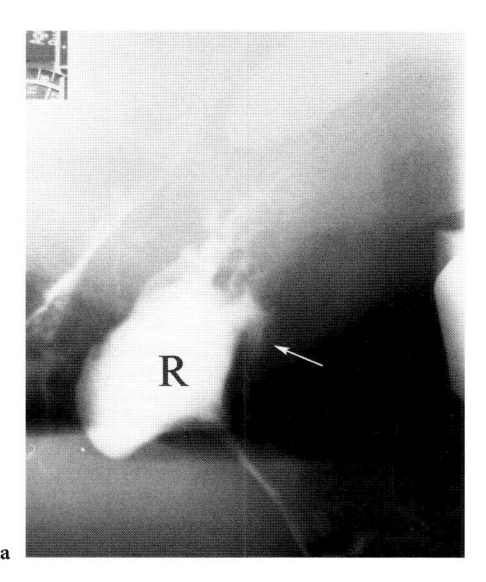

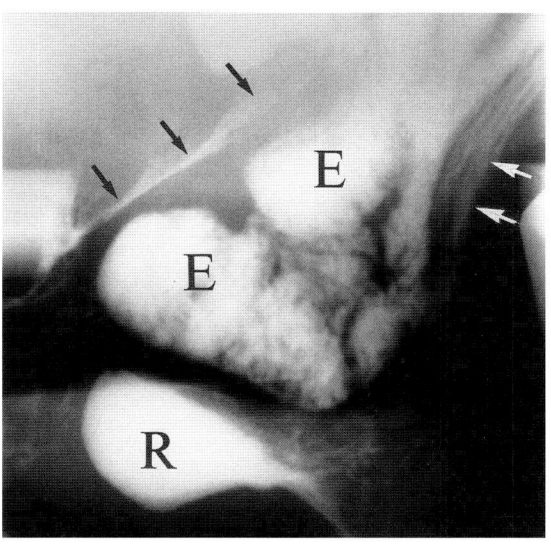

Fig. 4.2.3a, b. Importance of post-toilet state for demonstration of enterocele. a Post-evacuation image shows large rectocele (*R*) with considerable barium trapping. Note also a posterior rectocele (*arrow*) due to herniation through the levator anus. The rectovaginal space is widened, consistent with a peritoneocele. b Following evacuation in bathroom, the rectocele (*r*) has almost completely emptied. The rectovaginal space is now filled by a large enterocele (*E*) (reprinted with permission from KELVIN and MAGLINTE 1997)

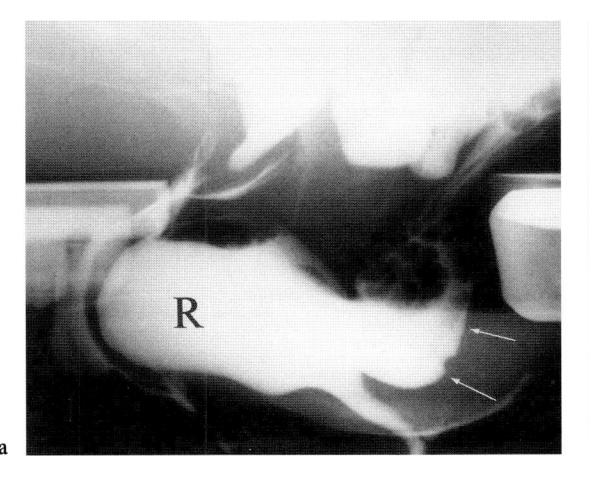

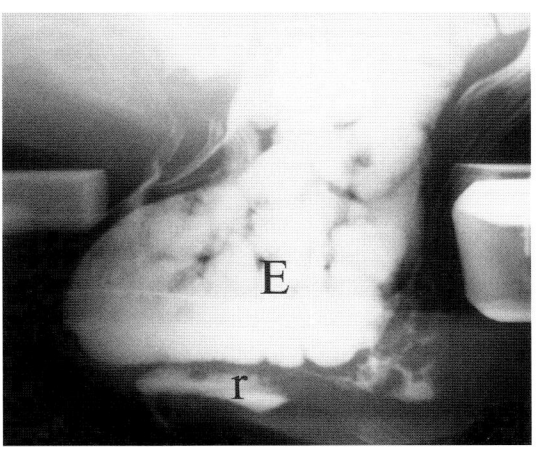

Fig. 4.2.4a, b. Enterocele in rectovaginal space only visualized on straining maximally. a Post-evacuation image taken without straining shows no evidence of enterocele. Note barium trapping in rectocele (*R*). b On maximal straining, small bowel loops have descended between the vagina and collapsed upper rectum indicating an enterocele (*E*) in the rectovaginal space. Note descent of rectocele (*R*) on straining (reprinted with permission from KELVIN and MAGLINTE 1997)

Both enteroceles and rectoceles are well demonstrated by either DCP or MR imaging. Recently, detection of enteroceles by the technique of dynamic anorectal endosonography has also been described (KARAUS et al. 2000). In a small series, all enteroceles found in the Pouch of Douglas by this endoluminal technique were confirmed by subsequent proctography. Anorectal endosonography is easier to perform and less cumbersome for the patient than proctography, and is deserving of further evaluation.

Enteroceles have long been held responsible for causing pressure on the rectum and thereby obstructing rectal evacuation, so-called "defecation block" (WALLDEN 1952). A much more recent proctographic study has shown that enteroceles do not impair rectal evacuation (HALLIGAN et al. 1996).

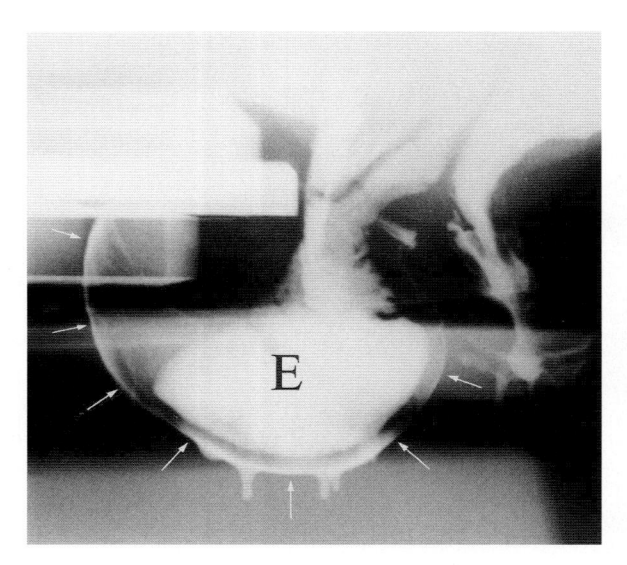

Fig. 4.2.5. Intravaginal enterocele and competing cystocele. Post-evacuation image shows external vaginal prolapse. The everted vagina is coated with contrast material (*arrows*). A large enterocele (*E*) is present posteriorly within the prolapsed vagina, while the anterior half of the vagina is occupied by non-opacified cystocele

4.2.2.3.3
Peritoneocele

The combination of proctography and simultaneous peritoneography demonstrates the location and extent of the posterior peritoneal cul-de-sac. The term "peritoneocele" has been applied to herniation of the cul-de-sac (BREMMER et al. 1997). BREMMER et al. defined a peritoneocele as an extension of the rectouterine excavation to below the upper third of the vagina (BREMMER et al. 1997).

When peritoneography is performed, only approximately 50% of peritoneoceles are found to contain bowel (BREMMER et al. 1997; HALLIGAN et al. 1996). In our experience, however, peritoneoceles usually contain small bowel; this probably reflects our routine use of imaging in the post-toilet phase (Fig. 4.2.3) (KELVIN et al. 2000). Peritoneoceles have been classified as rectal, septal or vaginal, depending on their location: rectal peritoneoceles are located within an associated rectal intussusception; septal peritoneoceles descend within the rectovaginal space; and vaginal peritoneoceles bulge into the vagina itself (BREMMER et al. 1997). Recognition of a peritoneocele, whether by peritoneography or MR imaging, is important because it predisposes to enterocele formation and suggests the need for operative closure of the cul-de-sac if pelvic floor reconstructive surgery is undertaken (KELVIN et al. 2000).

The presence of a peritoneocele should be suspected at routine DCP if there is unexplained widening of the rectovaginal space (Fig. 4.2.3); in our experience, this is found in 9% of DCPs (KELVIN et al. 1999).

4.2.2.3.4
Sigmoidocele

A sigmoidocele is a redundancy of the sigmoid colon that extends caudally into the cul-de-sac (Fig. 4.2.6) (JORGE et al. 1994). Sigmoidoceles, even when large, are usually not detected on physical examination (FENNER 1996; KELVIN et al. 2000). They are less common than enteroceles and are found in approximately 5% of proctograms (FENNER 1996; JORGE et al. 1994; KELVIN et al. 1999). As with other organ prolapses, there is no unanimity of definition. FENNER et al. defined a sigmoidocele as sigmoid colon extending more than 4 cm below the pubococcygeal line, but according to our definition (see above), such a finding would constitute a moderately sized sigmoid herniation (FENNER 1996; KELVIN et al. 2000).

Large sigmoidoceles are often associated with constipation (FENNER 1996; JORGE et al. 1994). The redundant colon may compress the rectum and obstruct defecation. This is more likely to occur with a sigmoidocele than an enterocele because the colon contains more solid contents and is of greater caliber (FENNER 1996).

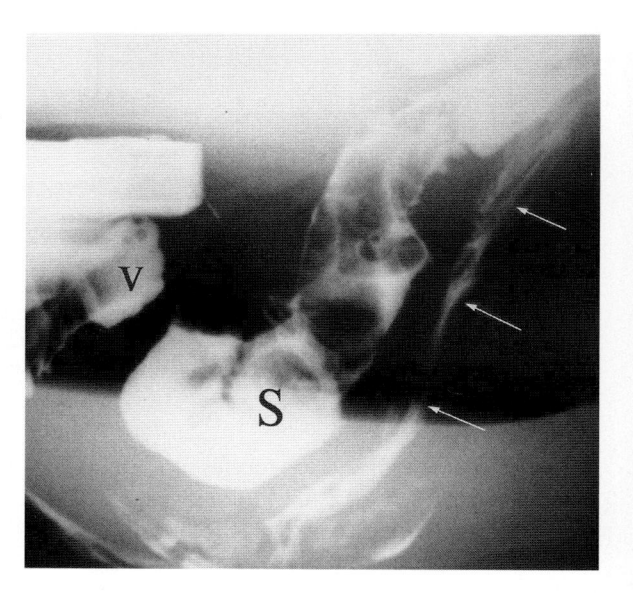

Fig. 4.2.6. Sigmoidocele. Post-evacuation image demonstrates a stool-filled loop of sigmoid colon (*S*) that has descended into the rectovaginal space, indicating a sigmoidocele (*V* vagina, *arrows* collapsed rectum)

4.2.2.3.5
Vaginal Vault Prolapse

Vaginal vault prolapse involves prolapse of the apex of the vagina toward, through, or beyond the introitus (TIMMONS and ADDISON 1996). External vaginal prolapse (Fig. 4.2.5) or vaginal prolapse to the introitus is usually clinically obvious. Vaginal vault prolapse is often associated with an enterocele. This association usually reflects loss of support at the level of the vaginal apex due to damage to the uterosacral-cardinal complex.

Despite adequate vaginal opacification, the precise location of the vaginal apex may be difficult to determine on the postevacuation and post-toilet images. With marked vaginal descent or external vaginal prolapse, however, clinical inspection is usually self-evident.

4.2.2.3.6
Cystocele

Cystoceles are the result of defects in the attachments of the pubocervical fascia to the pelvic walls. They are defined radiologically by descent of the bladder base below the pubococcygeal line. Contrast opacification is not essential for the recognition of cystoceles, as they can be inferred by downward displacement of the vagina provided that the vagina is well opacified. Cystocele size is frequently greater after rectal evacuation than during cystography, and is therefore often optimally assessed by the depth of the displacement of the anterior vaginal wall at the end of the proctographic phase (KELVIN et al. 1999). However, even if cystography is not performed, it is often nevertheless necessary to catheterize the bladder in order to facilitate bladder drainage. If this is not done, the large area occupied by an undrained cystocele may prevent detection of a coexistent enterocele or rectocele (Fig. 4.2.1).

Retention of the catheter within the bladder is also useful during filming as it indicates the axis of the urethra and identifies the region of the bladder neck. The urethral axis is normally less than 30° to the vertical; a horizontally inclined urethra indicates a urethrocele. The degree of mobility of the bladder neck can be measured at cystography by comparing its position at rest and on maximal strain. Urethral hypermobility is often associated with stress urinary incontinence although there is considerable overlap between normal and abnormal findings (ALA-KETOLA 1973). Funneling of the bladder neck at rest where contrast occupies the upper portion of the urethra may indicate intrinsic sphincter deficiency but is a non-specific sign and may also be seen in continent women (PANNU et al. 2000).

4.2.2.4
Comparison with Physical Examination

Early experience with evacuation proctography suggested that this radiologic technique detected enteroceles and sigmoidoceles that were not identified by physical examination (KELVIN et al. 1992). Subsequent comparative studies have confirmed the relative insensitivity of physical examination. The latter approach appears to identify only approximately 50% of enteroceles, but fares better in the recognition of rectoceles and cystoceles (ALTRINGER et al. 1995; KELVIN et al. 1999; VANBECKEVOORT et al. 1999).

Insensitivity of the physical examination is almost certainly related to the patient's inability to strain maximally while being examined but also because the nature of the intestine in the protruding bulge cannot be always determined by palpation. Complete relaxation of pelvic floor muscles occurs only during defecation (and micturition), thereby allowing pelvic organ prolapse to manifest itself to the fullest extent. The degree of straining achieved by the patient while encumbered by an examining digit (with or without a vaginal speculum) is clearly less than that achieved during defecation.

A more fundamental benefit of imaging is that it directly visualizes the organs at the site of prolapse, whereas the positions of these organs can only be inferred on physical examination. Incorrect inferences may lead to a lack of correlation between the two methods of examination. It must be emphasized, however, that these two diagnostic approaches are based upon entirely different reference points: the hymeneal ring and the pubococcygeal line. A common reference system would be enormously beneficial (KELVIN and MAGLINTE 2000) and findings in the normal asymptomatic population are also needed.

It appears likely that the limitations of physical examination have contributed to the frequent need for reoperation. One study found that the diagnosis of rectocele, enterocele and cystocele was changed in 75% of patients in whom DCP was performed (ALTRINGER et al. 1995). More recently, the complementary contributions of both DCP and MR imaging to the physical examination have been emphasized (KAUFMAN et al. 2001). Prolapse almost invariably involves multiple organs. Indeed, 95% of patients investigated radiologically for prolapse have abnormalities in all three pelvic compartments (Maglinte et al. 1997, 1999). It is advisable to identify all the areas of prolapse preoperatively because they may all require surgical correction, and ideally this is done at one operative setting (Benson 1992).

4.2.3
Dynamic MR Imaging of the Pelvic Floor

MR imaging can be used as an alternative or complementary technique to other imaging modalities for the evaluation of pelvic organ prolapse. The chief advantages of MR imaging are superior soft tissue contrast and lack of ionizing radiation. The supine position of the patient is a drawback but can be addressed by the administration of rectal contrast followed by patient defecation to ensure adequate increase in abdominal and pelvic pressure during the study. The role of MR imaging is evolving and the optimal techniques for performing and interpreting the study are being refined.

4.2.3.1
Technique

The technique for MR imaging is not standardized. One of the main variables relates to the administration of rectal contrast. Adequate increase in abdominal pressure is necessary to avoid false-negative MR imaging studies and may be more reliably achieved if there is evacuation of rectal contrast. Although the pelvic soft tissues are well seen without luminal contrast, the rectum may not be adequately distended if its lumen is not opacified. Furthermore, abnormalities of rectal evacuation such as intussusception are difficult to appreciate without contrast administration. One of the reasons that MR imaging has not replaced fluoroscopy is the concern that suboptimal straining in the supine position masks clinically relevant pelvic floor defects (Brubaker and Heit 1993) This must be balanced, however, with the possibility of false-positive results because an abnormality that exists only in the seated, defecatory position may not be responsible for symptoms that occur during the remainder of the day.

Rectal contrast usually consists of semisolid material such as ultrasound gel or mashed potatoes mixed with gadolinium. Reports in the literature have shown that patients are able to defecate while supine and the magnet is very rarely contaminated if absorbent pads are placed under the patient to contain the semisolid contrast. In addition to rectal contrast, contrast is also placed within the vagina to facilitate its identification. The small bowel and bladder are identified by natural contrast in the form of fluid and gas in the bowel and urine in the bladder. The patient is usually asked to void prior to the study since overdistension of the bladder may prevent uterine and small bowel descent.

Dynamic imaging of the pelvis is performed with gradient echo or single shot fast spin echo sequences which have short image acquisition times in the range 1–2 s. Contrast between the pelvic viscera is excellent with the single shot T2-weighted technique (Unterweger et al. 2001). Rest, straining and defecating images are obtained. Sagittal images are essential (Fig. 4.2.7). Coronal and axial images provide supplemental information. Sample protocols are: (1) single shot fast spin echo sequence with TR infinite, TE 60 ms, NEX 0.5, FOV 28 cm, slice thickness 6 mm, gap 2 mm, matrix 256+256, bandwidth 32 kHz, and echo train length 16; and (2) gradient echo sequence with TR/TE 31/13 and flip angle 60° (Tunn et al. 2000).

4.2.3.2
Evolution of Dynamic MR Imaging

The role of MR imaging as a problem-solving technique for uterine and ovarian pathology has been recognized for several years, and static imaging of the urogenital tract is common. However, pelvic organ prolapse often is only evident during patient straining when abdominal pressure rises. Yang et al. reported on a novel method to study organ prolapse on MR imaging by imaging patients while straining and documenting organ descent (Yang et al. 1991). They carried out dynamic MR imaging examinations with rest and strain images in 26 women with prolapse and 16 asymptomatic women, and then formulated guidelines for the normal range of organ descent during straining. The technique proposed by Yang et al. has subsequently been modified to include administration of rectal and vaginal contrast, as well as imaging during defecation (Lienemann et al. 1997). With this protocol, the technique of MR imaging parallels that of the fluoroscopic examination.

Upright MR imaging with the patient seated on a commode combines the advantages of MR imaging and fluoroscopy. The effects of gravity and defecation optimize the detection of prolapse, rectal dysfunction can be evaluated during defecation, and the soft tissues of the pelvic floor can also be assessed. However,

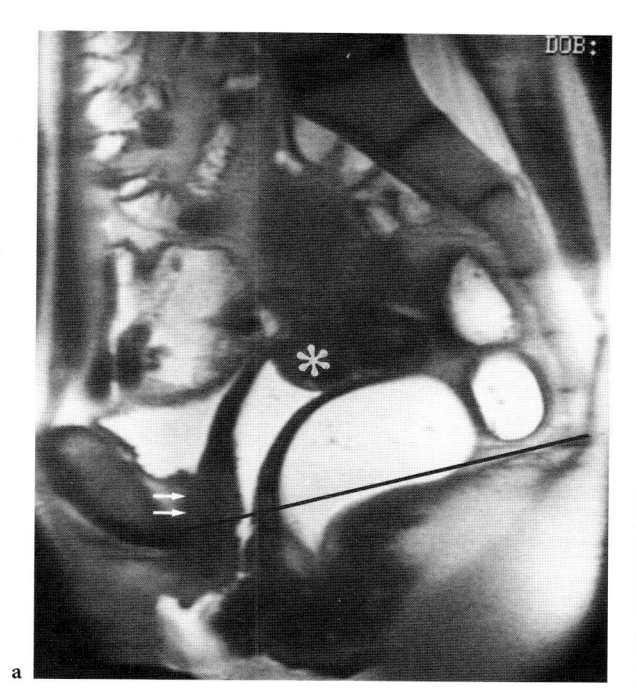

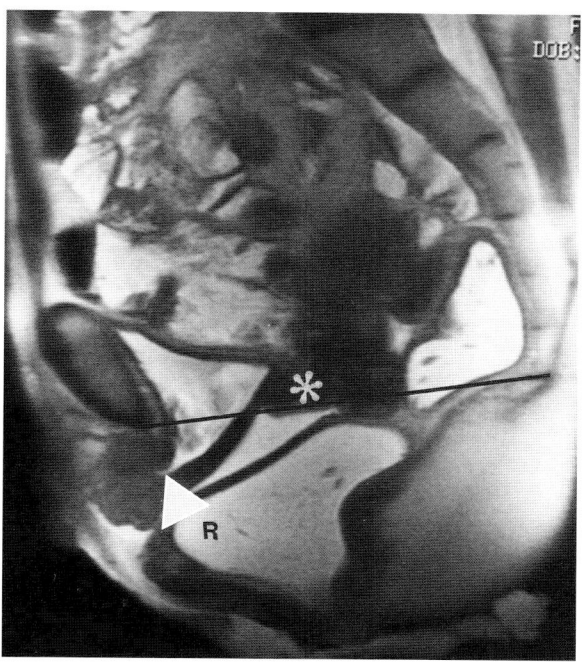

Fig. 4.2.7a, b. Pelvic organ prolapse on sagittal images. Urethral mobility and funneling, cystocele, cervical prolapse, and anterior rectocele in a 42-year-old woman with stress urinary incontinence and pelvic floor laxity on physical examination. Sagittal T2 weighted MR images of the pelvis with the patient at rest (**a**) and during evacuation (**b**). Gel has been placed in the vagina and rectum. At rest, the urethra (*double arrows*) is normal in orientation but becomes horizontal when the patient strains due to urethral hypermobility. The urethrovesical junction is closed at rest but opens with straining (*arrowhead*) and there is descent of the bladder consistent with a small cystocele. The cervix (*asterisk*) also descends with straining from above the level of the pubis to the inferior margin. An anterior rectocele (*R*) also develops when the patient strains. The anal canal is open as the patient is defecating for the study. The *straight line* indicates the pubococcygeal line

a vertical configuration magnet is required which has a central gap into which the commode can be placed. Although a magnet of this design may be structurally ideal for imaging prolapse, it is a research machine that is currently available in only a limited number of institutions worldwide and is predominantly used for interventional MR imaging. A few investigators have reported patient studies using such magnets with visualization of rectal abnormalities such as rectoceles, anismus and rectal intussusception as well as anterior pelvic prolapse (HILFIKER et al. 1998; LAMB et al. 2000; SCHOENENBERGER et al. 1998). In another study involving 102 women it was shown that the positions of the pelvic organs are lower at rest, straining and contraction in multiparous women when compared to nulliparous women (LAW et al. 2001). Additionally, bladder descent has been found to be greater in the seated than in the supine position (FIELDING et al. 1998). In both seated and supine MR imaging studies, alteration in levator muscle morphology with contraction and straining has been demonstrated (Bo et al. 2001; CHRISTENSEN et al. 1995a,b).

The literature on supine MR imaging studies is more extensive and includes descriptions of the changes in the pelvis following vaginal delivery. Initially, probably due to edema, the signal intensity of the levator muscle is increased relative to the obturator internus muscle on T2-weighted images (TUNN et al. 1999). With time, the signal intensity of muscle and size of the pelvic hiatus decrease. Increased signal intensity of the levator muscle has also been reported in women with urinary incontinence and pelvic organ prolapse and may be due to replacement of the muscle by fat or connective tissue (TUNN et al. 1998). Loss of muscle fiber may be the cause of the focal eventrations which are sometimes seen on MR imaging.

The multiplanar imaging capability of MR is well suited to demonstrating the complex anatomy of the levator muscle and also allows three-dimensional modeling of the muscle (FIELDING et al. 2000; FROHLICH et al. 1997; STROHBEHN et al. 1996a). Normally, the levator ani has a dome-shaped appearance at rest due to the continuous tone provided by slow twitch fibers (Fig. 4.2.8) (HJARTARDOTTIR et al. 1997). With strain-

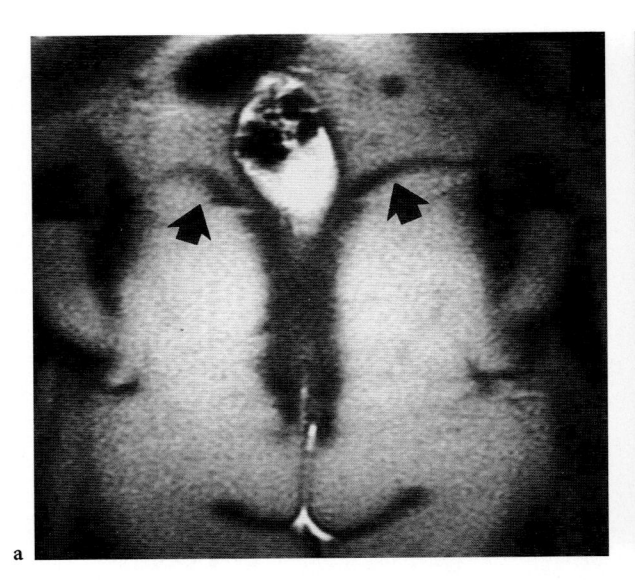

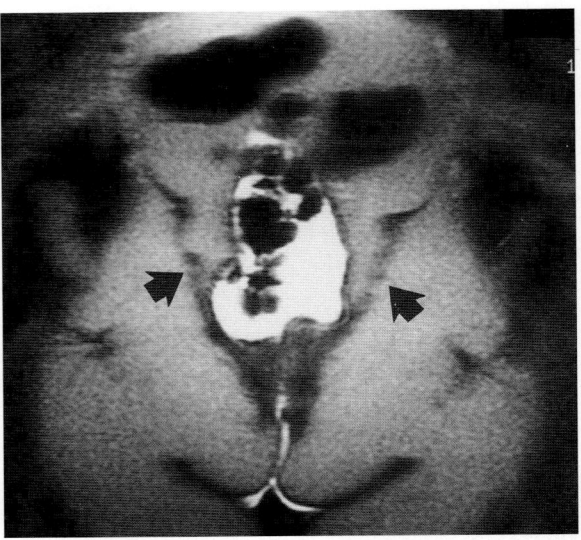

Fig. 4.2.8a, b. Bulging of the levator ani muscle in a 66-year-old woman with vaginal prolapse and anal sphincter defect. Coronal T2-weighted MR images of the pelvis with the patient at rest (**a**) and on straining (**b**). At rest, the levator muscle has a dome-shaped appearance (*arrows*). The levator bulges (*arrows*) when the patient strains, resulting in a basin-shaped configuration. This corresponds to the increase in the pelvic hiatus area seen on the axial images

ing, this configuration changes to a basin shape which is more pronounced in women with prolapse. On sagittal images, a line drawn through the levator plate lies inferior to the pubis due to caudal angulation of the muscle (Osaza et al. 1992). Caudal angulation and ballooning of the muscle is known to occur in constipated patients with resultant increase in the pelvic hiatus (Healy et al. 1997a). Greater attention to MR imaging of the levator muscle is likely to provide important information on the factors that predispose patients to prolapse.

Specific findings on MR imaging in women with prolapse are descent of the bladder and uterus in constipated patients and predominantly anorectal descent in patients with fecal incontinence (Healy et al. 1997b). After surgical repair, a decrease in the amount of organ prolapse can be documented (Goodrich et al. 1993; Lienemann et al. 2001). However, caudal angulation of the levator muscle and the width of the pelvic hiatus may not be altered by surgery.

A study of the levator ani in nulliparous volunteers concluded that the muscle is composed of two main components, the iliococcygeus which is best seen in the coronal plane, and the puborectalis which is optimally visualized on axial sections (Singh et al. 2002). These authors concluded that the main function of the iliococcygeus is supportive, whereas the inferomedially located puborectalis serves to maintain pelvic floor closure. Gaps were identified in the normal iliococcygeus and asymmetry of the puborectalis, which was thinner on the right, was also found.

4.2.3.3
Specific Sites of Prolapse on MR Examination

4.2.3.3.1
Urethra and Vagina

Change in the urethral axis is easily seen on sagittal MR images in patients with urethral hypermobility. The axis can change from the normal vertical position to a horizontal lie as abdominal pressure increases (Fig. 4.2.7). A urethral angle greater than 30° from the vertical and a posterior urethrovesical angle greater than 115° are traditionally considered abnormal (Comiter et al. 1999; Fielding et al. 1996) but findings in normal women are needed. Differential mobility of the walls of the urethra has been described on ultrasound. This is due to greater movement of the posterior than the anterior urethral wall with resultant funneling of the proximal urethral lumen (Mostwin et al. 1995).

In addition to dynamic information on urethral mobility, MR imaging can provide information on urethral and vaginal support as well as urethral abnormalities such as diverticula. Deficient urethral and vaginal support occurs with tears in the lateral portion of the endopelvic fascia; these are referred to as paravaginal defects. The evidence for such tears is usually indirect on MR imaging and is suggested by loss of the normal "H" shape of the vagina as the lateral insertions of the endopelvic fascia overlying the anterior vaginal wall are believed to be responsible for this vaginal shape on axial MR sections (Fig. 4.2.9) (ARONSON et al. 1995; HUDDLESTON et al. 1995). However, lack of an "H" shape has also been described in normal nulliparous volunteers; consequently the reliability and significance of this finding require clarification (FIELDING et al. 2000). Direct demonstration of a ligamentous abnormality would provide more reliable evidence of a paravaginal tear. Attenuation or absence of ligaments from the posterior pubic symphysis to the anterior vaginal wall has been seen in a small series of patients with incontinence imaged by endovaginal MR (ARONSON et al. 1995). There is controversy in the literature regarding the existence and course of urethral support ligaments to the pelvic side wall (FIELDING et al. 2000; KIRSCHNER-HERMANNS et al. 1993; KLUTKE et al. 1990; TAN et al. 1997, 1998). Urethral support is provided by a combination of connective and muscular support, and evaluation of both the levator ani muscle and the fascial connections to the pelvic sidewall will be needed to understand these support abnormalities (DELANCEY 1994). Further investigation of normal and abnormal supporting pelvic floor structures shows both muscle and connective tissue abnormalities (DELANCEY 2002) and MR would soon contribute to our understanding of the pathophysiology of pelvic floor dysfunction by identifying these abnormalities.

In addition to lateral detachments of the vaginal fascia, the retropubic space is also enlarged in patients with incontinence (ARONSON et al. 1995). Other findings on MR imaging are descent of the vaginal apex and loss of the normal posterior angulation of the proximal vagina due to deficient superior support (OSAZA et al. 1992). With severe prolapse, the vaginal mucosa is everted.

Urethral and vaginal morphology and, to a lesser extent, their support ligaments are evaluated on MR imaging. Due to the high soft tissue contrast, abnormalities of the urethral wall such as diverticula are easily diagnosed. As opposed to fluoroscopy, catheterization is not necessary and the diverticula appear as fluid filled sacs adjacent to the lumen of the urethra (KIM et al. 1993; NEITLICH et al. 1998; ROMANZI et al. 2000). Similar to reports on the anal sphincter, the submucosal and muscular components of the urethra can be distinguished on MR imaging (TAN et al. 1998). The mucosa and submucosa are hypointense, the smooth muscle is hyperintense and the outer striated muscle is hypointense (STROHBEHN et al. 1996b). Investigational work with endourethral

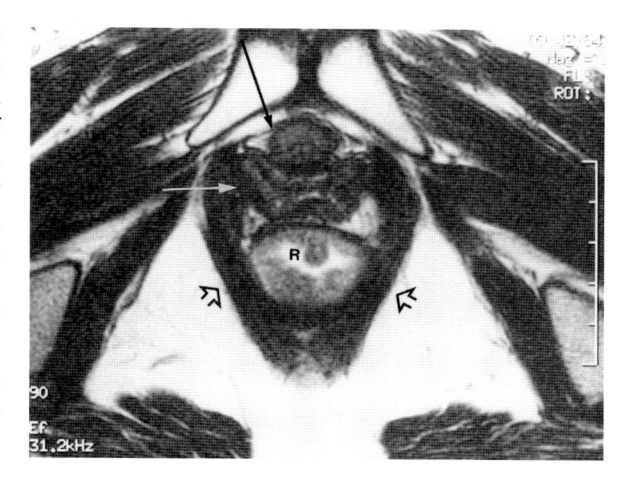

Fig. 4.2.9. Normal anatomy. The patient is a 42-year-old woman with a history of rectocele. High resolution axial T2-weighted image of the pelvis at the level of the pubic symphysis. Urethra (*black arrow*) with outer hypointense striated muscle and inner hyperintense smooth muscle layers. The normal "H" shape of the vagina (*white arrow*) is seen (R rectum). The levator ani muscles (*open arrows*) are normal in configuration

MR imaging and ultrasound may provide important information regarding alteration in muscle bulk with aging (QUICK et al. 2001). Another application of MR imaging is in the monitoring of patients treated with submucosal intraurethral collagen injections (CARR et al. 1996).

4.2.3.3.2
Bladder, Uterus and Cul-De-Sac

Cystoceles appear as posterior bulges of the bladder into the anterior vaginal wall as seen on sagittal images or as descent of the bladder base below the pubococcygeal line (Fig. 4.2.10). Axial images can be helpful to determine if the cystocele is midline and if there is a focal defect in the support of the pubocervical fascia. With large cystoceles, the urethrovesical junction may be kinked. Uterine prolapse appears as descent of the uterus into the vaginal canal. If the uterus prolapses completely out of the pelvic cavity, it is referred to as procidentia (Fig. 4.2.11). Defects in the superior portion of the rectovaginal fascia allow peritoneal fat, small bowel or sigmoid colon to prolapse into the rectovaginal space (Fig. 4.2.12). An enterocele may be missed if the bladder is distended and the patient has a cystocele. This can lead to recurrent prolapse after surgery if it is not recognized. Therefore, having the patient void prior to the study or obtaining postvoid images is essential.

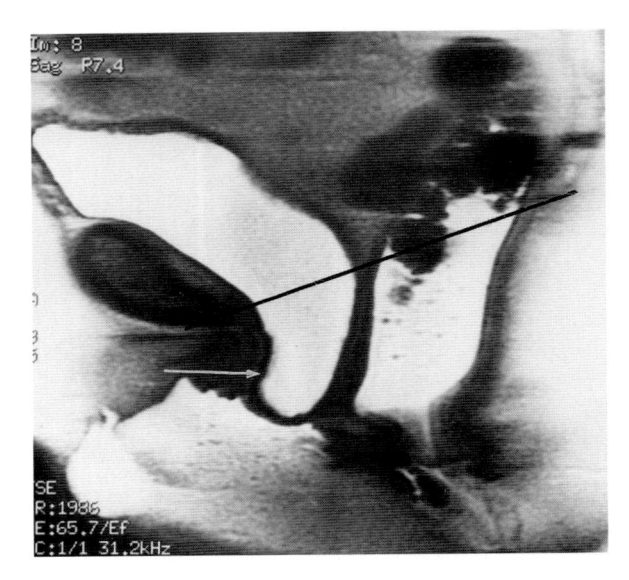

Fig. 4.2.10. Cystocele. Typical cystocele on a sagittal T2-weighted image of the pelvis of a 66-year-old woman with a history of vaginal prolapse and prior repair. The patient is straining and there is descent of the bladder (*arrow*). The rectum appears normal. The *straight line* indicates the pubococcygeal line

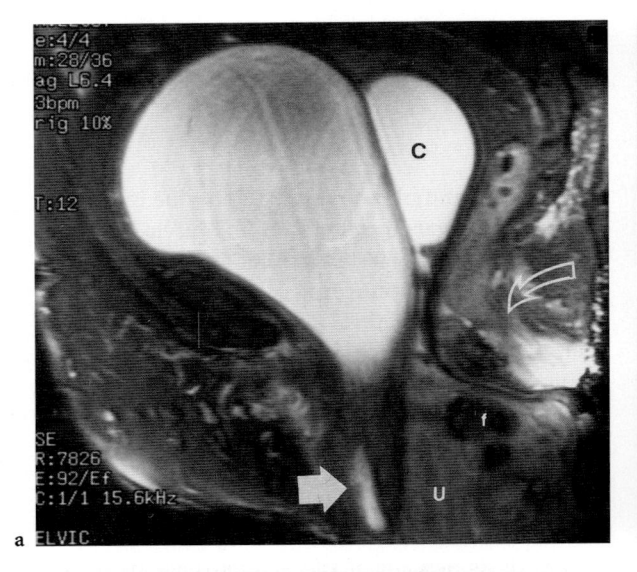

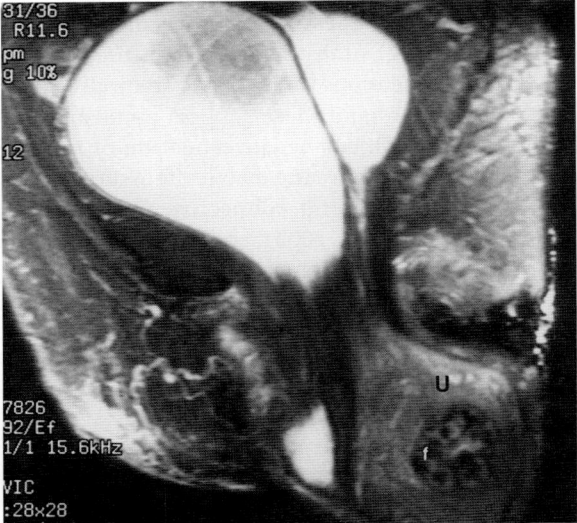

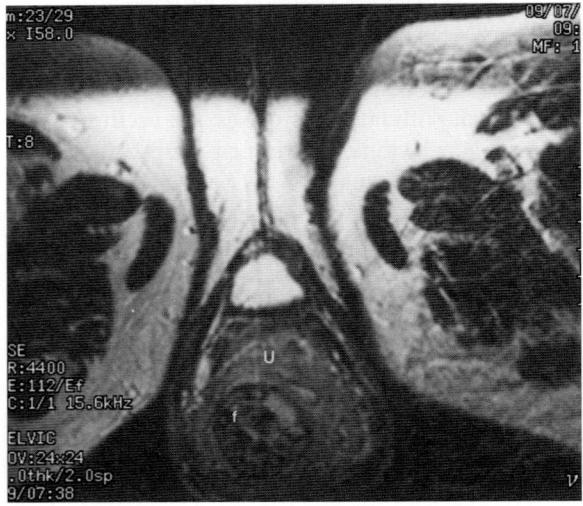

Fig. 4.2.11a–c. Uterine prolapse in a 92-year-old woman with a history of a cystic adnexal mass. **a** Sagittal T2-weighted MR image of the pelvis with the patient at rest. The midsagittal image shows a low-lying bladder consistent with cystocele (*solid arrow*). The anus is normal in position (*open arrow*). The protruding structure between the bladder and the anus is the prolapsed uterus (*U*) containing fibroids (*f*). There is also an ovarian cyst (*C*), lying posterior to the bladder secondary to uterine prolapse. **b** A parasagittal image shows the uterus (*U*) more clearly (*f* contained fibroids). **c** Axial image in the same patient showing the uterus (*U*) lying low below the confines of the pelvis, indicating procidentia (*f* fibroids)

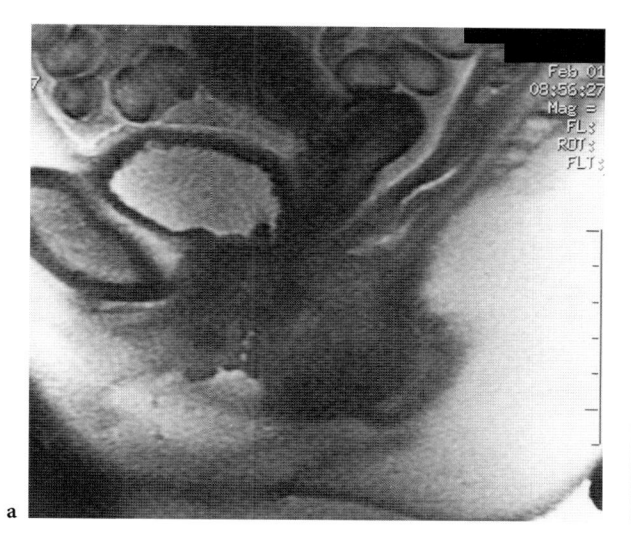

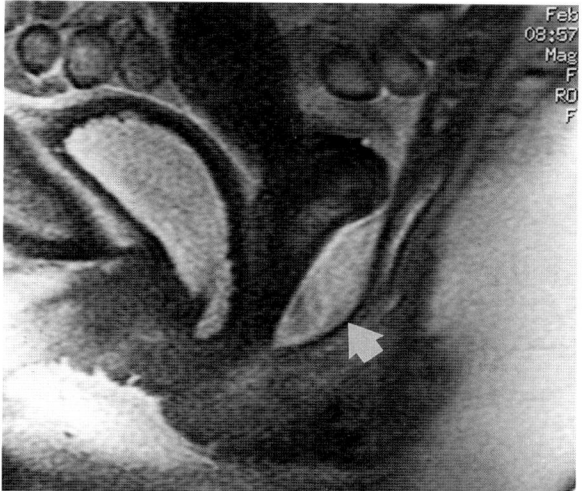

Fig. 4.2.12a,b. Peritoneocele and cystocele in a 66-year-old woman with a history of pelvic relaxation. **a** Sagittal T2-weighted MR image of the pelvis with the patient at rest shows normal appearances. **b** When the patient strains, there is widening of the rectovaginal space by peritoneal fat (*arrow*). The findings are compatible with a defect in the rectovaginal fascia and peritoneocele

4.2.3.3.3
Rectum

The rectum can bulge anteriorly or posterolaterally. Defects in the rectovaginal fascia lead to anterior rectoceles (Figs. 4.2.7, 4.2.13), which are by far the commonest type of rectocele. Posterior or lateral bulges of the rectum occur when there is deficient support by the levator ani muscle. The lateral component of a rectocele is not demonstrated on fluoroscopic DCP confined to the lateral projection.

Other primary abnormalities of the rectum, in particular rectal prolapse and rectal intussusception, can be visualized on MR imaging if rectal contrast is administered and the patient defecates during the study. Imaging of the anal sphincter can be performed by ultrasound or MR. Both modalities show the anal wall and tears in the sphincter (Hussain et al. 1995; Stoker and Rociu 1999; Stoker et al. 2001).

4.2.3.4
Criteria for Diagnosing Pelvic Organ Prolapse on MR Imaging

As with the fluoroscopic technique, there is no consensus as to the criteria for diagnosing organ prolapse on MR imaging. The pubococcygeal line is usually used as a reference on sagittal images. The line is drawn from the last coccygeal joint to the inferior pubic symphysis (Yang et al. 1991). This reference line is much easier to identify on MR images than the fluoroscopic study.

A combination of the guidelines provided by Yang et al. in their initial article and fluoroscopic criteria are used to diagnose prolapse. In general, if the bladder base, uterine cervix and vaginal apex descend below the pubococcygeal line, there is abnormal organ descent or prolapse (Lienemann et al. 1997; Goh et al. 2000; Yang et al. 1991). Peritoneocele, enterocele or sigmoidocele are diagnosed when there is widening of the rectovaginal space by peritoneal fat, small bowel or sigmoid colon. Rectocele is defined above (section 4.2.2.3.1). In all cases, the findings on imaging have to be correlated with patient symptoms since there is wide variation in the range of normal organ descent and only symptomatic patients are treated.

In distinction to most measurement schemes which use the pubococcygeal line as a reference, there is also a separate "HMO" classification for measuring prolapse on sagittal images (Comiter et al. 1999). These authors draw an "H" line from the pubis to the posterior anal canal to measure the width of the levator hiatus, and an "M" line to measure the descent of the levator plate relative to the pubococcygeal line. Organ descent ("O" line) is then measured relative to the "H" line. Additional measurements that can be performed on MR imaging are the width and area of the pelvic hiatus on axial images. The transverse diameter of the levator muscle on axial images measures the extent of its ballooning (Fig. 4.2.14). The use of standardized criteria on MR images will facilitate comparison between studies.

A more recent MR imaging study used the midpubic line drawn through the longitudinal axis of the

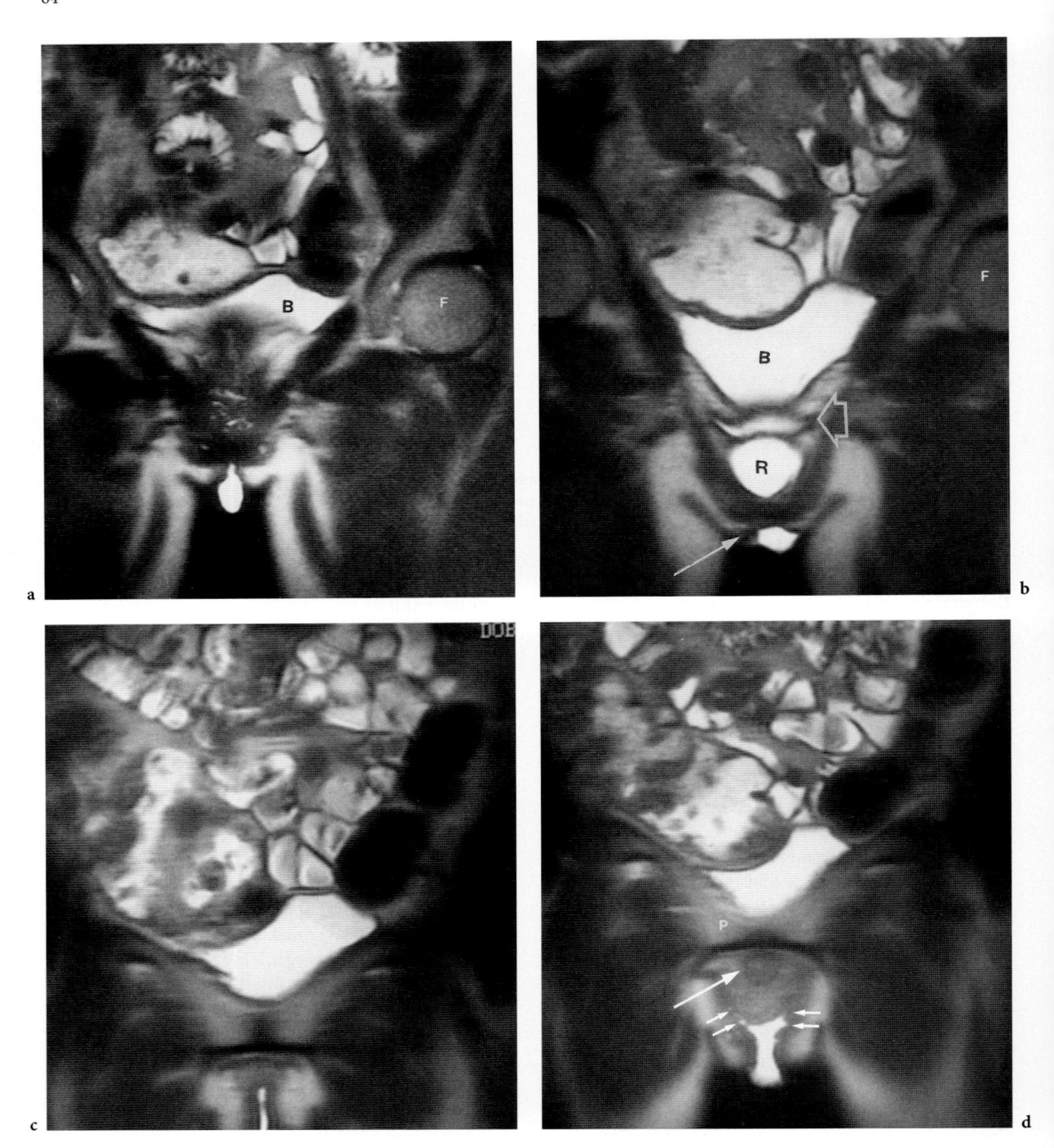

Fig. 4.2.13a–d. Pelvic organ prolapse on coronal images. Cystocele, vaginal prolapse, and anterior rectocele. Same patient as in Fig. 4.2.7. **a** Coronal T2-weighted MR image of the pelvis at rest. Gel is seen in the vagina and rectum. The posterior portion of the bladder (*B*) is seen to be normal in position (*F* femoral head). **b** With the patient straining, the bladder (*B*) descends below the level of the femoral heads (*F*). The anterior and inferior displacement of the vagina (*open arrow*) results in the vagina being seen inferior to the bladder. Similarly, anterior and inferior displacement of the rectum (*R*) results in anterior bulging of the rectum, indicating a rectocele (*solid arrow* labia). **c** A more anterior coronal image shows the normal appearance of the pelvic structures at rest. **d** On straining, a coronal image at thee same level as in **c** shows anterior and inferior displacement of the urethra (*long arrow*) below the pubis (*P*). The anterior soft tissues bulge into the vagina (*short arrows*)

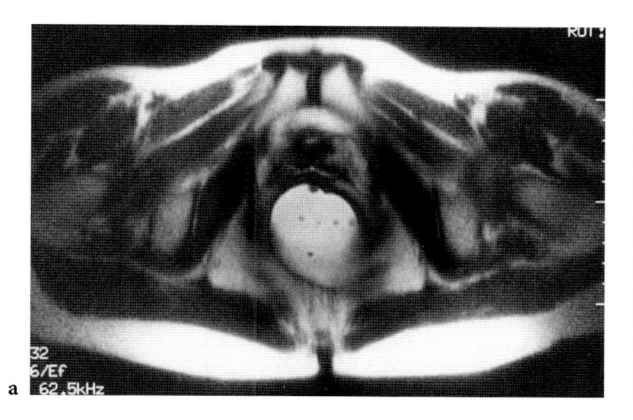

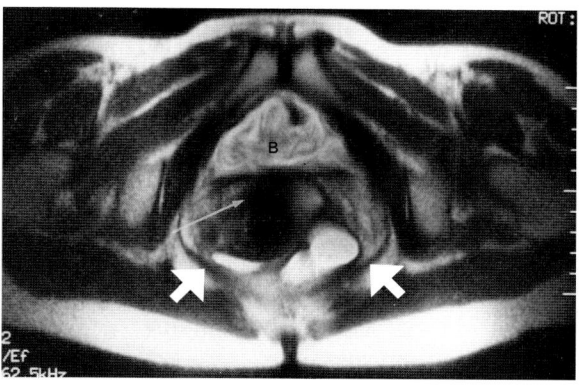

Fig. 4.2.14a, b. Pelvic organ prolapse on axial images. Cystocele, cervical prolapse, and bulging levator ani muscles. Same patient as in Fig. 4.2.7. **a** Axial T2-weighted MR image of the pelvis at rest at the level of the pubic symphysis. Gel is present in the rectum and vagina. **b** On straining, an axial image at the same level shows descent of the bladder (*B*). The cervix (*long arrow*) is also seen to descend into the vagina. The area of the pelvic hiatus increases with straining as a result of bulging of the levator ani muscle (*short arrows*)

pubic bone as the reference line (SINGH et al. 2001). This more caudad reference line has been shown in cadaveric studies by these authors to correspond to the level of the hymeneal ring. In their study of 20 patients with prolapse, the MR imaging staging based on the midpubic line correlated with the clinical staging in 75% of patients (SINGH et al. 2001). This new reference line on MR images seems to be a promising advance that requires further assessment and validation with the findings on pelvic organ prolapse quantification (POPQ) used by clinicians on physical examination.

Each of these systems has its advantages. They are, however, provisional. Whether or not a fetus is large for gestational age is based on samples of large numbers of normal fetuses. We must recognize that this is the proper way to define the ranges of normal. At present, these data on large populations of normal women are not available. Until these data are available care should be exercised in assigning a clinical diagnosis to a radiographic finding. This is especially important because a larger portion of the normal curve lies at the dividing line between normal and abnormal than farther out on the tail. Small changes in where this line is drawn will affect large numbers of women and lead to the inclusion of those women who are most likely to be asymptomatic from their prolapse. The radiologists long-learned and appropriate desire to avoid missing a diagnosis of cancer, for example, does not apply to this issue, since this is not a life-threatening condition.

4.2.4
Comparison of MR and Fluoroscopic Techniques

MR imaging is an advantageous way to study pelvic organ prolapse as the pelvis can be imaged in multiple planes and the entire urogenital tract evaluated (RODRIGUEZ and RAZ 2001). The uterus, pelvic floor muscles and urethral/anal walls are directly visualized; this is not possible with fluoroscopy, which is regarded currently as the gold standard. The two modalities have been compared in small series with differing results; these are likely due to variability in both the MR and fluoroscopic techniques (GUFLER et al. 1999; KELVIN et al. 2000; LIENEMANN et al. 1997). When a triphasic approach using cystographic, proctographic, and post-toilet phases was used for both examinations, the number of pelvic floor defects detected by the two studies was similar in a study of ten patients (KELVIN et al. 2000). In another study of 44 patients who evacuated rectal contrast during the examination, comparison of MR imaging and fluoroscopy showed that the number of abnormal compartments was greater on MR imaging than on fluoroscopy (LIENEMANN et al. 1997). The higher soft tissue contrast on MR imaging allowed more frequent detection of uterine prolapse and enterocele. A defect in the rectovaginal fascia results in herniation of peritoneal fat (peritoneocele) and small bowel (enterocele) into the rectovaginal space. If there is no contained small bowel, the diagnosis of a peritoneocele on the fluoroscopic study is only inferential unless concomitant peritoneography is performed, whereas peritoneal fat in the rectovaginal space is readily visible on MR imaging. Prolapse of bladder or sigmoid colon into this space can also be identified; these findings may influence surgical planning. One study comparing MR imaging with the surgical diagnosis of defects found high sensitivities ranging from 76% for rectocele to 100% for cystocele (GOUSSE et al. 2000). The detection of incidental pelvic pathology also affected the management of some of these patients.

However, other studies have found that fluoroscopy is more accurate than MR imaging (DELEMARRE et al. 1994; VANBECKEVOORT et al. 1999). The first study found that rectocele size was smaller on MR imaging than on fluoroscopy and in the second of these studies more abnormalities were found on fluoroscopy than on MR imaging. Both these studies appear to have been done without patient defecation during MR imaging, which may have accounted for the false-negative findings. It is only during rectal evacuation (or micturition) that full relaxation of the pelvic floor musculature occurs, thereby enabling the complete extent of pelvic organ prolapse to be shown.

The accuracy of MR imaging compared with that of fluoroscopy will require studies in larger groups of women with pelvic organ prolapse with both examinations being performed with optimized protocols. However, imaging of patients with predominantly rectal dysfunction will still likely require imaging in a seated position on a commode. This is routinely done on fluoroscopy and is possible with research MR scanners.

References

Ala-Ketola L (1973) Roentgen diagnosis of female stress urinary incontinence. Roentgenological and clinical study. Acta Obstet Gynecol Scand Suppl 23:1–59
Altringer WE, Saclarides TJ, Dominguez JM, et al (1995) Four-contrast defecography: pelvic "floor-oscopy." Dis Colon Rectum 38:695–699
Aronson MP, Bates SM, Jacoby AF, et al (1995) Periurethral and paravaginal anatomy: an endovaginal magnetic resonance imaging study. Am J Obstet Gynecol 173:1702–1710
Bartram CI, Turnbull GK, Lennard-Jones JE (1988) Evacuation proctography: an investigation of rectal expulsion in 20 subjects without defecatory disturbance. Gastrointest Radiol 13:72–80
Benson JT (1992) Female pelvic floor disorders. Investigation and management (Preface). Norton, New York
Bethoux A, Bory S, Huguier M, Cheo Seang Lan (1965) Une technique radiologique d'exploration des prolapsus genitaux et des incontinences d'urine: le colpocystogramme. Ann Radiol (Paris) 8:809–828
Bo K, Lilleas F, Talseth T, et al (2001) Dynamic MRI of the pelvic floor muscles in an upright sitting position. Neurourol Urodyn 20:167–174
Bremmer S, Mellgren A, Holmstrom B, et al (1997) Peritoneocele: visualization with defecography and peritoneography performed simultaneously. Radiology 202:373–377
Brubaker L, Heit MH (1993) Radiology of the pelvic floor. Clin Obstet Gynecol 36:952–959
Brubaker L, Retzky S, Smith C, et al (1993) Pelvic floor evacuation with dynamic fluoroscopy. Obstet Gynecol 82:863–868
Carr LK, Herschorn S, Leonhardt C (1996) Magnetic resonance imaging after intraurethral collagen injected for stress urinary incontinence. J Urol 155:1253–1255
Christensen LL, Djurhuus JC, Constantinou CE (1995a) Imaging of pelvic floor contractions using MRI. Neurourol Urodyn 14:209–216
Christensen LL, Djurhuus JC, Lewis MT, et al (1995b) MRI of voluntary pelvic floor contractions in healthy female volunteers. Int J Urogynecol 6:138–152
Comiter CV, Vasavada SP, Barbaric ZL, et al (1999) Grading pelvic prolapse and pelvic floor relaxation using dynamic magnetic resonance imaging. Urology 54:454–457
DeLancey JOL (1994) Structural support of the urethra as it relates to stress urinary incontinence: the hammock hypothesis. Am J Obstet Gynecol 170:1713–1720
DeLancey JOL (2002) Fascial and muscular abnormalities in women with urethral hypermobility and anterior vaginal wall prolapse. Am J Obstet Gynecol 187:93–98
Delemarre JBVM, Kruyt RH, Doornbos J, et al (1994) Anterior rectocele: assessment with radiographic defecography, dynamic magnetic resonance imaging, and physical examination. Dis Colon Rectum 37:249–259
Fenner DE (1996) Diagnosis and assessment of sigmoidoceles. Am J Obstet Gynecol 175:1438–1442
Fielding JR, Versi E, Mulkern RV, et al (1996) MR imaging of the female pelvic floor in the supine and upright positions. J Magn Reson Imaging 6:961–963
Fielding JR, Griffiths DJ, Versi E, et al (1998) MR imaging of pelvic floor continence mechanisms in the supine and sitting positions. Am J Roentgenol 171:1607–1610
Fielding JR, Dumanli H, Schreyer AG, et al (2000) MR-based three-dimensional modeling of the normal pelvic floor in women: quantification of muscle mass. Am J Roentgenol 174:657–660
Frohlich B, Hotzinger H, Fritsch H (1997) Tomographical anatomy of the pelvis, pelvic floor, and related structures. Clin Anat 10:223–230
Goh V, Halligan S, Kaplan G, et al (2000) Dynamic MR imaging of the pelvic floor in asymptomatic subjects. Am J Roentgenol 174:661–666
Goodrich MA, Webb MJ, King BF, et al (1993) Magnetic resonance imaging of pelvic floor relaxation: dynamic analysis and evaluation of patients before and after surgical repair. Obstet Gynecol 82:883–891
Gousse AE, Barbaric ZL, Safir MH, et al (2000) Dynamic half Fourier acquisition, single shot turbo spin-echo magnetic resonance imaging for evaluating the female pelvis. J Urol 164:1606–1613
Greenberg T, Kelvin FM, Maglinte DDT (2001) Barium trap-

ping in rectoceles: are we trapped by the wrong definition? Abdom Imaging 26:587–590

Gufler H, Laubenberger J, DeGregorio G, et al (1999) Pelvic floor descent: dynamic MR imaging using a half-Fourier RARE sequence. J Magn Reson Imaging 9:378–383

Halligan S, Bartram CI (1995) Evacuation proctography combined with positive contrast peritoneography to demonstrate pelvic floor hernias. Abdom Imaging 20:442–445

Halligan S, Bartram CI, Park HJ, et al (1995) Proctographic features of anismus. Radiology 197:679–682

Halligan S, Bartram C, Hall C, et al (1996) Enterocele revealed by simultaneous evacuation proctography and peritoneography: does "defecation block" exist? Am J Roentgenol 167:461–466

Healy JC, Halligan S, Reznek RH, et al (1997a) Magnetic resonance imaging of the pelvic floor in patients with obstructed defecation. Br J Surg 84:1555–1558

Healy JC, Halligan S, Reznek RH, et al (1997b) Patterns of prolapse in women with symptoms of pelvic floor weakness: assessment with MR imaging. Radiology 203:77–81

Hilfiker PR, Debatin JF, Schwizer W, et al (1998) MR defecography: depiction of anorectal anatomy and pathology. J Comput Assist Tomogr 22:749–755

Hjartardottir S, Nilsson J, Petersen C, et al (1997) The female pelvic floor: a dome – not a basin. Acta Obstet Gynecol Scand 76:567–571

Ho LM, Low VHS, Freed KS (1999) Vaginal opacification during defecography: utility of placing a folded gauze square at the introitus. Abdom Imaging 24:562–564

Hock D, Lombard R, Jehaes C, et al (1993) Colpocystodefecography. Dis Colon Rectum 36:1015–1021

Huddleston HT, Dunnihoo DR, Huddleston PM, et al (1995) Magnetic resonance imaging of defects in DeLancey's vaginal support levels I, II, and III. Am J Obstet Gynecol 172:1778–1784

Hussain SM, Stoker J, Lameris JS (1995) Anal sphincter complex: endoanal MR imaging of normal anatomy. Radiology 197:671–677

Johansson CD, Nilsson BY, Holmstrom B, et al (1992) Association between rectocele and paradoxical sphincter response. Dis Colon Rectum 35:503–509

Jorge JMN, Yang Y-K, Wexner SD (1994) Incidence and clinical significance of sigmoidoceles as determined by a new classification system. Dis Colon Rectum 37:1112–1117

Karaus M, Neuhaus P, Wiedenmann B (2000) Diagnosis of enteroceles by dynamic anorectal endosonography. Dis Colon Rectum 43:1683–1688

Kaufman HS, Buller JL, Thompson JR, et al (2001) Dynamic pelvic magnetic resonance imaging and cystocolpoproctography alter surgical management of pelvic floor disorders. Dis Colon Rectum 44:1575–1584

Kelvin FM, Maglinte DDT (1997) Dynamic cystoproctography of female pelvic floor defects and their interrelationships. Am J Roentgenol 169:769–774

Kelvin FM, Maglinte DDT (2000) Radiologic investigation of prolapse. J Pelv Surg 6:218–220

Kelvin FM, Maglinte DDT, Hornback JA, et al (1992) Pelvic prolapse: assessment with evacuation proctography (defecography). Radiology 184:547–551

Kelvin FM, Hale DS, Maglinte DDT, et al (1999) Female pelvic organ prolapse: diagnostic contribution of dynamic cystoproctography and comparison with physical examination. Am J Roentgenol 173:31–37

Kelvin FM, Maglinte DDT, Hale DS, et al (2000) Female pelvic organ prolapse: a comparison of triphasic dynamic MR imaging and triphasic fluoroscopic cystocolpoproctography. Am J Roentgenol 174:8–88

Kim B, Hricak H, Tanagho EA (1993) Diagnosis of urethral diverticula in women: value of MR imaging. Am J Roentgenol 161:809–815

Kirschner-Hermanns R, Wein B, Niehaus S (1993) The contribution of magnetic resonance imaging of the pelvic floor to the understanding of urinary incontinence. Br J Urol 72:715–718

Klutke C, Golomb J, Barbaric Z, et al (1990) The anatomy of stress incontinence: magnetic resonance imaging of the female bladder neck and urethra. J Urol 143:563–566

Kuhn RJP, Hollyock VE (1982) Observations on the anatomy of the rectovaginal pouch and septum. Obstet Gynecol 59:445–447

Lamb GM, De Jode MG, Gould SW, et al (2000) Upright dynamic MR defaecating proctography in an open configuration MR system. Br J Radiol 73:152–155

Law PA, Danin JC, Lamb GM, et al (2001) Dynamic imaging of the pelvic floor using an open-configuration magnetic resonance scanner. J Magn Reson Imaging 13:923–929

Lienemann A, Anthuber C, Baron A, et al (1997) Dynamic MR colpocystorectography assessing pelvic-floor descent. Eur Radiol 7:1309–1317

Lienemann A, Sprenger D, Anthuber C, et al (2001) Functional cine magnetic resonance imaging in women after abdominal sacrocolpopexy. Obstet Gynecol 97:81–85

Maglinte DDT, Kelvin FM, Hale DS, et al (1997) Dynamic cystoproctography: a unifying diagnostic approach to pelvic floor and anorectal dysfunction. Am J Roentgenol 169:759–767

Maglinte DDT, Kelvin FM, Fitzgerald K, et al (1999) Association of compartment defects in pelvic floor dysfunction. Am J Roentgenol 172:439–444

Mostwin JL, Yang A, Sanders R, et al (1995) Radiography, sonography, and magnetic resonance imaging for stress incontinence. Urol Clin North Am 22:539–549

Neitlich JD, Foster HE, Glickman MG, et al (1998) Detection of urethral diverticula in women: comparison of a high resolution fast spin echo technique with double balloon urethrography. J Urol 159:408–410

Osaza H, Mori T, Togashi K (1992) Study of uterine prolapse by magnetic resonance imaging: topographical changes involving the levator ani muscle and the vagina. Gynecol Obstet Invest 34:43–48

Pannu HK, Kaufman HS, Cundiff GW, et al (2000) Dynamic MR imaging of pelvic organ prolapse: spectrum of abnormalities. Radiographics 20:1567–1582

Quick HH, Serfaty JM, Pannu HK, et al (2001) Endourethral MRI. Magn Reson Med 45:138–146

Rodriguez LV, Raz S (2001) Diagnostic imaging of pelvic floor dysfunction. Curr Opin Urol 11:423–428

Romanzi LJ, Groutz A, Blaivas JG (2000) Urethral diverticulum in women: diverse presentations resulting in diagnostic delay and mismanagement. J Urol 164:428–433

Schoenenberger AW, Debatin JF, Guldenschuh I, et al (1998) Dynamic MR defecography with a superconducting, open-configuration MR system. Radiology 206:641–646

Shorvon PJ, McHugh S, Diamant NE, et al (1989) Defecography in normal volunteers: results and implications. Gut 30:1737–1749

Singh K, Reid WMN, Berger LA (2001) Assessment and grading of pelvic organ prolapse by use of dynamic magnetic resonance imaging. Am J Obstet Gynecol 185:71-77

Singh K, Reid WMN, Berger LA (2002) Magnetic resonance imaging of normal levator ani anatomy and function. Obstet Gynecol 99:433-438

Stoker J, Rociu E (1999) Endoluminal MR imaging of diseases of the anus and rectum. Semin Ultrasound CT MR 20:47-55

Stoker J, Halligan S, Bartram CI (2001) Pelvic floor imaging. Radiology 218:621-641

Strohbehn K, Ellis JH, Strohbehn JA, et al (1996a) Magnetic resonance imaging of the levator ani with anatomic correlation. Obstet Gynecol 87:277-285

Strohbehn K, Quint LE, Prince MR, et al (1996b) Magnetic resonance imaging anatomy of the female urethra: a direct histologic comparison. Obstet Gynecol 88:740-756

Tan IL, Stoker J, Lameris JS (1997) Magnetic resonance imaging of the female pelvic floor and urethra: body coil vs endovaginal coil. Magma 5:59-63

Tan IL, Stoker J, Zwamborn AW, et al (1998) Female pelvic floor: endovaginal MR imaging of normal anatomy. Radiology 206:777-783

Timmons MC, Addison WA (1996) Vaginal vault prolapse. In: Brubaker LT, Saclarides TJ (eds) The female pelvic floor: disorders of function and support. Davis, Philadelphia, pp 262-268

Tunn R, Paris S, Fischer W, et al (1998) Static magnetic resonance imaging of the pelvic floor muscle morphology in women with stress urinary incontinence and pelvic prolapse. Neurourol Urodyn 17:579-589

Tunn R, DeLancey JOL, Howard D, et al (1999) MR imaging of levator ani muscle recovery following vaginal delivery. Int Urogynecol J 10:300-307

Tunn R, Paris S, Taupitz M, et al (2000) MR imaging in posthysterectomy vaginal prolapse. Int Urogynecol J 11:87-92

Unterweger M, Marincek B, Gottstein-Aalame N, et al (2001) Ultrafast MR imaging of the pelvic floor. Am J Roentgenol 176:959-963

Vanbeckevoort D, Van Hoe L, Oyen R, et al (1999) Pelvic floor descent in females: comparative study of colpocystodefecography and dynamic fast MR imaging. J Magn Reson Imaging 9:373-377

Van Dam JH, Ginai AZ, Gosselink M, et al (1997) Role of defecography in predicting clinical outcome of rectocele repair. Dis Colon Rectum 40:201-207

Wallden L (1952) Defecation block in cases of deep rectogenital pouch. Acta Chir Scand [Suppl] 165:1-121

Weidner AC, Low VHS (1998) Imaging studies of the pelvic floor. Obstet Gynecol Clin 25:826-848

Yang A, Mostwin JL, Rosenshein NB, et al (1991) Pelvic floor descent in women: dynamic evaluation with fast MR imaging and cinematic display. Radiology 179:25-33

4.3 Ultrasound

C. I. Bartram

CONTENTS

4.3.1   Introduction 69
4.3.2   Technique for Endoanal Ultrasonography 69
4.3.3   Normal Findings 70
4.3.4   Anatomical Differences Between Sexes 72
4.3.5   Morphological Details 72
4.3.6   Internal Anal Sphincter Abnormalities 72
4.3.7   External Anal Sphincter Abnormalities 74
4.3.8   Transvaginal Sonography for Imaging
        the Anal Sphincters 77
4.3.9   Perineal Ultrasound 77
        References 78

4.3.1
Introduction

Several different types of probes may be used to interrogate the pelvic floor. In women the anal sphincters may be viewed via a transvaginal approach, or the probe placed on the perineum to show the bladder base and rectovaginal region. These approaches have the advantage that standard ultrasound probes, available in any department, may be used, whereas endoanal ultrasound that specifically targets the anal sphincters, requires a specialized endoprobe.

Endosonography is only a minimally invasive procedure that yields high resolution images of the anus. The sphincters are circular structures that are best appreciated in cross section. This requires a 360° axial image at right angles to the longitudinal axis of the canal. Currently the only way to produce such an image is to use a mechanically rotated single crystal, and only a few manufacturers have maintained expertise in this field. One of the main contenders has been B-K Medical (Sandoften 9, 2820 Gentofte, Denmark), and much of the developmental work has been accomplished using their systems. Other ultrasound manufacturers include Kretztechnik (Tiefenbach 15, 4871, Zipf, Austria) and Aloka (11–13 Zandsteen, 2132 MZ Hoofddorp, The Netherlands). Some other manufacturers make sector probes that can scan axially at right angles, but have a limited field of view.

The B-K Medical endoprobe was designed specifically for rectal scanning, to be inserted high into the rectum via a short sigmoidoscope. Acoustic contact with the rectal wall is achieved using a water filled balloon. This was modified for use in the anal canal by replacing the balloon with a hard cone (Law and Bartram 1989), the walls of which are parallel to prevent deformity of the anus as the probe is moved within the canal (Fig 4.3.1). The width of the cone was minimized (17 mm) to reduce patient discomfort and undue stretching of the sphincters. With improvements in the electronics of the unit, a 10 MHz crystal was developed with near-field focusing tailored for use in the anal canal.

4.3.2
Technique for Endoanal Ultrasonography

The endoprobe needs to be prepared carefully, with all air bubbles removed from the cone. Boiled water should be used, as this removes gas from the water

C. I. Bartram, FRCS, FRCP, FRCR
Intestinal Imaging, Level 4V, St Mark's Hospital, Northwick Park, Harrow, HA1 3UJ, UK

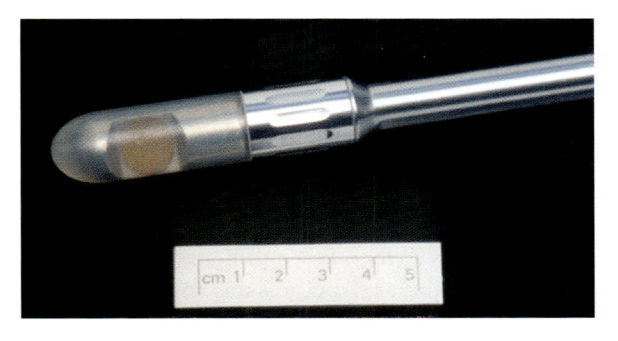

Fig. 4.3.1. B-K Medical 10-Hz endoprobe with 1.7-m plastic hard cone for anal endosonography

as well as sterilizing it. Distilled water is not recommended as over time this may erode the aluminium casing of the transducer, causing failure. The outer casing of the cone is covered liberally with ultrasound gel to ensure good acoustic contact, a protective cover placed over the probe and more gel coated on the outside of the cover.

The position in which the patient is examined is important. In men the left lateral is adequate, but in women either the prone or lithotomy position must be used, as in the left lateral position the anterior structures are deformed impairing diagnosis (FRUDINGER et al. 1998). A series of images should be taken on withdrawal of the probe to record the appearances of the canal at all levels, with detailed scanning of any abnormality.

4.3.3
Normal Findings

The reflectivity of muscle depends more on its fibroelastic content and the orientation of these fibres rather than on the type of muscle cells, as these on their own are all of low reflectivity. The internal sphincter has low fibroelastic content, and presents as a well-defined ring of low reflectivity. The external sphincter is more variable in fibre content. The puborectalis shows a typical fibrillated pattern that may be seen in any striated muscle within the body. In women the external sphincter may be similar, or of moderate reflectivity without any textured pattern. In men most of the external sphincter is of low reflectivity with a broad fibrillated pattern (BARTRAM and FRUDINGER 1997).

Boundaries between layers are highlighted by interface reflections when adjacent tissues are of different acoustic impedance. This acoustic mismatch is often enhanced by fat interspersed between layers. The axial view of the anus is therefore a complex of interface and layer reflections.

The anus is fundamentally a four-layer structure (Fig 4.3.2):
1. Subepithelium – moderately reflective. Thin crescents of the muscularis submucosae ani are often visible in the upper canal. The level of the dentate line is not discernible. Vascular channels may be seen at 6 and 12, with 12 orientated ventrally (with reference to a clock face and hours), and are low-reflective tubular structures that may be traced up the canal to the anal cushions.
2. Internal anal sphincter – a well-defined low-reflective ring about 2 mm thick. Usually symmetric in thickness, it is best measured at either 3 or 9. It may be slightly thicker just proximal to its termination, but often the thickest part is at the cranial end. High in the canal anteriorly there may be a central wedge that is reflective, suggesting a break in continuity of the sphincter. The cause of this is uncertain, but it is a normal variant.
3. Longitudinal layer – this is a complex layer incorporating an extension of smooth muscle from the outer longitudinal layer of the rectum, striated muscle from the puboanalis, with a fibroelastic mesh derived from endopelvic fascia that permeates throughout the sphincter anchoring it into the perineum (Fig. 4.3.3). The muscle components in the upper canal are seen as either low reflective bundles or sheets. In the lower canal the longitudinal layer is predominantly fibroelastic and more reflective, particularly in men. There are often thin layers of fat either side of this layer, more pronounced on the outer side between the longitudinal layer and the external sphincter, which create interface reflections. These fascial planes, and probably often the outer one, represent the

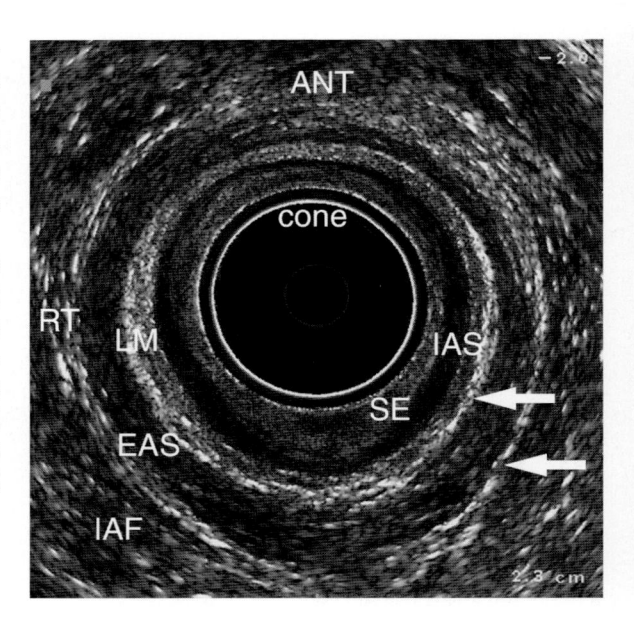

Fig. 4.3.2. Axial endosonographic image showing normal orientation with anterior uppermost (*ANT*) and right (*RT*) on the body right side (*IAF* ischioanal fossa, *EAS* external anal sphincter, *LM* longitudinal layer, *IAS* internal anal sphincter, *SE* subepithelial tissues). Two bright interface reflections are seen from the cone with other interface reflections at fascial planes between the longitudinal layer/external sphincter and external sphincter/ischioanal fossa (*arrows*)

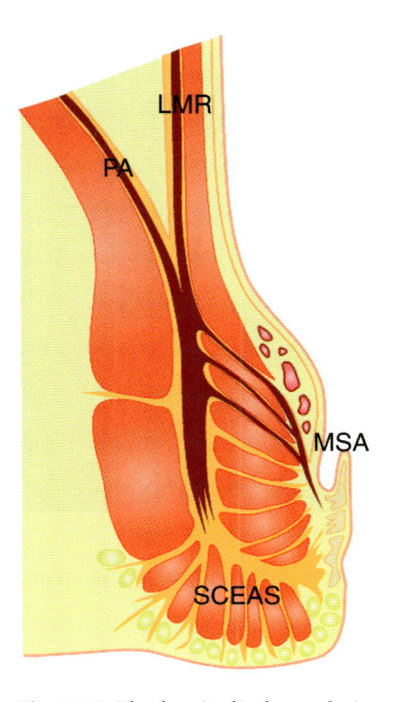

Fig. 4.3.3. The longitudinal muscle is a composite layer with smooth muscle from the longitudinal muscle of the rectum (*LMR*), striated from puboanalis (*PA*) and fibroelastic tissue from the endopelvic fascia. Slips from the longitudinal muscle run through the internal sphincter to the muscularis submucosae ani (*MSA*). Fibroelastic tissue also tracks through the subcutaneous external sphincter (*SCEAS*) to insert into the perianal skin

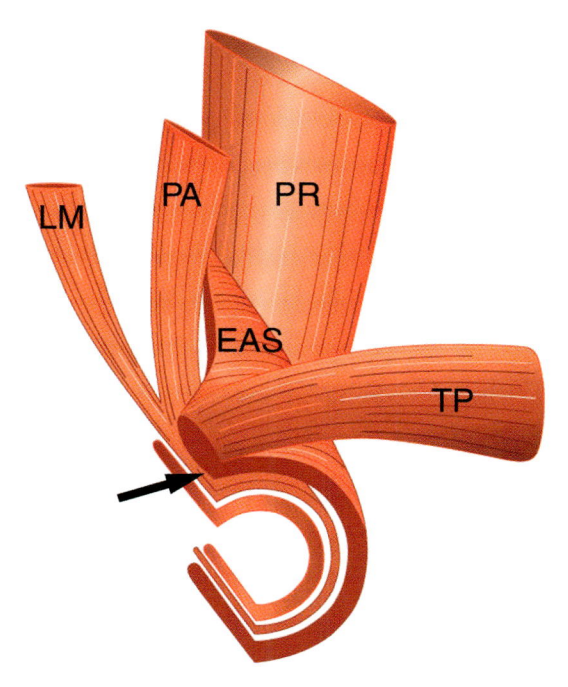

Fig. 4.3.4. The puboanalis (*PA*) rises from the medial border of the puborectalis (*PR*), joining the longitudinal muscle of the rectum (*LM*) to form the longitudinal layer (*arrow*). The transverse perinei is seen to fuse with the external anal sphincter

intersphincteric space, a surgical plane of dissection between the sphincters.
4. External anal sphincter – the deep part merges with the puborectalis dorsally, the superficial ends at the caudal extent of the internal sphincter, and the subcutaneous part hooks around fibroelastic bundles of the longitudinal layer, which penetrate through this part of the sphincter to insert into the perianal skin. The outer border of the external sphincter is demarcated from the ischioanal fossa by an interface reflection.

The junction of the anus to the striated muscles of the pelvic floor is complex. The puboanalis is an inner slip of the puborectalis that can be traced down into the longitudinal layer (Fig. 4.3.4). The fibre orientation is different and it is seen as a low-reflective triangular structure immediately medial to the puborectalis (Fig. 4.3.5). The transverse perinei come in from the side. In men these merge into the central point of the perineum with clear separation from the external sphincter (Fig. 4.3.6), in women they fuse into the external sphincter without a plane of dissection.

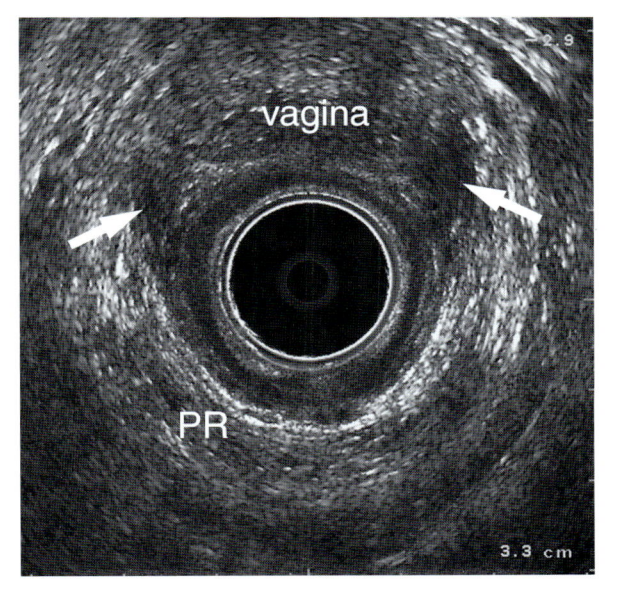

Fig. 4.3.5. The puboanalis (*arrows*) is a triangular low-reflective segment medial to the puborectalis (*PR*)

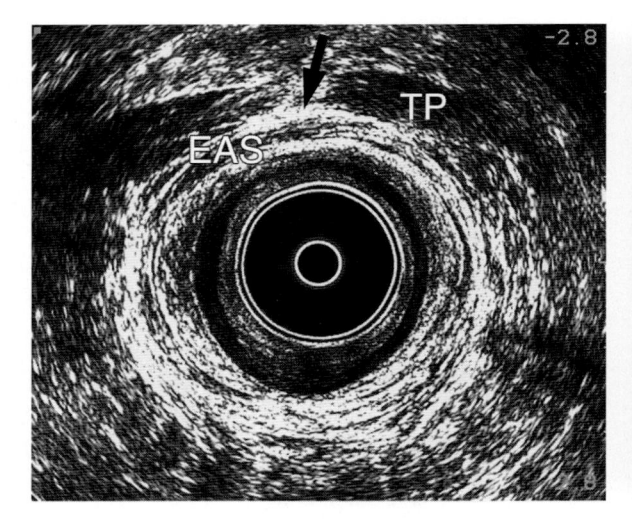

Fig. 4.3.6. The transverse perinei (*TP*) tend to be better defined in men and join the centre point of the perineum, creating a gap (*arrow*) between the transverse perinei and the external anal sphincter (*EAS*), whereas in women the transverse perinei fuse into the external sphincter directly

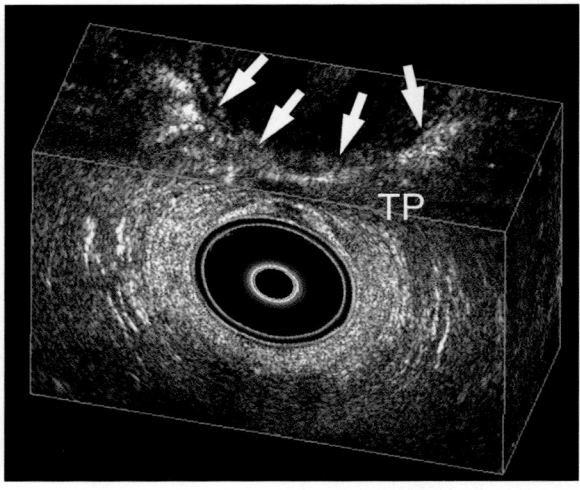

Fig. 4.3.7. 3-D view in a woman of the external sphincter sloping down to an intact anterior ring (*arrows*) with the transverse perinei (*TP*) fusing into this from each side

4.3.4
Anatomical Differences Between Sexes

There is a marked difference in the appearance of the external sphincter between the sexes. In men it is more symmetric, less reflective and easier to delineate. In women the perineal body seems devoid of any structure, as it is mainly fibroelastic in content. The edges of the anterior aspect of the external sphincter slope downwards to meet in the midline (Fig. 4.3.7). The puborectalis, measured on 3-D endoanal ultrasound studies (WILLIAMS et al. 2000) did not show any significant difference in length between the sexes (mean of 23.9 mm in men, 27.1 mm in women), neither did the internal sphincter (mean 34.4 mm, 33.2 mm, respectively), but there was a significant difference in the length of the external sphincter in all planes (anterior 30.1 vs 15.6 mm, coronal 31.6 vs 19.5 mm, posterior 29.3 vs 16.5 mm, respectively). This confirms that the sphincter is shorter anteriorly and that the general reduction in length of the external sphincter explains the shorter overall canal length.

4.3.5
Morphological Details

The internal anal sphincter is not constant in thickness during life. In neonates it is very thin (<1 mm), measuring 1–2 mm in young adults, 2–3 mm in middle age and 3–4 mm in the elderly. The internal sphincter termination is frequently asymmetric, so that irregularity in the last millimetre or so is a normal variant.

The thicknesses of various layers have been compared to those found with endocoil MRI, using 3-D to determine equivalent depth axial images. Using the layer characteristics described above, good intra- and interobserver correlation has been shown amongst experienced observers, and it may be concluded that, in young controls at least, endoanal ultrasound provides a reliable measurement of layer thickness.

4.3.6
Internal Anal Sphincter Abnormalities

The internal sphincter may show abnormalities of thickness, or of loss of integrity. The sphincter may be either too thick or too thin for the patient's age. An abnormally thick sphincter (Fig. 4.3.8) may be seen occasionally with uncomplicated constipation, but is invariably present in the solitary rectal ulcer syndrome (HALLIGAN et al. 1995) and associated with intraanal intussusception or rectal prolapse, to the extent that a thick sphincter is an indication for evacuation proctography to exclude rectal prolapse if the diagnosis has not been made clinically. The mechanism for this is uncertain; it may just be a secondary phenomenon from prolonged straining and intussusception into the anal canal. With rectal

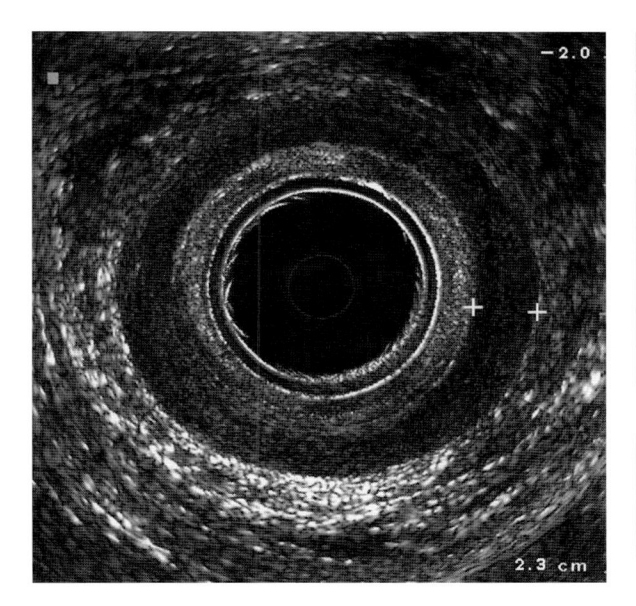

Fig. 4.3.8. Thick internal anal sphincter (4.3 mm between markers) in a 36-year-old woman with solitary rectal ulcer syndrome

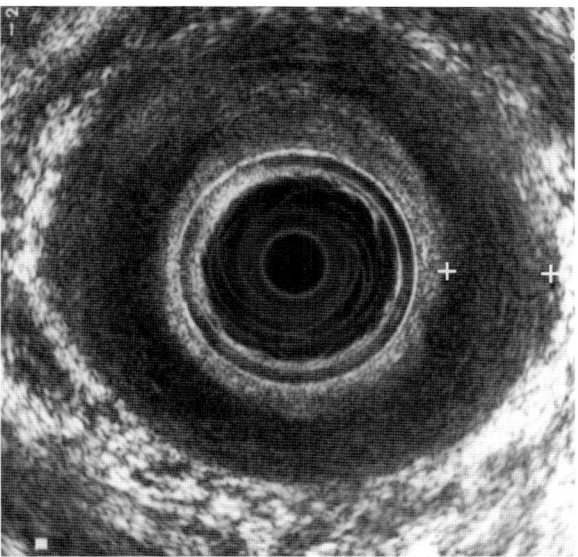

Fig. 4.3.9. Hereditary internal sphincter myopathy with a 7.6-mm internal sphincter thickness in a 76-year-old female with a long history of severe proctalgia fugax. Her mother had a similar history, and her daughter in her early 50s had just started having a similar pain

prolapse there may be secondary damage to the internal sphincter so that it is thinned or discontinuous in parts. A very rare condition is hereditary internal anal sphincter myopathy (KAMM et al. 1991), which produces a severe proctalgia fugax type syndrome with thickening of the internal sphincter (Fig. 4.3.9) by up to 1 cm.

The internal sphincter should become thicker with age, but it is notable that in many patients with passive incontinence that this does not occur and the internal sphincter is rather thin (Fig. 4.3.10). The cause of this is unknown, but an internal sphincter of less than 2 mm in thickness in a patient more than 50 years old is abnormal and primary degeneration of the internal sphincter has been used to describe this (VAIZEY et al. 1997).

Prior to pharmacological treatments for anal fissure, lateral internal anal sphincterotomy was performed commonly for this condition, and still is for chronic unresponsive cases. Classically only the lower third of the internal sphincter should be divided. The cut ends spring apart leaving a small gap in the lower part of the internal sphincter. If the entire internal sphincter is cut, the patient may not be totally incontinent but will certainly have some degree of incontinence. Unfortunately, as was shown on one study (SULTAN et al. 1994a), this is easily done in women (Fig. 4.3.11), as the shorter length of the external sphincter and the dentate line that is used as a reference point for the extent of the incision in men does not apply in women.

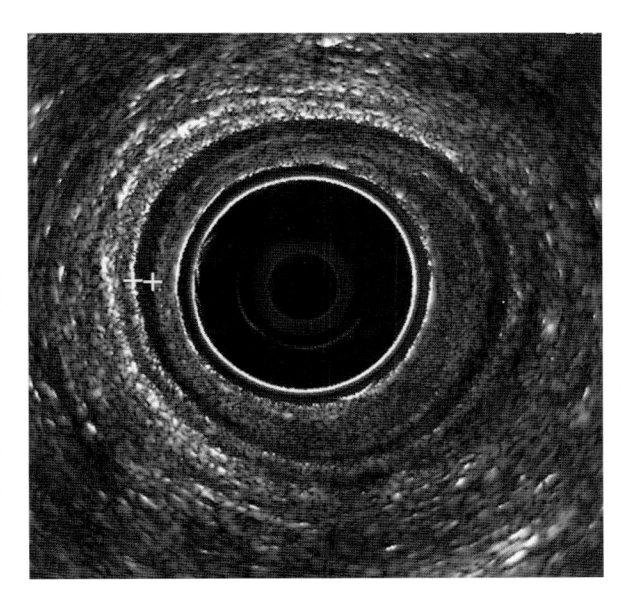

Fig. 4.3.10. A 70-year-old man with passive faecal incontinence. The sphincters are intact but the internal sphincter is abnormally thin for this age, measuring 1.1 mm, indicative of internal sphincter degeneration

Dilatation or stretch procedures of the internal sphincter may not be performed as regularly as they were some years ago, but evidence of damage to the internal sphincter following a stretch is still a relatively common finding (Fig. 4.3.12). A range

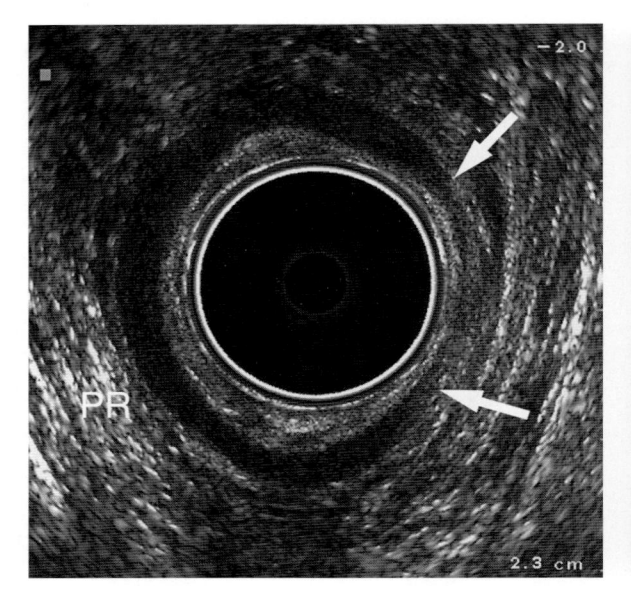

Fig. 4.3.11. Complete division of the internal anal sphincter with a defect (*arrows*) high in the canal at the level of the puborectalis (*PR*)

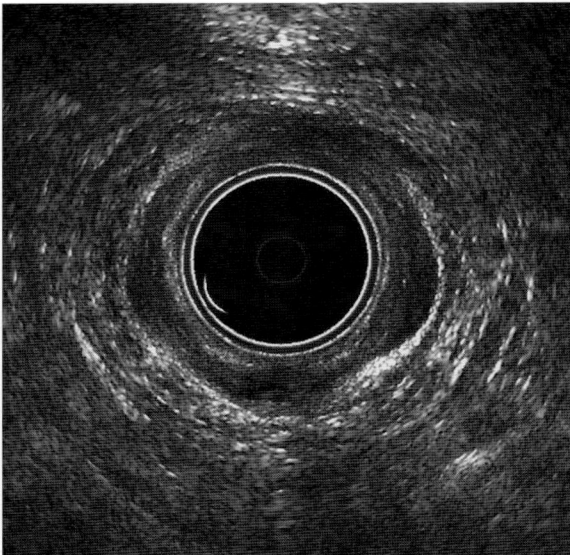

Fig. 4.3.12. Fragmentation of the internal anal sphincter following an anal stretch procedure

of changes indicates pathological damage: marked irregularity of the sphincter thickness, gross thinning of segments, or fragmentation where only irregular isolated remnants of sphincter remain. Dilatation from violent sexual abuse may result in internal sphincter tears (ENGEL et al. 1995), though homosexual men engaging in anoreceptive intercourse do not appear to have damaged sphincters (CHUN et al. 1997).

4.3.7
External Anal Sphincter Abnormalities

As with the internal anal sphincter, the external anal sphincter may be torn or abnormal in muscle fibre density. The latter is a complex issue, and one of the main indications for endoanal ultrasound is to determine whether the sphincter has been torn by childbirth. Direct trauma from penetrating injuries or road traffic accidents is quite rare by comparison (Fig. 4.3.13).

Tears from childbirth result either from overstretching, or extension from an adjacent rupture or episiotomy. Rupture of muscle fibres may be patchy, leading to an incomplete tear, or complete. The ruptured area heals with granulation tissue and fibrosis, which is relatively homogeneous and low in reflectivity. Tears are therefore indicated by the presence

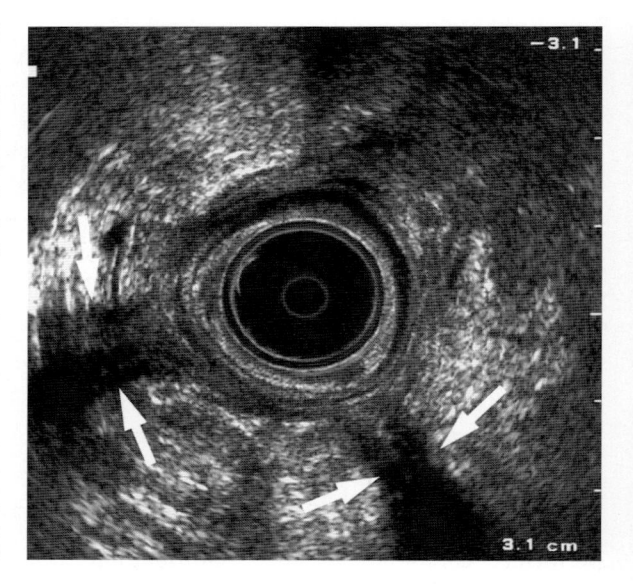

Fig. 4.3.13. Partial rupture of the sphincter with well-defined segmental scarring and acoustic shadowing (*arrows*) from this in a young boy who fell on a wooden stake

of a segment of low reflectivity within the external sphincter that usually crosses other layers, particularly the longitudinal layer and often the internal sphincter (Fig. 4.3.14).

Examination of women for suspected obstetric trauma should always be carried out in the prone (or lithotomy) position, and the internal sphincter

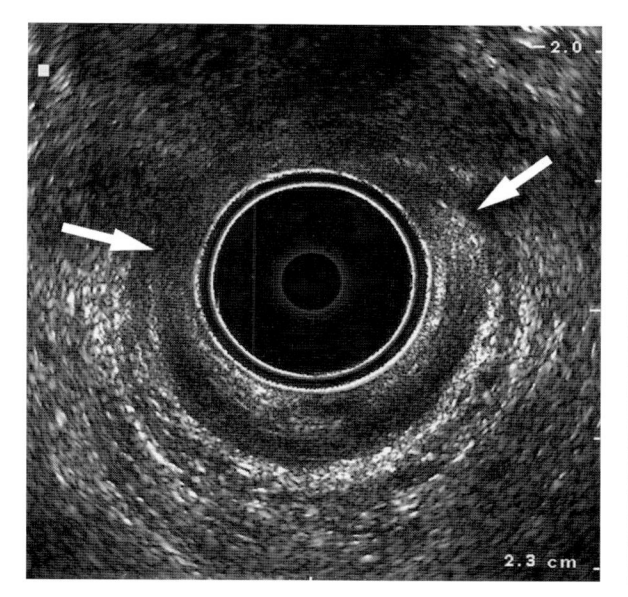

Fig. 4.3.14. Large obstetric tear between 10 and 2 o'clock (*arrows*) involving both the internal and external anal sphincters

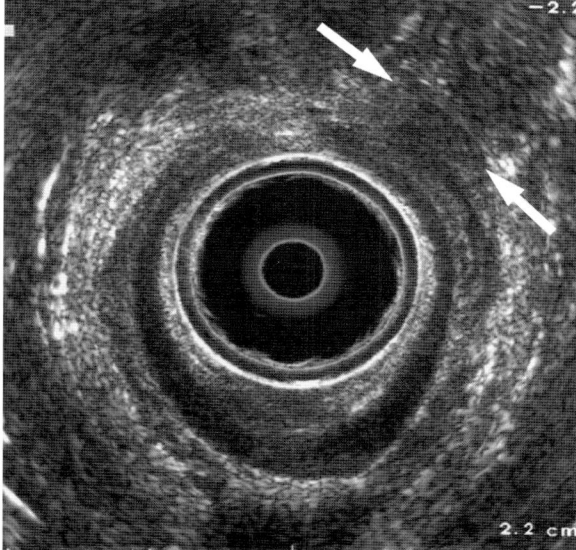

Fig. 4.3.15. Obstetric external sphincter tear between 1 and 2 o'clock. The internal sphincter is thinned anteriorly with a small defect at 12 o'clock

checked. If there is discontinuity high up, it should be in the anterior half of the sphincter. If in the posterior half, it is due to some other cause. The extent of internal anal sphincter discontinuity usually matches that of the external sphincter. Internal sphincter tears do not occur without external sphincter damage. External sphincter continuity is checked when the probe is slowly withdrawn, looking for the anterior parts coming together centrally. If this appears to be eccentric, this is a pointer for a tear. A tear is recognized by comparing one side to the other, searching for an abnormal segment of low reflectivity that has obliterated normal tissue planes (Fig. 4.3.15). The tear should be mapped out in hours and longitudinal extent. Many are just in the upper part of the external sphincter, but may extend down to the subcutaneous part. Major tears of the perineum produce a cloacal type defect (Fig 4.3.16).

An 11–35% incidence of external anal sphincter tears has been reported, but is probably in the region of 11% (WILLIAMS et al. 2001a). It is important to separate out tears to the puboanalis and to the transverse perinei, which are common. Tears to the puboanalis create an area of low reflective widening between the puborectalis and upper external sphincter (Fig. 4.3.17); tears to the transverse perinei are lower, just below the puborectalis and lateral to the external sphincter (Fig. 4.3.18). Manometric comparisons indicate that tears to these structures are not functionally significant (WILLIAMS et al. 2001a).

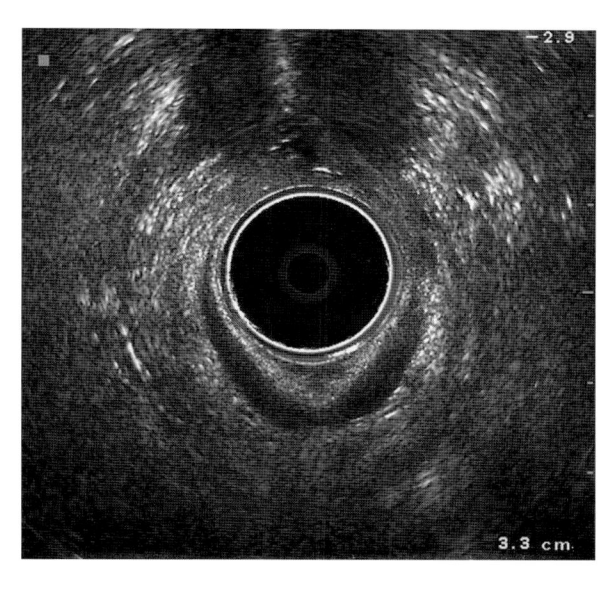

Fig. 4.3.16. Major obstetric tear with complete disruption of the perineum and only the posterior halves of the internal and external sphincters remaining, creating a cloacal defect

Caesarean section is not associated with any sphincter trauma. Damage is most frequent with forceps-assisted delivery. Tears are commonest during the first delivery, and are often termed "occult" as they are not apparent on clinical inspection. The perineum is often intact, and episiotomy does not appear to have a protective effect, although this has not been definitely studied. Third degree tears, where there is direct clini-

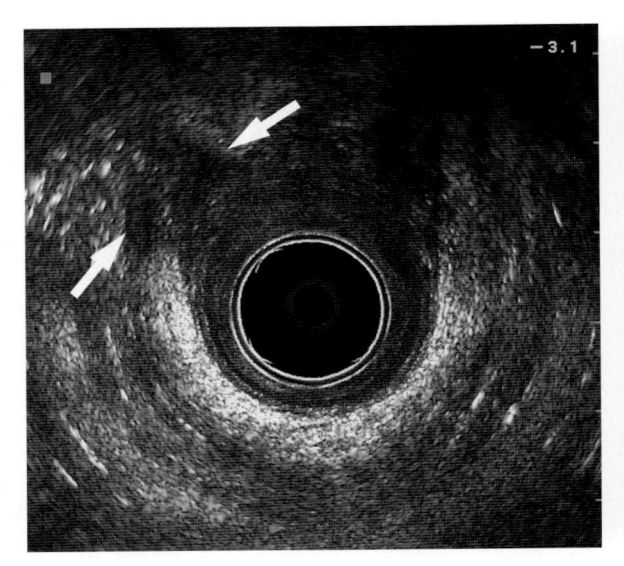

Fig. 4.3.17. Tear in the right puboanalis (*arrows*) causing widening compared to the left side

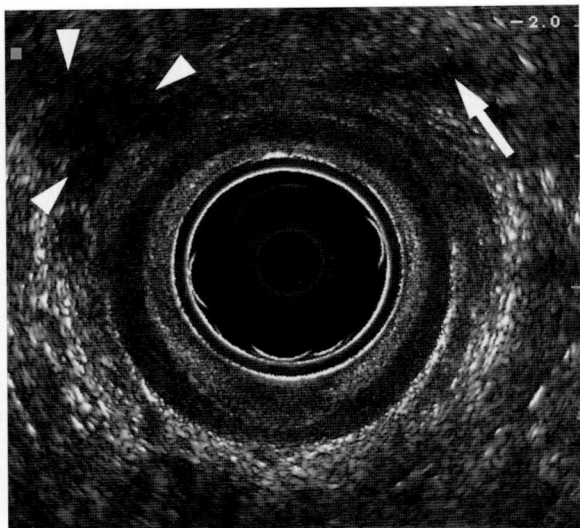

Fig. 4.3.18. Tear of the right transverse perinei (*arrowheads*) presenting with an amorphous area of low reflectivity from scar tissue compared to the normal left side (*arrow*)

cal evidence of external sphincter disruption are much less common with an incidence of about 1%. There may also be some permanent changes even when there is no tear. An initial study has suggested thinning of the anterior external sphincter (FRUDINGER et al. 1999) and other layers. However, this was not a matched pre- and post-delivery study. A later study that was matched and used 3D for more exact comparison (WILLIAMS et al. 2002) do not show any change in layer thickness. The only significant post-partum alteration was slight shortening of the external anal sphincter (21.7 mm vs 20.5 mm post-delivery) and increased angulation of anterior segment (10° vs 13.8° post-delivery). There was no structural abnormality on endosonography that could be related to the post-delivery fall in squeeze pressure.

Perhaps the commonest sphincter abnormality is the one that is most difficult to quantify on endosonography. External anal sphincter atrophy is related to neurological damage and secondary either to childbirth with damage from stretching of the pudendal nerves, spinal injury or simply the neuropathy of ageing. The endocoil MR imaging criteria for external anal sphincter atrophy are discussed in Chapter 4.4.2. The endosonographic diagnosis is difficult as fat replacement within the atrophied muscle causes loss of the normal muscle/fat interface border at the outer margin of the external sphincter. The outer border of the external sphincter is then not defined making it impossible to measure thickness. Loss of definition of the outer border of the external

sphincter is abnormal (Fig. 4.3.19), and coupled with a thin internal sphincter (<2 mm) gives a positive predictive value of 74% for atrophy (WILLIAMS et al. 2001b).

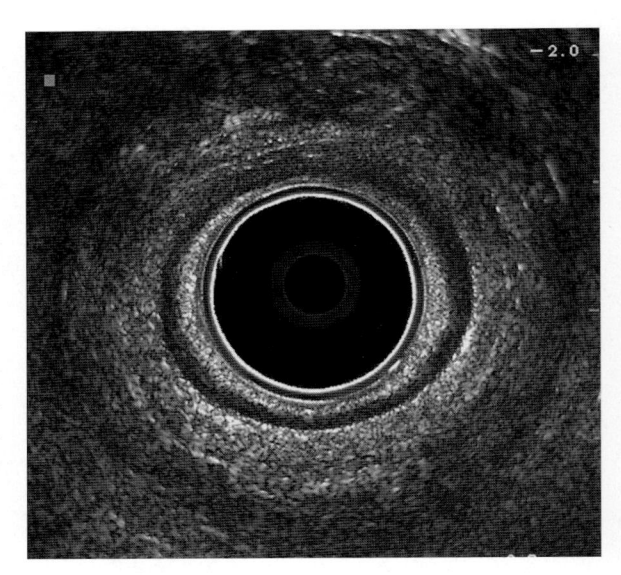

Fig. 4.3.19. External sphincter atrophy in a middle-aged woman with faecal incontinence. The sphincters are intact. The internal sphincter is thin (<2 mm) but the external sphincter is poorly defined, and the longitudinal layer and outer border of the sphincter cannot be differentiated

4.3.8
Transvaginal Sonography for Imaging the Anal Sphincters

Endosonography is not the only method for imaging the anal sphincters, particularly in women. A transvaginal endfire probe may be placed in the distal vagina/perineum and angled backwards to visualize the sphincters. This provides a unique view of the sphincter in its closed state. The anal cushions are seen (Fig. 4.3.20) and the subepithelial thickness may be measured. The internal sphincter is noted to be slightly thicker than on endoanal examination as it is not being stretched (Sultan et al. 1994b).

Good results have been reported for sphincter damage (Peschers et al. 1997a; Sandridge and Thorp 1995; Stewart and Wilson 1999). The perineal body thickness may be measured. This is also possible with endoanal examination using digital contact with the inner perineum (Zetterstrom et al. 1998), where the normal thickness has been found to be 12±3 mm.

Transvaginal ultrasound does show the anal sphincters, and is an alternative to endoanal examination. One study has indicated that this is unreliable (Frudinger et al. 1997) for demonstrating sphincter tears. The probe used may not have been ideal for this style of examination, but experimentation with a wide variety of probes suggests that although major tears may be seen, endoanal examination is more accurate in defining the extent of any tear and confirming that the sphincters are intact throughout their length.

Transvaginal examination of the bladder and urethra may also be performed either in the supine or sitting position, to assess change in position in relationship to the pubic symphysis and to image the consequences of provocative manoeuvres on the urinary continence mechanism (Quinn et al. 1988). Posteroinferior rotation of the urethrovesical junction (see Chapter 4.5) may be seen with opening of the bladder neck, urethra and urinary leakage in stress incontinence. This technique may be used to investigate postoperative appearances (Quinn et al. 1989). However, there is always the problem that the probe is stenting the vagina and limiting movement of the bladder neck. Bowel loops extending down into the rectovaginal septum implies the presence of an enterocoele and may be visible on transvaginal examination (Halligan et al. 1996).

4.3.9
Perineal Ultrasound

The pelvic floor may also be viewed by placing a probe on the perineum. The image quality of the urethrovesical junction is inferior to that achieved with transvaginal examination, but there is less interference by the probe to movement of the junction. With the probe placed over the vulva in the sagittal plane, good views of the bladder neck and pubic symphysis may be obtained at rest and during Valsalva (Fig. 4.3.21a, b). These have been shown to be reproducible, except for the posterior urethrovesical angle during Valsalva (Schaer et al. 1995). A more recent study (Alper et al. 2001) has confirmed that although the transperineal route is more accurate than transvaginal ultrasound, the reliability of measuring this angle by ultrasonography must be questioned. The imaging of bladder neck funnelling may be enhanced by using ultrasound contrast agents to increase urinary reflectivity (Schaer et al. 1996).

Bladder neck elevation, an index of levator ani function, is significantly reduced in the immediate postpartum period, but perineal ultrasound has shown a return to normal by 6–10 weeks (Peschers et al. 1997b), in keeping with MR imaging evidence for a morphological return to normality of the levators in this time (Tunn et al. 1999).

Dynamic transperineal ultrasound studies of the pelvic floor may be aided by opacifying the rectum and vagina with 50 ml of ultrasound coupling gel (Beer-Gabel et al. 2002). The patient is examined in the left lateral position with a full bladder. The probe is placed on the perineum, scanning in the sagittal and coronal planes with movement of the pelvic floor observed during straining and squeezing.

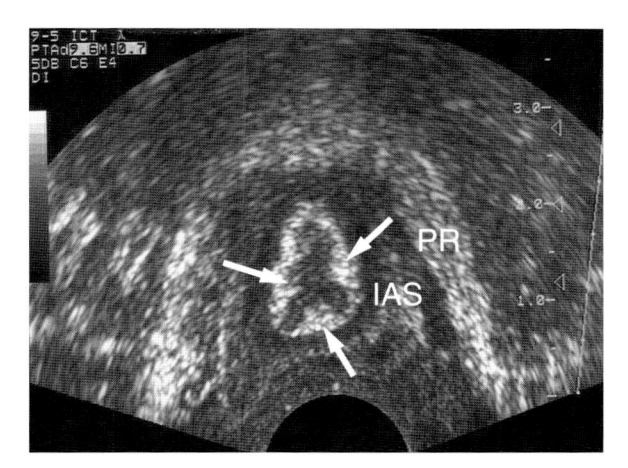

Fig. 4.3.20. Perineal ultrasound with a transvaginal probe held against the perineum, showing the puborectalis (*PR*), internal anal sphincter (*IAS*) and the anal cushions (*arrows*)

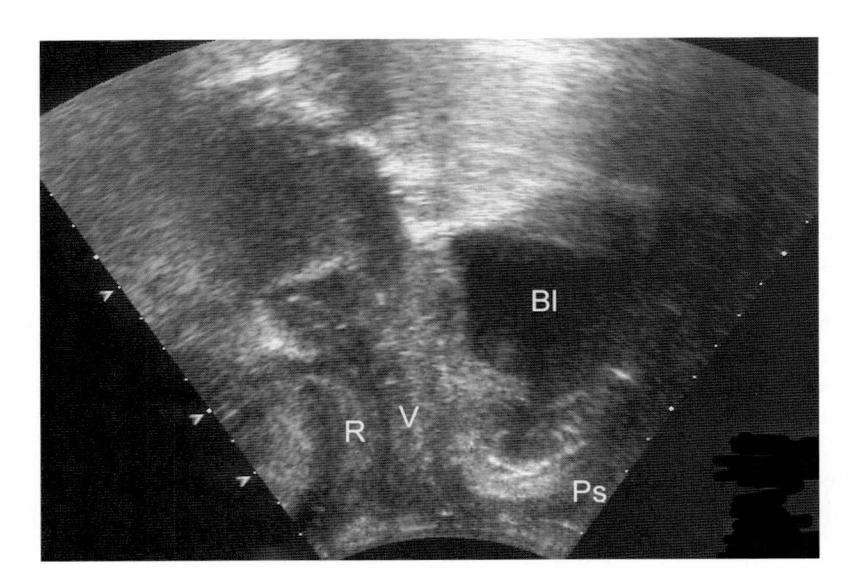

Fig. 4.3.21. Perineal ultrasound in the midline sagittal plane. *Bl* = baldder; *V* = vagina; *R* = rectum; *Ps* = pubic symphsis

The position of the puborectalis, bladder neck and anorectal angle may be measured. During straining, rectocoeles, cystocoeles and enterocoeles may be apparent and rectal intussusception imaged. Dynamic transperineal ultrasound has considerable potential as a simple, cheap and relatively noninvasive technique. Its relationship to other imaging methods and reliability await further assessment.

References

Alper T, Cetinkaya M, Okutgen S, et al (2001) Evaluation of urethrovesical angle by ultrasound in women with and without urinary stress incontinence. Int Urogynecol J Pelvic Floor Dysfunct 12:308–311

Bartram CI, Frudinger A (1997) A handbook of anal endosonography. Wrightson Biomedical Publishing, Petersfield (UK) Bristol (Pa.)

Beer-Gabel M, Teshler M, Barzilai N, et al (2002) Dynamic transperineal ultrasound in the diagnosis of pelvic floor disorders: pilot study. Dis Colon Rectum 45:239–245

Chun AB, Rose S, Mitrani C, et al (1997) Anal sphincter structure and function in homosexual males engaging in anoreceptive intercourse. Am J Gastroenterol 92:465–468

Engel AF, Kamm MA, Bartram CI (1995) Unwanted anal penetration as a physical cause of faecal incontinence. Eur J Gastroenterol Hepatol 7:65–67

Frudinger A, Bartram CI, Kamm MA (1997) Transvaginal versus anal endosonography for detecting damage to the anal sphincter. AJR Am J Roentgenol 168:1435–1438

Frudinger A, Bartram CI, Halligan S, et al (1998) Examination techniques for endosonography of the anal canal. Abdom Imaging 23:301–303

Frudinger A, Halligan S, Bartram CI, et al (1999) Changes in anal anatomy following vaginal delivery revealed by anal endosonography. Br J Obstet Gynaecol 106:233–237

Halligan S, Sultan A, Rottenberg G, et al (1995) Endosonography of the anal sphincters in solitary rectal ulcer syndrome. Int J Colorectal Dis 10:79–82

Halligan S, Northover J, Bartram CI (1996) Vaginal endosonography to diagnose enterocoele. Br J Radiol 69:996–999

Kamm MA, Hoyle CH, Burleigh DE, et al (1991) Hereditary internal anal sphincter myopathy causing proctalgia fugax and constipation. A newly identified condition. Gastroenterology 100:805–810

Law PJ, Bartram CI (1989) Anal endosonography: technique and normal anatomy. Gastrointest Radiol 14:349–353

Peschers UM, DeLancey JO, Schaer GN, et al (1997a) Exoanal ultrasound of the anal sphincter: normal anatomy and sphincter defects. Br J Obstet Gynaecol 104:999–1003

Peschers UM, Schaer GN, DeLancey JO, et al (1997b) Levator ani function before and after childbirth. Br J Obstet Gynaecol 104:1004–1008

Quinn MJ, Beynon J, Mortensen NJ, et al (1988) Transvaginal endosonography: a new method to study the anatomy of the lower urinary tract in urinary stress incontinence. Br J Urol 62:414–418

Quinn MJ, Beynon J, Mortensen NN, et al (1989) Vaginal endosonography in the post-operative assessment of colposuspension. Br J Urol 63:295–300

Sandridge DA, Thorp JM (1995) Vaginal endosonography in the assessment of the anorectum. Obstet Gynecol 86:1007–1009

Schaer GN, Koechli OR, Schuessler B, et al (1995) Perineal ultrasound for evaluating the bladder neck in urinary stress incontinence. Obstet Gynecol 85:220–224

Schaer GN, Koechli OR, Schuessler B, et al (1996) Usefulness of ultrasound contrast medium in perineal sonography for visualization of bladder neck funneling – first observations. Urology 47:452–453

Stewart LK, Wilson SR (1999) Transvaginal sonography of the anal sphincter: reliable, or not? AJR Am J Roentgenol 173:179–185

Sultan AH, Kamm MA, Nicholls RJ, et al (1994a) Prospective study of the extent of internal anal sphincter division during lateral sphincterotomy. Dis Colon Rectum 37:1031–1033

Sultan AH, Loder PB, Bartram CI, et al (1994b) Vaginal endosonography. New approach to image the undisturbed anal sphincter. Dis Colon Rectum 37:1296–1299

Tunn R, DeLancey JO, Howard D, et al (1999) MR imaging of levator ani muscle recovery following vaginal delivery. Int Urogynecol J Pelvic Floor Dysfunct 10:300–307

Vaizey CJ, Kamm MA, Bartram CI (1997) Primary degeneration of the internal anal sphincter as a cause of passive faecal incontinence. Lancet 349:612–615

Williams AB, Cheetham MJ, Bartram CI, et al (2000) Gender differences in the longitudinal pressure profile of the anal canal related to anatomical structure as demonstrated on three-dimensional anal endosonography. Br J Surg 87:1674–1679

Williams AB, Bartram CI, Halligan S, et al (2001a) Anal sphincter damage after vaginal delivery using three-dimensional endosonography. Obstet Gynecol 97:770–775

Williams AB, Bartram CI, Modhwadia D, et al (2001b) Endocoil magnetic resonance imaging quantification of external anal sphincter atrophy. Br J Surg 88:853–859

Williams AB, Bartram CI, Halligan S, et al (2002) Alteration of anal sphincter morphology following vaginal delivery revealed by multiplanar anal endosonography. BJOG 109:942–946

Zetterstrom JP, Mellgren A, Madoff RD, et al (1998) Perineal body measurement improves evaluation of anterior sphincter lesions during endoanal ultrasonography. Dis Colon Rectum 41:705–713

4.4 Endoanal Magnetic Resonance Imaging

E. Rociu and J. Stoker

CONTENTS

4.4.1 Introduction 81
4.4.2 Technique 81
4.4.2.1 Coil and Patient Preparation 81
4.4.2.2 Sequences and Protocol 82
4.4.3 Normal Presentation, Variances and Pitfalls 82
4.4.4 Lesions of the Anal Sphincter Muscles 84
4.4.4.1 Internal Sphincter 84
4.4.4.2 External Sphincter 85
4.4.5 Role of Endoanal MRI in Pelvic Floor Disorders 87
References 87

4.4.1
Introduction

Magnetic resonance imaging (MRI) has an important role in visualizing the anal sphincter. High-resolution techniques are preferable, and endoanal MRI has been evaluated for both clinical use and research.

Anal sphincter lesions have been shown to be a major cause of faecal incontinence (Burnett et al. 1991; Sultan et al. 1993). High definition of the sphincter has become an essential part of diagnosis and treatment of this condition. The high intrinsic contrast resolution of endoanal MRI results in an accurate delineation of the integrity of the sphincter complex, while the multiplanar capabilities demonstrate the sphincter in surgically relevant planes.

E. Rociu, MD; J. Stoker, MD
Department of Radiology, Academic Medical Center, University of Amsterdam, 22700, 1100 DE, Amsterdam, The Netherlands

4.4.2
Technique

4.4.2.1
Coil and Patient Preparation

For endoanal MRI several strategies can be used. Here general guidelines are given.

No bowel preparation is necessary but patients are asked to fast 4 h prior to the examination to reduce artefacts from bowel motion. Patients should empty their bladder before the study in order to prevent discomfort from a distended bladder and consequent motion artefacts. Patients are then familiarized with the procedure. Care is taken to make the procedure as comfortable as possible and stress the importance of minimizing motion (e.g. not contracting the anal sphincter). Before imaging, a smooth muscle relaxant, for example 1 ml butylscopolamine bromide, Buscopan, 20 mg/ml (Boehringer Ingelheim, Germany) or 1 mg glucagon hydrochloride (GlucaGen, Bagsvaerd, Denmark), may be injected intramuscularly to reduce peristalsis, though the need for this has not been proven.

Dedicated endoanal coils are preferred over rectal coils, as the design of rectal coils makes these less suitable for endoanal imaging. Some rectal coils, developed for prostate imaging, are sensitive in only one plane. Three types of endoanal coils are currently available, with outer coil holder diameters ranging from 7 to 19 mm, with the coil itself 1–2 mm smaller in diameter (Stoker et al. 1999; DeSouza et al. 1996). Coil diameter is a compromise between effective volume and compression of adjacent structures.

The device is covered with a condom, and lubricant is applied to the surface. The amount of lubricant should be minimized to reduce high signal intensity by near field effect. The endocoil is introduced in the left lateral position and the patient then turned supine, with sandbags or other supportive material used to secure the position of the coil. Endoanal MR imaging is well tolerated and easily performed (Stoker et al. 1999). Discomfort is comparable to that of endoanal ultrasonography, although the procedure is more time-consuming (approximately 30 min vs 5 min).

4.4.2.2
Sequences and Protocol

A T2-weighted sequence (e.g. turbo spin-echo) is used as a basic sequence. For a 1.5 T magnet the following T2-weighted turbo spin-echo (SE) parameters may be used: TR 2.800 ms; TE (effective) 90 ms; echo train length 10; echo spacing 21.8 ms; field of view 120+90 mm; imaging matrix 512+256; section thickness 2.0–3.0 mm; and eight signals acquired, giving an acquisition time of 5 min. The parameters should be optimized for contrast resolution, and moderate T2 weighting is preferable. Contrast resolution is evaluated by checking the difference in signal intensity between internal sphincter (relatively hyperintense) and external sphincter and puborectalis (relatively hypointense). Fat suppression techniques are not helpful in T2-weighted imaging for faecal incontinence. T1-weighted sequences, either standard or dynamic with contrast medium, increase the cost without any particular benefit. The transverse or axial plane, oriented at right angles to the axis of the anal canal, is the most relevant, and should be supplemented by at least one longitudinal plane, with coronal preferred over sagittal. The coronal plane reduces partial-volume effects and provides additional information on the extent of disorder. Phase-encoding direction should be adjusted to prevent artefacts in the anterior part of the anal sphincter.

Lesions may be described axially in hours and longitudinally in distance (centimetres) from the lower edge of the external sphincter.

4.4.3
Normal Presentation, Variances and Pitfalls

In the axial plane (Fig. 4.4.1a, b) the following layers are recognized by their different signal intensities:
1. The muscularis submucosae ani (SM) as a band of low signal in the relatively high subepithelial tissues.
2. The inner ring of internal sphincter (IS) with a characteristic high signal intensity.
3. The relatively hypointense longitudinal muscle (LM) lying within the intersphincteric space between the internal and external sphincters,

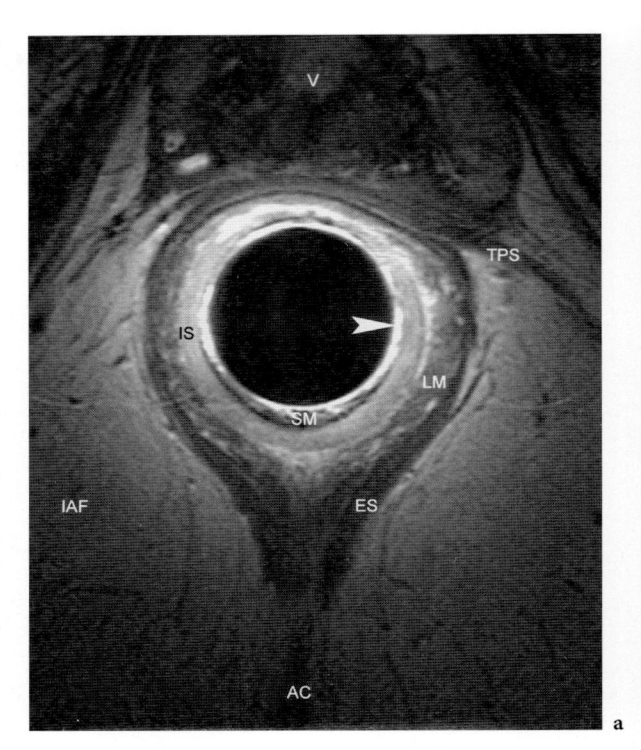

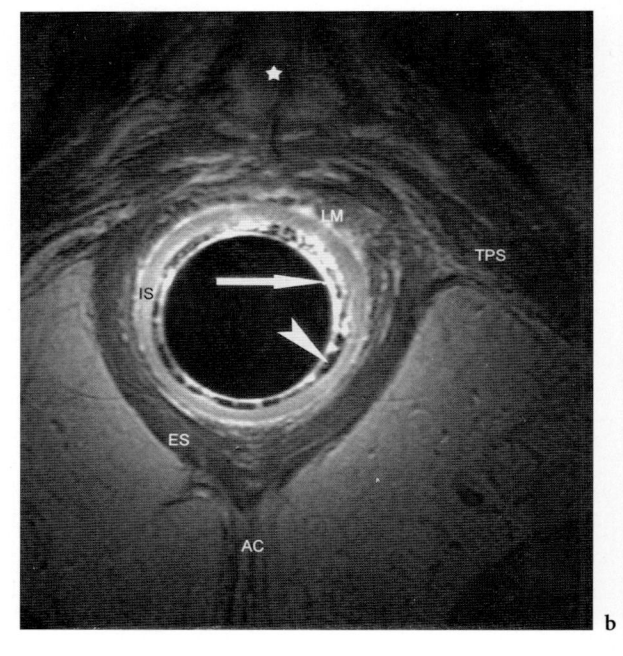

Fig. 4.4.1. a Axial T2-weighted image. Normal female anatomy in the mid anal canal (*arrowhead* coil surface, *ES* external sphincter, *IS* internal sphincter, *V* vagina, *TP* transverse perinei, *LM* longitudinal muscle, *SM* submucosa and muscularis mucosa, *IAF* ischioanal fossa, *AC* anococcygeal ligament). **b** Axial T2-weighted image. Normal male anatomy in the mid-anal canal (*arrow* directly on the coil surface submucosa, *arrowhead* muscularis mucosa, *ES* external sphincter, *IS* internal sphincter, *TP* transverse perinei, *LM* longitudinal muscle, *AC* anococcygeal ligament, *star* corpus spongiosum)

which is otherwise of relatively high signal from fibroelastic tissue.
4. The outer ring of external sphincter, which is striated muscle of low signal intensity.

In the coronal plane (Fig. 4.4.2), the external sphincter has a characteristic "J" shape. Often a thin fat plane can be seen between the deep part and the puborectalis. Below this the superficial part is seen as a separate component. The subcutaneous part of the external sphincter curves around to form the bottom of the "J". The entire sphincter complex is embedded in the fatty ischioanal fossa (IAF), and is therefore relatively hyperintense.

Evaluation of the sphincter in the axial plane should start from the lower border, moving upwards to find where the ring becomes complete. Below this level, discontinuity of the ring does not necessarily imply a defect, and may be just asymmetry of the anterior ends of the external sphincter (Fig. 4.4.3). The most caudal slices, below the level of the internal sphincter and longitudinal muscle, contain only the external sphincter. The internal sphincter begins above the level of the subcutaneous external sphincter, and the longitudinal muscle ramified in many thin septa that are too delicate to be visualized.

The anterior aspect of the deep external sphincter may cause problems in evaluation, particularly in the female, at the transition from deep external sphincter to the puborectalis where separation of the muscle groups is not clear, with fibres intermixing, inserting into the perineal body, and others continuing forward and anteriorly. The resulting open shape can be misdiagnosed as an anterior defect. The subcutaneous external sphincter may appear to have a posterior defect as it runs along both sides of the anococcygeal ligament (AC), which is a normal variant (Fig. 4.4.1a). On higher images the external sphincter fibres will be seen to merge symmetrically posteriorly reestablishing the sphincteric ring. Lacerations by comparison are asymmetric, irregular and bordered with scar tissue.

Sex-related differences should also be taken into account. The anterior edge of the external sphincter is shorter and closer to the horizontal in women (14 mm average) than in men (27 mm average) (Rociu et al. 2000). In women, the longitudinal muscle terminates just cranial to the external sphincter, whereas in men it extends to the caudal part of the external sphincter. The transverse perinei (TP) also have a different relationship to the external sphincter. In women, the TP fuse with the external sphincter, whereas in men they insert into the central point of the perineum (Fig. 4.4.1a, b).

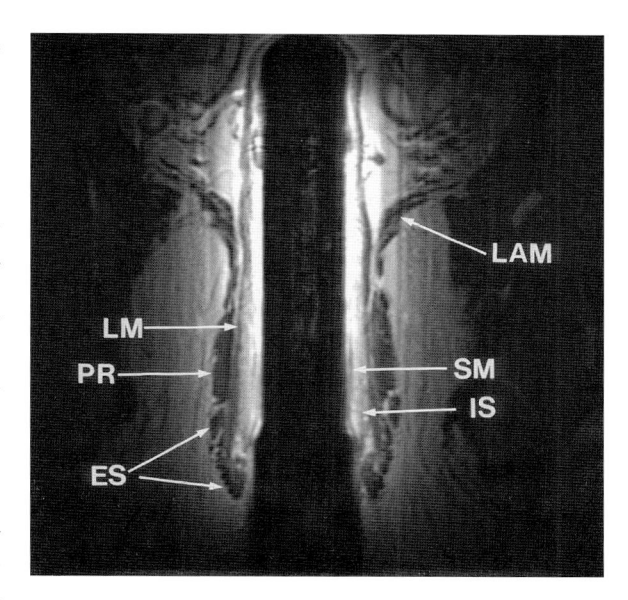

Fig. 4.4.2. Mid coronal T2-weighted image. Normal anatomy, coil in the anal canal (*ES* external sphincter, *IS* internal sphincter, *SM* submucosa and muscularis mucosa, *PR* puborectal muscle, *LAM* levator ani muscle, *LM* longitudinal muscle). Motion artefacts create lines parallel to the long axis of the coil

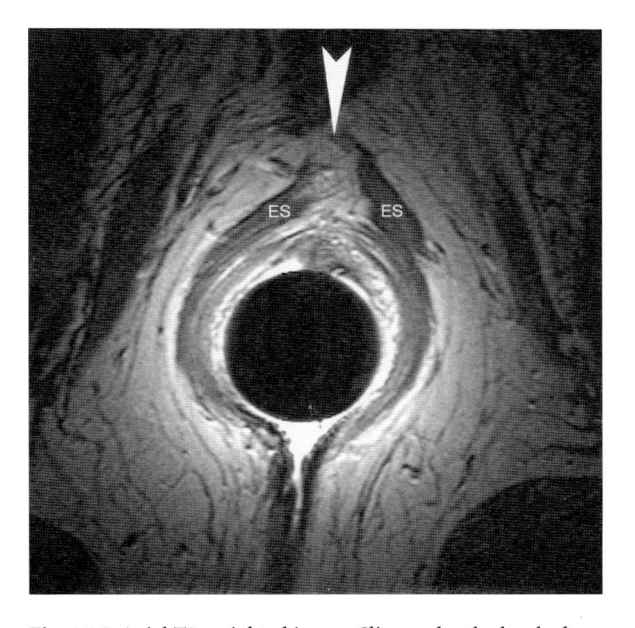

Fig. 4.4.3. Axial T2-weighted image. Slice under the level where the external sphincter (*ES*) forms a complete ring. Ring discontinuity (*arrowhead*) is caused by longer edges of the sphincter on the lateral sides and it does not represent a defect. At this level the internal sphincter and longitudinal muscle are not yet visible

The anal canal is angulated posteriorly to the table. With the patient supine, this may cause some compression of the internal sphincter. Normally the internal sphincter shows only a slight calibre change (Fig. 4.4.1a), but if thinned by compression it retains the normal high signal intensity, unlike a tear where it is disrupted, asymmetric and of lower signal intensity.

4.4.4
Lesions of the Anal Sphincter Muscles

Abnormalities of the sphincteric muscles comprise disruption (also called tears or defects) and volume changes. Muscle volume anomalies include generalized thinning or thickening of the muscle regardless of the integrity of the muscle ring.

4.4.4.1
Internal Sphincter

4.4.4.1.1
Tears

Disruption of the internal sphincter may be isolated (Fig. 4.4.4) or accompanied by external sphincter disruption (Fig. 4.4.5). Tears cause an asymmetric disruption of the sphincteric ring, and are associated with scar tissue, which is of relatively low signal, at the borders of the tear and crossing tissue planes if other structures have been torn.

4.4.4.1.2
Muscle Volume Anomalies

Normal Values: The average thickness of internal sphincter in healthy volunteers is 2.7 mm.

Thinning (<2 mm): A pathological entity, named internal sphincter degeneration, is the generalized thinning of the internal sphincter observed in patients over 50 years of age with passive incontinence (VAIZEY et al. 1997).

Thickening (>3.5 mm): In the elderly an internal sphincter thickness of 3 mm is normal but is abnormal in a patient under 35 years of age. Denervation of the external sphincter in idiopathic faecal incontinence is reported to lead to thinning of the external sphincter muscle and compensatory generalized thickening of the internal sphincter muscle. The internal sphincter has been reported to be thickened in other defecation disorders, such as obstructed defecation (NIELSEN et al. 1993).

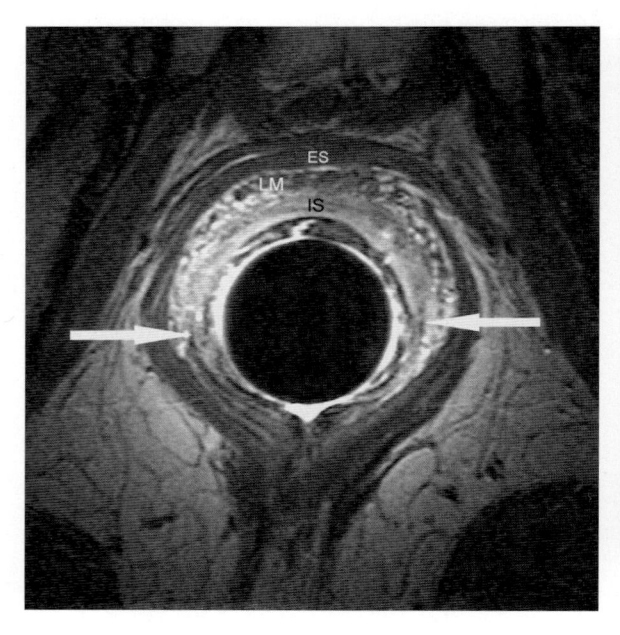

Fig. 4.4.4. Axial T2-weighted image (*arrows* internal sphincter defect, *IS* internal sphincter, *ES* external sphincter, *LM* longitudinal muscle)

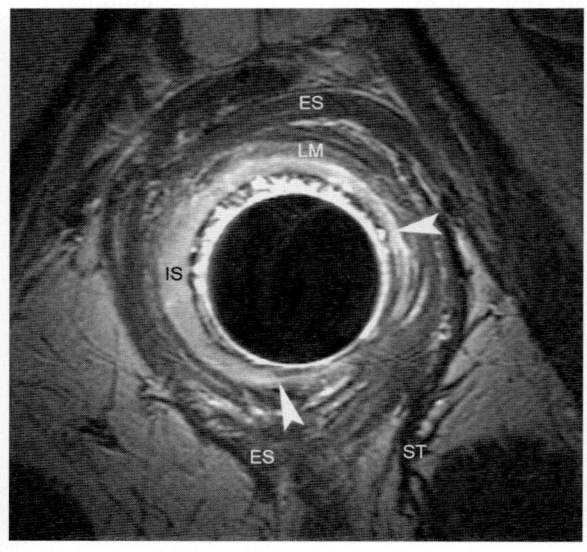

Fig. 4.4.5. Axial T2-weighted image. Complex lesion involving external sphincter defect, internal sphincter defect (*arrowheads*) and scar tissue (*ST*) between the margins of the sphincter defect. Longitudinal muscle (*LM*) also shows ring disturbance and asymmetry

4.4.4.2
External Sphincter

4.4.4.2.1
Tears

Obstetric trauma involves the anterior half of the external sphincter and when the internal sphincter is also torn, this usually involves the same segment. Continuity of the muscles is partially or completely destructed (Fig. 4.4.5). An area of mixed signal intensity replaces the muscle and low signal fibrous scars may be seen as late sequelae (Figs. 4.4.5). Tears of the external sphincter also can be seen after surgery or unwanted anal penetration. This may result in fragmentation of the whole sphincter ring (Fig. 4.4.6). The overall interobserver agreement for assessment of sphincter integrity using endoanal MR imaging is strongest if the sphincters are either both intact or both disrupted (Malouf et al. 2001). The full extent of the damage is best appreciated in longitudinal plane sequences (Fig. 4.4.7).

Secondary changes to the architecture of adjacent structures (longitudinal muscle, perianal fat) provide supportive evidence of a tear. The opposite side may be atrophic, but if normal it may compared with the torn side.

4.4.4.2.2
Muscle Volume Anomalies

Normal Values: Average thickness in healthy volunteers is 4 mm.

External sphincter atrophy (<2 mm) comprises generalized thinning and reduction of the striated muscle with fatty replacement. Reinnervation, as evidence of external sphincter atrophy, is most accurately detected by single fibre EMG studies. The popularity of endosonography emphasizes the detection of sphincter tears rather than atrophy, as it is not a reliable indicator for this (Gold et al. 1999). However, endocoil MRI does allow the thickness and fat content of the external sphincter to be assessed accurately (Figs. 4.4.8, 4.4.9). In a study with histological comparison, endoanal MRI has been shown to be able to determine the presence or absence of external sphincter atrophy with a sensitivity of 89% and a specificity of 94% (Briel et al. 2000). In a comparative study (Briel et al. 1999) of endoanal ultrasonography and endoanal MRI in 20 women with faecal incontinence due to obstetric trauma, external sphincter atrophy was not identified at ultrasonography but was present at endoanal MRI in eight women.

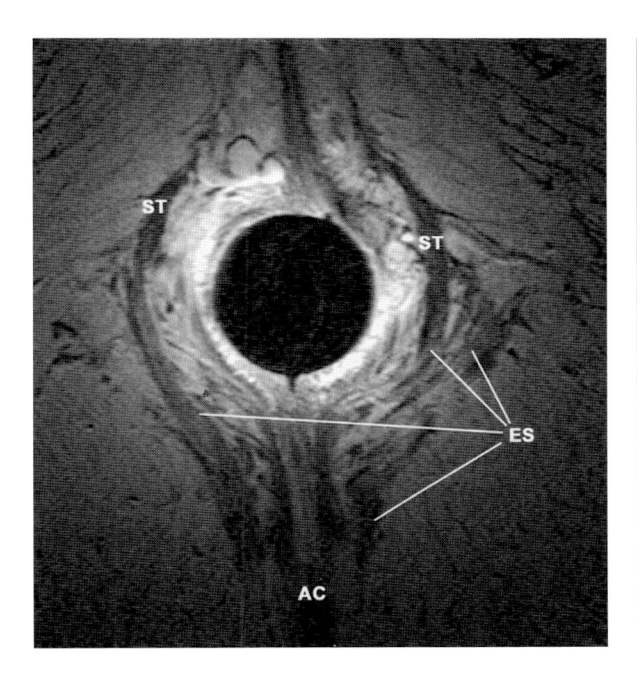

Fig. 4.4.6. Axial T2-weighted image. Traumatic fragmentation of external sphincter (*ES*) (*ST* scar tissue, *AC* anococcygeal ligament)

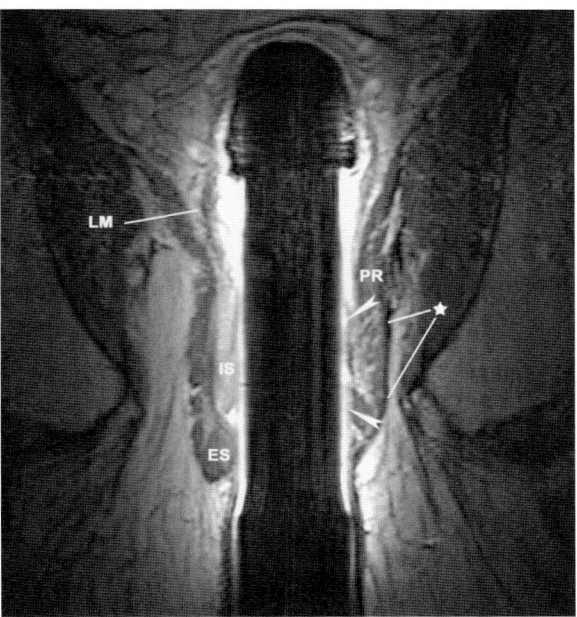

Fig. 4.4.7. Coronal T2-weighted image. Internal sphincter (*IS*) normal on the right side. Internal sphincter defect on the left side (*arrowheads*), and scar tissue (*star*) deforming the right side of the external sphincter (*ES*) (*LM* longitudinal muscle, *PR* puborectalis)

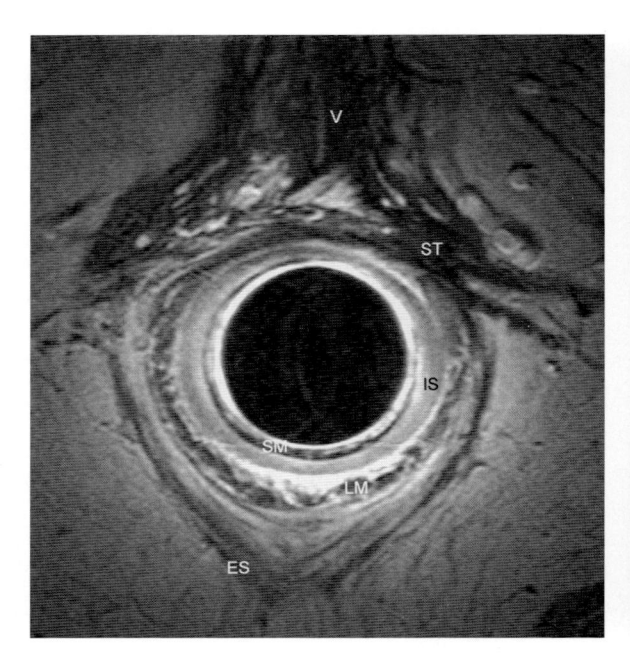

Fig. 4.4.8. Axial T2-weighted image. External sphincter (*ES*) atrophy with scar tissue (*ST*) after episiotomy (*LM* longitudinal muscle, *IS* internal sphincter, *SM* submucosa/muscularis mucosa, *V* vagina)

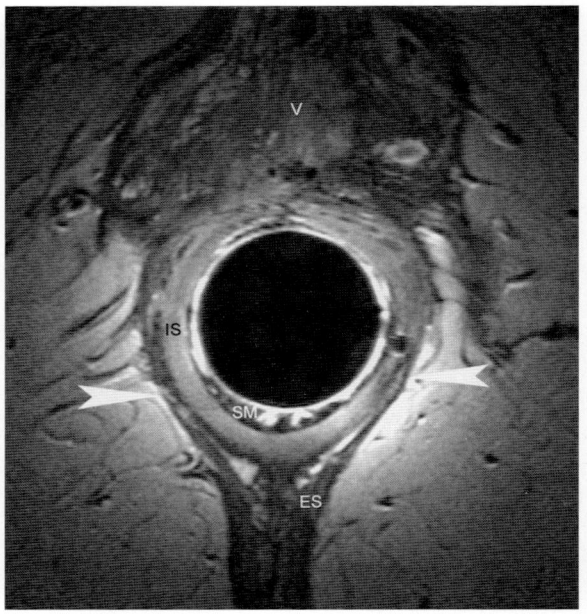

Fig. 4.4.9. Axial T2-weighted image. External sphincter (*ES*) atrophy. The external sphincter is extremely thin (*arrowheads*) and the longitudinal muscle can no longer be recognized (*IS* internal sphincter, *SM* submucosa/muscularis mucosa, *V* vagina)

A diagnosis of atrophy may be made at a workstation by visual assessment of the muscle mass, as well as by measurement of the area of the remaining muscle (BRIEL et al. 1999). Endoanal MRI is strongly recommended prior to sphincter repair to exclude significant atrophy the presence of which correlates ($P=0.004$) with poor outcome after anal repair. Endoanal MRI has the advantage of simultaneously evaluating external sphincter atrophy and the presence of anterior external sphincter lacerations.

Although atrophy is visible in all planes, the coronal plane gives the best indication of overall sphincteric volume and allows comparison of each side (Fig. 4.4.10). When analysing the volume of the external sphincter it is important to remember that women have a shorter external anterior sphincter than men. On longitudinal images the lateral side of the external sphincter averages 27 mm in length in women and 28.6 mm in men, but the anterior aspect averages 14 mm in women compared to 27 mm in men. On mid axial images, in young women (£35 years of age) the external sphincter is thinner (4.32 mm average) than in young men (5.21 mm average) (ROCIU et al. 2000).

A recent study delineated the external sphincter with endoanal MRI and found a relationship between function (e.g. squeeze pressure) and external sphincter bulk (WILLIAMS et al. 2001). There is a decrease of external sphincter thickness with age. In women from an average of 4.3 mm to 3.9 mm in the elderly, and in men from 5.2 mm to 3.45 mm. This is part of the ageing process, and should be differentiated from atrophy causing incontinence, where the muscle is <2 mm (ROCIU et al. 2000).

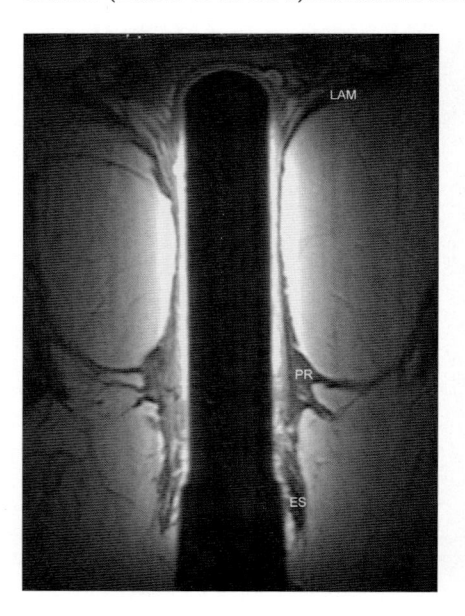

Fig. 4.4.10. Mid-coronal T2-weighted image. Atrophic anal sphincter (*ES* external sphincter, *PR* puborectal muscle, *LAM* levator ani muscle). The internal sphincter can barely be seen. Compare with normal anal sphincter on coronal images as seen in Fig. 4.4.2

4.4.5
Role of Endoanal MRI in Pelvic Floor Disorders

When conservative treatment fails, faecal incontinence is most often due to local sphincter dysfunction. The local high spatial resolution multiplanar endoanal MRI makes this technique particularly suitable for diagnosis. Moreover, imaging has become central in the work-up of faecal incontinence, since physical examination is not accurate, electromyography too painful and manometry only indicates the functional status without information on sphincter integrity.

The role of phased-array-coil MRI has not been evaluated yet. Promising results regarding visualization of the pelvic floor anatomy have been published (Beets-Tan et al. 2001), but the local spatial resolution of this technique is inferior to that of endoluminal techniques. It remains to be demonstrated whether phased-array-coil MRI does allow enough delineation of pelvic muscles for accurate detection of sphincter defects and atrophy. Phased array MRI has the potential advantage of a simpler examination. Endovaginal sonography and endovaginal MRI are not ideal alternatives as the distance between transducer/coil and the sphincter is increased.

Endoanal MRI and endosonography are competitive techniques in the work-up of faecal incontinence. Two studies have been published addressing this issue. A retrospective study of 22 patients with sphincter defects compared anal endosonography and endoanal MRI to surgery, and found MRI to be the most accurate. External sphincter defects were detected with sonography and endoanal MRI in, respectively, 16 patients (73%) and 20 patients (91%), and internal sphincter defects in, respectively, 15 (68%) and 17 (77%) (Rociu et al. 1999). A second, prospective study in 52 consecutive patients with faecal incontinence suggested that endoanal ultrasonography and endoanal MRI are comparable for detection of external sphincter defects and that endoanal ultrasonography is superior for detection of internal sphincter defects (Malouf et al. 2000). The differences between the results of both studies are at least partly related to differences in patient populations, study design and experience with the two techniques. Major difference between the techniques is in the detection of external sphincter atrophy. In a comparative study of endosonography and endoanal MRI in 20 women with faecal incontinence due to obstetric trauma, external sphincter atrophy was not identified at endosonography, when it was present at endoanal MRI in eight women (Briel et al. 1999).

The present consensus is that endoanal MRI is preferable for external sphincter disorders and endoanal ultrasonography preferable in cases of internal sphincter disorders. In the current work-up, local expertise remains very important in the choice between the endoanal imaging modalities. From a practical point of view, endoanal ultrasonography can be used as the primary technique and endoanal MRI as the second-line technique, depending on local expertise and availability. Nevertheless, when surgical repair is considered after ultrasonographic diagnosis of external sphincter tear endoanal MRI should be performed. This is mandatory to exclude atrophy of the external sphincter, a predicting factor for negative outcome. Most likely, other surgical techniques such as artificial sphincter implants or dynamic graciloplasty should be considered in patients with considerable external sphincter atrophy.

References

Beets-Tan RG, Morren GL, Beets GL, et al (2001) Measurement of anal sphincter muscles: endoanal US, endoanal MR imaging, or phased-array MR imaging? A study with healthy volunteers. Radiology 220:81–89

Briel JW, Stoker J, Rociu E, et al (1999) External anal sphincter atrophy on endoanal magnetic resonance imaging adversely affects continence after sphincteroplasty. Br J Surg 86:1322–1327

Briel JW, Zimmerman DD, Stoker J, et al (2000) Relationship between sphincter morphology on endoanal MRI and histopathological aspects of the external anal sphincter. Int J Colorectal Dis 15:87–90

Burnett SJ, Spence-Jones C, Speakman CT, et al (1991) Unsuspected sphincter damage following childbirth revealed by anal endosonography. Br J Radiol 64:225–227

deSouza NM, Puni R, Zbar A, et al (1996) MR imaging of the anal sphincter in multiparous women using an endoanal coil: correlation with in vitro anatomy and appearances in fecal incontinence. AJR Am J Roentgenol 167:1465–1471

Gold DM, Halligan S, Kmiot WA, et al (1999) Intraobserver and interobserver agreement in anal endosonography. Br J Surg 86:371–375

Malouf AJ, Williams AB, Halligan S, et al (2000) Prospective assessment of accuracy of endoanal MR imaging and endosonography in patients with fecal incontinence. AJR Am J Roentgenol 175:741–745

Malouf AJ, Halligan S, Williams AB, et al (2001) Prospective assessment of interobserver agreement for endoanal MRI in fecal incontinence. Abdom Imaging 26:76–78

Nielsen MB, Rasmussen OO, Pedersen JF, et al (1993) Anal endosonographic findings in patients with obstructed defecation. Acta Radiol 34:35–38

Rociu E, Stoker J, Eijkemans MJ, et al (1999) Fecal incontinence: endoanal US versus endoanal MR imaging. Radiology 212:453–458

Rociu E, Stoker J, Eijkemans MJ, et al (2000) Normal anal sphincter anatomy and age- and sex-related variations at high-spatial-resolution endoanal MR imaging. Radiology 217:395–401

Stoker J, Rociu E, Zwamborn AW, et al (1999) Endoluminal MR imaging of the rectum and anus: technique, applications, and pitfalls. Radiographics 19:383–398

Sultan AH, Kamm MA, Hudson CN, et al (1993) Anal sphincter disruption during vaginal delivery. N Engl J Med 329:1905–1911

Vaizey CJ, Kamm MA, Bartram CI (1997) Primary degeneration of the internal anal sphincter as a cause of passive faecal incontinence. Lancet 349:612–615

Williams AB, Malouf AJ, Bartram CI, et al (2001) Assessment of external anal sphincter morphology in idiopathic fecal incontinence with endocoil magnetic resonance imaging. Dig Dis Sci 46:1466–1471

4.5 Urodynamics

K. STROHBEHN

CONTENTS

4.5.1 Introduction 89
4.5.1.1 When to Perform Urodynamics 90
4.5.1.2 Definitions 90
4.5.2 Storage Studies 90
4.5.2.1 Bladder Function 90
4.5.2.2 Urethral Function 93
4.5.3 Emptying/Flow Studies 95
4.5.3.1 Postvoid Residual 95
4.5.3.2 Simple Uroflowmetry 95
4.5.3.3 Complex Uroflowmetry 95
4.5.3.4 Pressure-Flow Studies 96
4.5.4 Other Studies 96
4.5.4.1 Electromyography 96
4.5.4.2 Imaging 96
4.5.5 Summary 97
References 98

4.5.1 Introduction

The term "urodynamic" is defined as "pertaining to the flow and motion of fluids in the urinary tract" (TAYLOR 1988). The term "urodynamic study" or "urodynamics" refers to the study of lower urinary tract function (bladder and urethra). Urodynamics are performed on subjects with disorders of bladder storage or emptying to further elucidate the etiology of the disorder and their symptoms. Urodynamic study is "any test which provides objective information about lower urinary tract function" (WALL et al. 1993). Using this definition, even tests such as a urinalysis and bladder intake/voiding diaries can be included in the spectrum of urodynamic studies.

K. STROHBEHN, MD, FACOG, FACS
Associate Professor, Dartmouth Medical School, Department of Obstetrics and Gynecology; Director, Division of Urogynecology/Reconstructive Pelvic Surgery, Dartmouth-Hitchcock Medical Center, One Medical Center Drive, Lebanon, NH 03756, USA

In this chapter the concepts of each method of examination are briefly reviewed, starting with the simplest to measure the specific bladder function, followed by more complex testing. In general, the more complex the testing, the higher the accuracy, but also the higher the cost to determine that function. For example, urodynamics can refer to simple tests, such as checking the amount of residual urine left in the bladder after micturition or timing of the average speed at which the bladder empties a measured volume of urine using a stopwatch. Urodynamics also refers to more complex testing of the bladder, such as pressure-flow studies to more accurately measure the bladder emptying function and multichannel cystometry to more accurately study bladder storage function. Table 4.5.1 summarizes most of the specific tests available for determining storage and emptying functions of the bladder.

There is no consensus on the utility of urodynamics in the optimal management of patients, nor is there consensus on the methodology and which tests are indicated for specific symptoms. Recently, WEBER and WALTERS (2000) examined the cost effectiveness of performing complex urodynamic testing on women with pelvic organ prolapse and stress urinary incontinence. They found that cure rates were similar for patients undergoing basic office evaluation versus urodynamic testing and that the testing markedly increased expense. In this respect, urodynamics are best utilized as an adjunct to a careful history and physical examination with basic evaluations such as measuring a postvoid residual volume, and not as a substitute for these (WALL et al. 1993).

Storage disorders can result in urinary incontinence or frequency, which are discussed in more detail in Chapter 5.2. Emptying disorders include problems of urinary retention or incomplete emptying of the bladder with micturition. Some subjects with emptying disorders have urinary incontinence because the bladder is overdistended, resulting in urine overflow and urinary incontinence.

Table 4.5.1. Types of urodynamic tests

	Simple	Medium	Complex
Storage functions			
Bladder function	1. Bladder diary	1. Pressure sensor cystometry	Ambulatory cystometrometry
	2. Urinalysis	2. Complex multichannel cystometrogram	
	3. Simple water cystometrogram		
	4. Bladder capacity		
Urethral support/ function	1. Mobility testing: Q-tip test, Visual inspection	Leak point pressures	1. Urethral pressure profilometry
	2. Cough or Valsalva stress test		2. Video fluoroscopic urodynamics
			3. Electromyography (EMG)
Emptying disorders			
	1. Bladder diary	Simple uroflowmetry	Complex uroflowmetry (pressure-flow studies)
	2. Postvoid residual		

4.5.1.1
When to Perform Urodynamics

As mentioned above, there is no consensus on how to perform urodynamics, nor is there consensus on the utility of urodynamic testing for specific disorders. Urodynamic testing can be a useful adjunctive study, because the symptoms and subjective history for patients with lower urinary tract disorders do not always predict the specific disorder that a woman has (CUNDIFF et al. 1997; SUMMITT et al. 1992; WALTERS and SHIELDS 1988). Recommendations for urodynamic testing have ranged from using these studies when the history and examination do not correspond, to any patient undergoing surgery, to those subjects who have failed prior therapies. In the United States, The Agency for Health Care Policy and Research have set up guidelines for the evaluation of incontinent patients (FANTL et al. 1996; URINARY INCONTINENCE GUIDELINE PANEL 1992). WEIDNER et al. (2001) recently looked at the AHCPR guidelines and found that using these guidelines improves the accuracy of diagnosis in comparison to history of stress incontinence alone. They also note, however, that fewer than 1 in 12 women who presented with incontinence was eligible for surgical repair of stress incontinence based on the AHCPR guidelines without first undergoing urodynamic testing (WEIDNER et al. 2001).

4.5.1.2
Definitions

The terminology of lower urinary tract dysfunction and testing has been standardized in several consensus documents produced by the International Continence Society (ABRAMS et al. 2002; GRIFFITHS et al. 1997; ROWAN et al. 1987; STOHRER et al. 1999; VAN KERREBROECK et al. 2002; VAN WAALWIJK VAN DOORN et al. 2000). These documents are extensive and a review is beyond the scope of this chapter. References are provided for the interested reader. The International Continence Society website is: *http://www.icsoffice.org*. Of interest to this readership, there is a subcommittee of the ICS Standardization Committee that is currently investigating standardization of imaging for the evaluation of incontinent subjects.

4.5.2
Storage Studies

4.5.2.1
Bladder Function

There are many helpful techniques for establishing the ability of the bladder to normally store urine. Voiding diaries are a good place to start and many incontinence centers mail these to the patient to complete prior to their first visit.

4.5.2.1.1
Bladder Diary

Bladder voiding and intake diaries are an integral part of the evaluation of patients with urinary incontinence. They supplement the history and it is not infrequent that a woman will identify her own problem once she undertakes the task of writing down her voids, her intake and her symptoms when she has incontinence. An example of one type of bladder diary for a woman with stress incontinence is shown in Fig. 4.5.1 (Fig 3.9 from WALL et al. 1993 p. 56). The bladder diary assists in determining daytime urinary frequency, nocturia, volume of urine per void, intake volume, bladder irritants and timing of incontinent episodes in relation to events such as external stimuli or coughing.

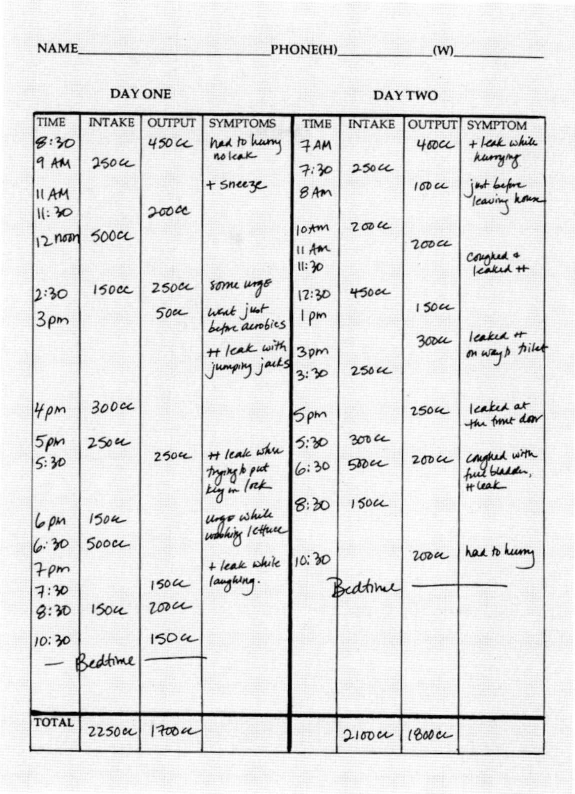

4.5.2.1.2
Urinalysis

Urinalysis is a helpful tool to assure there is not a subacute occult urinary tract infection, which is a rare cause of urinary incontinence (WALL et al. 1993). Any bacteriuric infection should be treated prior to proceeding with cystometry. In addition to eliminating a subclinical infection as the cause of incontinence, urinalysis can rule out hematuria which would need additional evaluation if found.

4.5.2.1.3
Cystometry

Cystometry is a test of detrusor function which measures the sensation, compliance, pressure and capacity of the bladder. Indirectly these measurements assess the neuromuscular integrity of the bladder.

4.5.2.1.3.1
Simple Cystometry

The easiest method to perform cystometry is to measure the bladder pressure during filling with a catheter by looking at the pressure seen on a column of water. The vesical pressure can be plotted against volume as the bladder is filled at a constant rate (COATES 1998). One way to measure this is by "eyeball cystometry", in which the water column is assessed from the same filling vessel that is connected to the catheter that is filling the bladder. This is the least accurate measurement of the true bladder pressure, but the easiest to perform. This measurement can be performed in any office setting. The only equipment required is a catheter, a catheter-tipped syringe and a sterile solution to fill the bladder. During bladder filling, the subject is instructed to relax and to avoid any activities that would increase the intraabdominal pressure, such as coughing, laughing or talking. Any activities such as those mentioned will cause a simultaneous rise in the intravesical pressure that cannot be distinguished from a true bladder contraction with simple cystometry.

Fig. 4.5.1. Bladder diary (frequency/volume chart) from a patient with normal fluid intake and normal urinary output, but with symptoms of stress and urge incontinence (with permission, Wall et al. 1993, p 56)

Intravesical pressure can also be measured with a catheter that is connected to a commercially available cystometric tubing set and thus the column of water can be more accurately assessed for the intravesical pressure without interruption of bladder filling (Fig. 4.5.2; from WALL et al. 1993, Fig. 4.1, p 91). During filling, the volume at first sensation in the bladder, sensation of urge to void and full capacity are recorded.

Cystometry can also be performed with more precise catheter pressure sensors such as fiberoptic catheters and microtip pressure transducers. In general, these sensors are more commonly used with multichannel cystometry. Cystometry can be performed with liquid or gas medium to fill the bladder.

4.5.2.1.3.2
Complex (Multichannel) Cystometry

Multichannel cystometry (also called subtracted cystometry) provides a more accurate measurement

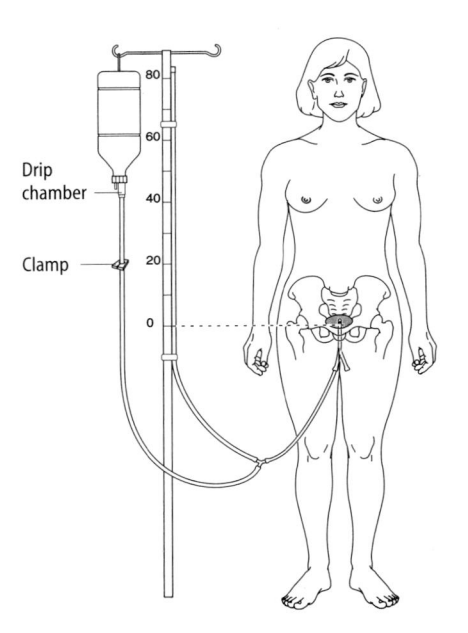

Fig. 4.5.2. Setup for simple water cystometry (with permission, WALL et al. 1993, p 91)

of bladder capacity and pressures. The abdominal pressure is measured with a second pressure catheter, placed within the rectum or vagina (Fig. 4.5.3; from WALTERS and SHIELDS 1988, p 57). The second pressure catheter allows for the abdominal pressure to be subtracted from the bladder pressure, thus giving a true bladder pressure, also called the "detrusor pressure". The formula format for this is:

$$P_{det} = P_{ves} - P_{abd}$$

where P_{det} is the true detrusor pressure generated by the bladder, P_{ves} is the bladder pressure measured with a catheter in the bladder and P_{abd} is the abdominal pressure. These pressures are plotted graphically against volume during filling.

Similar to simple cystometry, several events are recorded during filling, including the volume at which the patient first has sensation in the bladder, the volume that she would void and then the maximum volume or "maximum cystometric capacity". During filling, the pressure within the bladder is monitored to see if there are changes in the pressure. Usually the bladder pressure remains stable throughout filling with a small terminal rise in pressure at near bladder capacity (Fig. 4.5.4; from WALL et al. 1993 p 92, Fig. 4.5.4.2). A rise in the intravesical pressure is consistent with a bladder detrusor muscle contraction, which would correspond to a diagnosis of detrusor instability or urge incontinence (Fig. 4.5.5; from WALL et al. 1993 p 92, Fig. 4.5.4.3).

At different volume intervals during filling, the patient is instructed to perform Valsalva maneuvers and cough to look for stress urinary incontinence. This will be described in more detail under the section covering leak point pressures. The study is most accurately performed standing and the sensitivity increases with maneuvers such as running water and having the patient heel bounce and cough.

The sensitivity of cystometry is improved with subtracted cystometry in comparison to single channel cystometry (FANTL et al. 1996).

4.5.2.1.3.3
Ambulatory Cystometry

The premise of ambulatory urodynamics is that one can capture bladder events over a longer period and in a more normal environment than conventional cystometry can. The patient wears urodynamic catheters with an ambulatory monitor to record bladder pressures over

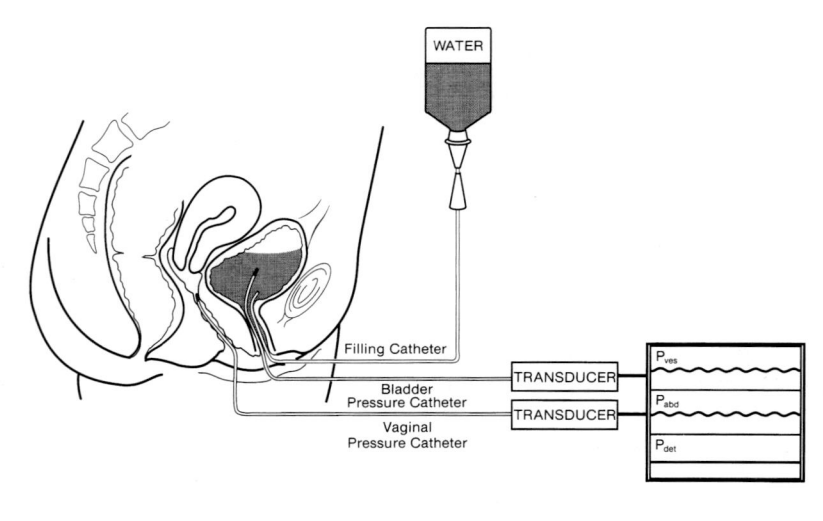

Fig. 4.5.3. Subtracted cystometry. Intravesical (P_{ves}) and intraabdominal (P_{abd}) pressures are measured and true detrusor pressure (P_{det}) is electronically derived ($P_{ves}-P_{abd}=P_{det}$) (with permission, KARRAM 1999, p 57)

Urodynamics

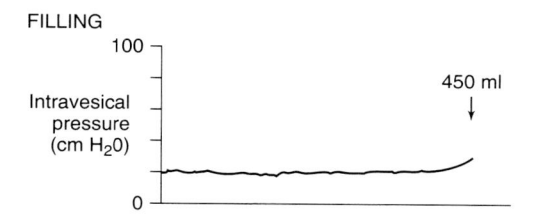

Fig. 4.5.4. Normal simple cystometrogram tracing. There are no fluctuations in bladder pressure and the capacity is 450 ml (with permission, WALL et al. 1993, p 92)

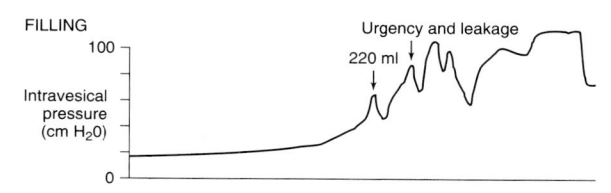

Fig. 4.5.5. Simple cystometrogram showing phasic fluctuations in bladder pressure due to detrusor overactivity (with permission, WALL et al. 1993, p 92)

a longer period of time. The concept is similar to that of a 24-h Holter monitor to record cardiac events such as arrhythmias that may not occur in a limited time frame. The sensitivity of cystometry improves further with ambulatory cystometry (RADLEY et al. 2001), but the false-positive rate also increases (FANTL et al. 1996). In one study where ambulatory cystometric evaluation was performed in 22 asymptomatic women, 68% had evidence of detrusor instability on ambulatory testing and 18% by conventional cystometry (HESLINGTON and HILTON 1996). Other drawbacks of ambulatory testing include inconvenience and expense, especially when empiric therapy for urge incontinence or sensory urgency conditions is a reasonable initial approach in the setting of a normal postvoid residual.

4.5.2.2
Urethral Function

Another important concept in the study of storage disorders is the integrity of the outlet of the bladder, namely the urethra. There are two methods to study urethral function in women with incontinence. Urethral pressures can be measured with a catheter in the urethral lumen. Alternatively, leak point pressures assess the pressure at which the bladder overcomes urethral resistance and causes urinary leakage.

4.5.2.2.1
Urethral Pressure Profilometry

Resting and dynamic urethral pressures can be assessed with a pressure catheter that is withdrawn through the urethral lumen at a constant rate. As the catheter is withdrawn from the bladder to the urethra and then out of the urethral meatus, a pressure curve is generated, as depicted in Figs. 4.5.6 and 4.5.7 (OSTERGARD and BENT 1996 p 128, Figs. 10.12 and 10.13). This pressure curve provides information regarding the location of the highest pressure within the urethra, corresponding to the urethral rhabdosphincter. The maximum urethral closure pressure (mUCP) is defined as the maximum urethral pressure (P_{ura}) minus the vesical pressure (P_{ves}). In addition to the urethral closure pressure, the pressure profile provides information regarding the functional length of the urethra.

The pressure transducer or catheter starts in the bladder, along with the bladder transducer. Dual tip catheters allow simultaneous measurement of the intravesical pressure and the intraurethral pressure.

4.5.2.2.1.1
Urethral Closure Pressure

The urethral pressure profile is one method to evaluate for stress urinary incontinence in women. Urethral closure pressures normally decline with age (RUD 1980). It has been frequently reported in the gynecologic literature as a tool that is useful in determining

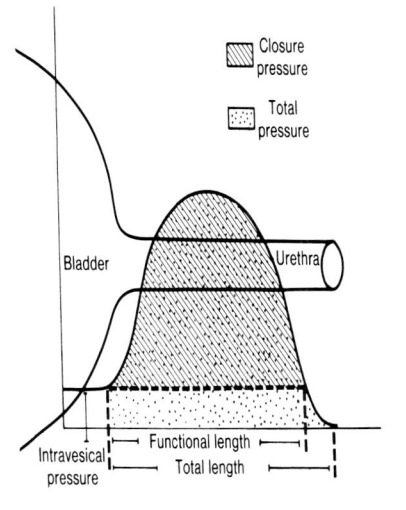

Fig. 4.5.6. The urethral closure pressure profile of a normal subject. The *hatched area* represents the area of closure pressure and the *dotted area* represents the area of total urethral pressure (with permission, JENSEN 1996, p 128)

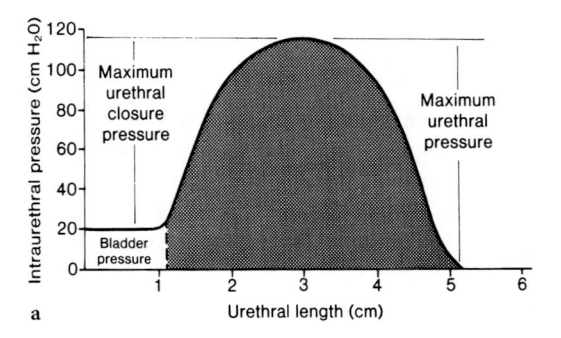

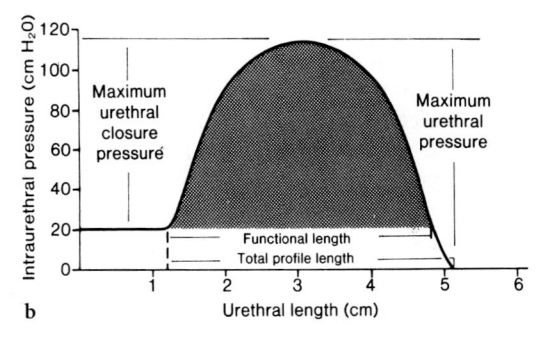

Fig. 4.5.7a, b. Integrated urethral closure profile. **a** The *shaded area* indicates the integrated total urethral pressure. **b** The *shaded area* indicates the integrated closure pressure (also called the continence area) (with permission, JENSEN 1996, p 128)

the appropriate incontinence procedure to treat stress urinary incontinence. Typically, stress incontinence is described as a problem of support of the bladder outlet ("hypermobility" or "type II stress incontinence") versus a problem with the sphincter of the urethra ("intrinsic sphincter deficiency" or "type III stress incontinence"). There have been several reports in the literature indicating that a low urethral closure pressure (urethral closure pressure <20 cm H_2O) correlates with patients who are more likely to fail a standard support operation (BOWEN et al. 1989; SAND et al. 1987). These patients have traditionally been recommended to undergo an operation to compensate for a weak urethral sphincter mechanism, using a "sling operation" or using bulking agents within the urethra. MCGUIRE et al. (1993) identified that urethral closure pressures are not a useful clinical measurement of urethral strength as there are some women who have incontinence at normal or high maximum urethral closure pressures. The opposite finding has been established by others, identifying a good correlation between closure pressures and the severity of incontinence (COATES 1998; HILTON and STANTON 1983; THEOFRASTOUS et al. 1995).

4.5.2.2.2
Leak Point Pressures

Sphincter function can also be assessed by measuring the abdominal or vesical pressure that overcomes urethral resistance and results in urinary leakage. Leak point pressures were first described by MCGUIRE (1981) as a tool to identify the risk of ureteral reflux in patients with neurologic disease who have poor emptying function. Patients in whom the detrusor pressure reaches a significantly high pressure (over 40 cm H_2O) without leakage are at risk for subsequent ureteral reflux and renal damage (MCGUIRE et al. 1981; WANG et al. 1988). MCGUIRE later used the leak point pressure as a measure of urethral resistance at the bladder outlet among patients with stress urinary incontinence (MCGUIRE et al. 1993). The concept is that subjects with a poorly functioning outlet are women who need a more durable, effective operation to treat the outlet, namely a sling-type procedure.

4.5.2.2.2.1
Valsalva Leak Point Pressure

Valsalva leak point pressures are obtained by measuring the pressure at which leakage will occur during a Valsalva maneuver. The subject is asked to strain until leakage is observed and the pressure within the bladder is measured. The volume at which these measurements are obtained has not been well standardized, and depends upon catheter size, and bladder volume during testing (BUMP et al. 1995; COATES 1998; SWIFT and OSTERGARD 1995; SWIFT and UTRIE 1996), but most examiners will check a Valsalva leak point pressure at 150–300 ml filling. The pressure measurements can be obtained using a bladder catheter transducer, or by measuring abdominal pressure via a catheter in the rectum or vagina. Leak point pressures were more commonly reported first in the urological literature, but are now commonly used by urogynecologists and specialists in reconstructive pelvic surgery as well. There is consensus that a Valsalva leak point pressure of less than 60 cm H_2O at a volume of 150 ml filling correlates with intrinsic sphincter deficiency (COATES 1998).

Correlation between Valsalva leak point pressures and urethral closure pressures are poor (BUMP et al. 1995, 1997; COATES 1998; SWIFT and OSTERGARD 1995). MCGUIRE emphasizes that the information gleaned by measuring static urethral closure pressures is clinically unimportant in comparison to the information gained from Valsalva leak point pressures regarding urethral resistance as abdominal pressure rises (COATES 1998; MCGUIRE et al. 1993).

4.5.2.2.2.2
Cough Leak Point Pressure

The technique of measuring cough leak point pressures is similar to that of obtaining Valsalva leak point pressures, except the patient is asked to cough with gradually higher cough intensities until leakage is observed. The leak point is that pressure generated by a cough that results in leakage of urine. In general, the intensity of a cough is more difficult to control and the actual leak point is more difficult to measure. Based on this, the utility of cough leak point pressures is less well established. However, there may be different mechanisms for maintaining continence with a sudden cough than there are with gradually straining and increasing the abdominal pressure in a more controlled fashion.

4.5.3
Emptying/Flow Studies

Bladder emptying disorders are usually due to either an atonic bladder (bladder dysnergia) or because of obstruction at the outlet of the bladder. Outlet obstruction is more common in men than women, due to prostatism, benign prostatic hypertrophy or other causes of enlargement. In women, obstruction is usually due to iatrogenic causes after surgery at the bladder outlet, or from prolapse of the upper vagina and bladder that can result in kinking at the urethra. Aging causes a decline in most voiding parameters measured, including postvoid residuals, average flow rates, peak flow rates, voided volumes and bladder capacity (MADERSBACHER et al. 1998). The options for study of bladder emptying disorders are described below.

4.5.3.1
Postvoid Residual

A postvoid residual (PVR) volume measurement is a simple and useful tool to establish the bladder's ability to properly empty. This provides preliminary information regarding the neuromuscular integrity of the bladder. A PVR can be obtained with a catheter, or by using ultrasound. The method of determining PVR with ultrasound is to measure the transverse breadth (b), anteroposterior height (h) with a probe frequency range of 3.5–5.0 MHz in the transverse direction and then to change the probe to the sagittal orientation and measure length (l). The volume is then calculated by the following equation, with a correlation coefficient of 0.982 when compared to catheter volumes (ROEHRBORN and PETERS 1988):

Volume (ml) = 0.52 (h + b + l)

More recently, commercial ultrasound technology has become available to check PVRs with an ultrasound probe (bladder scanner) that calculates the volume without taking individual measurements.

There is not a consensus regarding the normal PVR volume, but most agree that volumes greater than 60 ml identify some element of bladder dysfunction. The PVR also depends upon the voided volume. In general, voided volumes of less than 150 ml make the PVR unreliable (WALL et al. 1993). However, a normal PVR does not mean that the bladder emptying is effected via a normal bladder detrusor contraction, as some patients empty with abdominal straining or manually pushing on the suprapubic area.

4.5.3.2
Simple Uroflowmetry

Uroflowmetry is the measurement of the flow rate of the bladder during micturition. One simple way to obtain information regarding bladder emptying is to perform a stopwatch test. This test obtains an average flow rate for emptying. The patient is instructed to void into a collecting hat in private, but informed that there will be someone listening for the onset and end of voiding outside the room. A stopwatch is started with the initiation of the void and stopped at the conclusion. The urine collected is measured and the average rate of flow (ml/s) is measured by dividing the voided volume by the time to void. Normal flow rates are dependent upon the volume voided but a rate of less than 10 ml/s is below the tenth percentile for most subjects (HAYLEN et al. 1989). The flow of urine should be heard as a steady increase and decline. Any sound of "spurts" of urine suggests voiding dysfunction and could represent obstruction or use of abdominal straining to void rather than using the detrusor muscles.

4.5.3.3
Complex Uroflowmetry

A more complex uroflowmetry measurement can be obtained using a scale and a collection system, with the patient voiding into a commode place over the collection system (Fig. 4.5.8). The rate of flow is measured as the subject urinates, and is shown graphically (Fig. 4.5.9; Wall et al. 1993, Fig. 4.15, p 106). The volume, rate and peak flow can be obtained, as well as an assessment of whether or not there are abnormalities in the normal curve. Abnormalities can include spike in pressure caused by abdominal straining, or a low amplitude flow rate when there is obstruction at the outlet or a poorly functioning detrusor muscle.

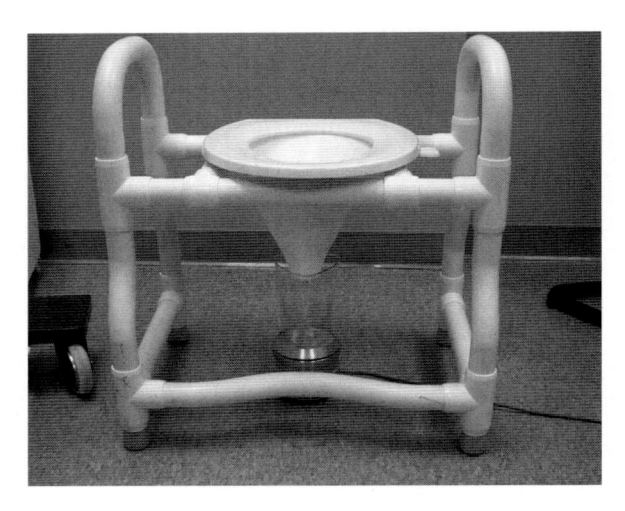

Fig. 4.5.8. Typical setup for a complex uroflowmetry with electrically calibrated urine flowmeter

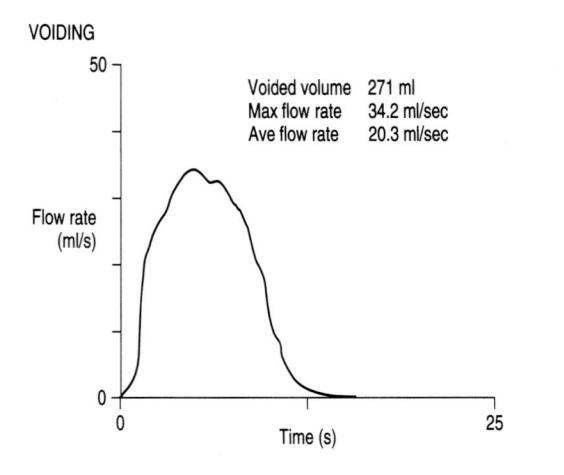

Fig. 4.5.9. Normal complex urine flow study from an electrically calibrated urine flowmeter (with permission, Wall et al. 1993, p 106)

4.5.3.4
Pressure-Flow Studies

Pressure-flow studies combine complex voiding studies with complex voiding cystometry (Wall et al. 1993). Similar to a complex cystometrogram, catheters are placed in the bladder and rectum to provide a subtracted measurement of the true bladder pressure P_{det}. The patient voids with the catheters in place while complex uroflowmetry is performed. This technique allows simultaneous evaluation of all pressure activity in relation to the urine flow pattern and provides information to help differentiate whether a patient voids with detrusor contraction, pelvic relaxation, or abdominal straining (Wall et al. 1993). There are some patients who are unable to "perform" in the setting of a urodynamic laboratory with catheters in place, so the results may be unreliable. Useful information can be obtained when a patient is found to void using their abdominal muscles or by relaxing the urethra or pelvic floor muscles. These patients are more likely to have voiding dysfunction after surgical repair of stress incontinence and may need prolonged catheterization (Wall et al. 1993).

4.5.4
Other Studies

4.5.4.1
Electromyography

Electrophysiologic studies such as electromyography (EMG) are an additional tool to study the pelvic floor muscles and external urethral sphincters. EMG has been performed with cystometry and uroflowmetry testing. It can be useful to determine the ability of the urethral sphincter muscle to appropriately contract with stimuli that increase abdominal pressures, such as a cough, and to determine the ability of the sphincter to relax during voiding (Coates 1998; Wall et al. 1993).

4.5.4.2
Imaging

Several imaging techniques have been proposed for adjunctive study of the bladder and urodynamic testing. The most utilized have been fluoroscopic study of the bladder and more recently, perineal ultrasound which both provide information regarding urethra and bladder neck mobility. Intraurethral ultrasound has recently been reported to calculate the cross-sectional area of the urethra and its muscle layers (HEIT 2000; MAJOR et al. 2002). There are few normative data on this new technology, but it may provide additional information about urethral integrity and its correlation with urethral resistance.

4.5.4.2.1
Fluoroscopy

Fluoroscopy provides additional information regarding the function of the bladder outlet and bladder contour. There are many who advocate its use for any complex evaluation (MCGUIRE and WOODSIDE 1981), in order to have a complete assessment of the bladder integrity, including whether or not there is ureteral reflux. Radiocontrast dye is instilled into the bladder during the cystometrogram rather than a saline solution. The diagnosis of stress urinary incontinence is established when leakage of the dye is seen with associated cough or Valsalva, in the absence of a detrusor contraction. Additional information gleaned from fluoroscopy includes the presence of bladder diverticula, as well as an assessment of the bladder outlet. The bladder outlet can be considered hypermobile if there is rotation of the urethrovesical neck (Fig. 4.5.10). Beaking of the urethrovesical neck or a funnel shape to the bladder outlet suggest a diagnosis of "intrinsic sphincter deficiency", or "type III" stress urinary incontinence (Fig. 4.5.11).

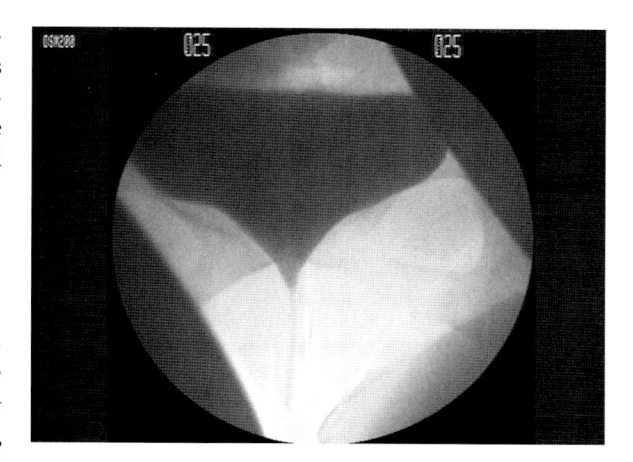

Fig. 4.5.11. Fluoroscopic view of the bladder neck of a subject with intrinsic sphincter deficiency. Beaking and funnel shape are seen at the bladder neck

4.5.4.2.2
Ultrasound

Perineal ultrasound has also been reported to assess the mobility of the urethrovesical neck. The benefits of ultrasound are that it provides a relatively noninvasive alternative to assessing mobility of the bladder neck in comparison to using a cotton swab (SCHAER et al. 1999). In addition, it avoids the drawback of ionizing radiation exposure with fluoroscopic video urodynamics. Intraurethral ultrasound has recently been under investigation to study intrinsic sphincter deficiency of the urethra in women with stress incontinence (HEIT 2000), and in women with detrusor instability (MAJOR et al. 2002). At this juncture, there is little standardization with this technology and it is considered investigational.

4.5.5
Summary

There are many studies available in which urinary incontinence and the normal functions of bladder storage and emptying have been investigated. While urodynamics has been accepted by many as the standard of care for treatment of subjects with urinary incontinence, it is important to recognize that there are many different tests that comprise urodynamic testing. Many of the simple tests can be easily performed in the office setting and can be thought of as adjunctive tests to confirm the diagnosis and assist in planning treatment. On the other hand, more expen-

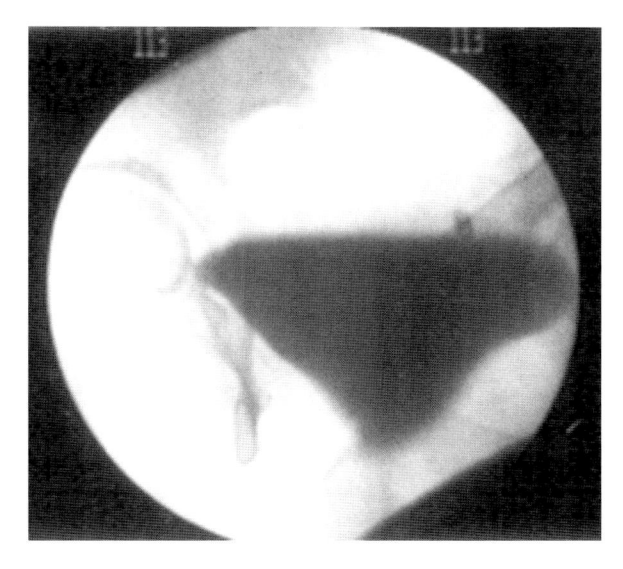

Fig. 4.5.10. Fluoroscopic view of the bladder neck of a subject with hypermobility and stress incontinence

sive and more invasive testing may be useful adjuncts for patients with very complex incontinence problems, or those who have failed initial treatment.

References

Abrams P, Cardozo L, Fall M, et al (2002) The standardisation of terminology of lower urinary tract function: report from the Standardisation Sub-Committee of the International Continence Society. Neurourol Urodyn 21:167–178

Bowen L, Sand P, Ostergard D, et al (1989) Unsuccessful Burch retropubic urethropexy: a case-controlled urodynamic study. Am J Obstet Gynecol 160:452–458

Bump R, Elser D, Theofrastous J, et al (1995) Valsalva leak point pressures in women with genuine stress incontinence: reproducibility, effect of catheter caliber, and correlations with other measurements of urethral resistance. Am J Obstet Gynecol 173:551–557

Bump R, Coates K, Cundiff G, et al (1997) Diagnosing intrinsic sphincter deficiency: comparing urethral closure pressures, urethral axis, and Valsalva leak point pressures. Am J Obstet Gynecol 177:303–310

Coates K (1998) Physiologic evaluation of the pelvic floor. Obstet Gynecol Clin North Am 25:805–824

Cundiff G, Harris R, Coates K, et al (1997) Clinical predictors of urinary incontinence in women. Am J Obstet Gynecol 177:262–267

Fantl J, Newman D, Colling J, et al (1996) Urinary incontinence in adults: acute and chronic management. In: Clinical practice guideline. Agency for Health Care Policy and Research, Public Health Service, US Department of Health and Human Services, Rockville, pp 1–154

Griffiths D, Hofner K, van Mastrigt R, et al (1997) Standardization of terminology of lower urinary tract function: pressure-flow studies of voiding, urethral resistance, and urethral obstruction. International Continence Society Subcommittee on Standardization of Terminology of Pressure-Flow Studies. Neurourol Urodyn 16:1–18

Haylen B, Ashby D, Sutherst J, et al (1989) Maximum and average urine flow rates in normal male and female populations – the Liverpool nomograms. Br J Urol 64:30–38

Heit M (2000) Intraurethral ultrasonography: correlation of urethral anatomy with functional urodynamic parameters in stress incontinent women. Int Urogynecol J 11:204–211

Heslington K, Hilton P (1996) Ambulatory monitoring and conventional cystometry in asymptomatic female volunteers. Br J Obstet Gynaecol 103:434–441

Hilton P, Stanton S (1983) Urethral pressure measurements by microtransducer: the results in symptom-free women and in those with genuine stress incontinence. Br J Obstet Gynaecol 90:919–933

Jensen JK (1996) Urodynamic evaluation. In: Ostergard DR, Bent AE (eds) Urogynecology and urodynamics: theory and practice. Williams and Wilkins, Baltimore

Karram MM (1999) Urodynamics: cystometry. In: Walters MD, Karram MM (eds) Urogynecology and reconstructive pelvic surgery. Mosby, St Louis

Madersbacher S, Pycha A, Schatzl G, et al (1998) The aging lower urinary tract: a comparative urodynamic study of men and women. Urology 51:206–212

Major H, Culligan P, Heit M (2002) Urethral sphincter morphology in women with detrusor instability. Obstet Gynecol 99:63–68

McGuire E (1981) Urodynamic findings in patients after failure of stress incontinence operations. Prog Clin Biol Res 78:351–360

McGuire E, Woodside J (1981) Diagnostic advantages of fluoroscopic monitoring during urodynamic evaluation. J Urol 125:830–834

McGuire E, Woodside J, Borden T, et al (1981) Prognostic value of urodynamic testing in myelodysplastic patients. J Urol 126:205–209

McGuire E, Fitzpatrick C, Wan J, et al (1993) Clinical assessment of urethral sphincter function. J Urol 150:1452–1454

Ostergard DR, Bent AE (eds) (1996) Urogynecology and urodynamics: theory and practice. Williams and Wilkins, Baltimore

Radley S, Rosario D, Chapple C, et al (2001) Conventional and ambulatory urodynamic findings in women with symptoms of bladder overactivity. J Urol 166:2253–2258

Roehrborn C, Peters P (1988) Can transabdominal ultrasound estimation of postvoiding residual replace catheterization? Urology 16:445–449

Rowan D, James E, Kramer A, et al (1987) Urodynamic equipment: technical aspects. Produced by the International Continence Society Working Party on Urodynamic Equipment. J Med Eng Technol 11:57–64

Rud T (1980) Urethral pressure profile in continent women from childhood to old age. Acta Obstet Gynecol Scand 59:331–335

Sand P, Bowen L, Panganiban R, et al (1987) The low pressure urethra as a factor in failed retropubic urethropexy. Obstet Gynecol 69:399–402

Schaer G, Perucchini D, Munz E, et al (1999) Sonographic evaluation of the bladder neck in continent and stress-incontinent women. Obstet Gynecol 93:412–416

Stohrer M, Goepel M, Kondo A, et al (1999) The standardization of terminology in neurogenic lower urinary tract dysfunction: with suggestions for diagnostic procedures. International Continence Society Standardization Committee. Neurourol Urodyn 18:138–158

Summitt RJ, Stovall T, Bent A, et al (1992) Urinary incontinence: correlation of history and brief office evaluation with multichannel urodynamic testing. Am J Obstet Gynecol 166:1835–1840

Swift S, Ostergard D (1995) A comparison of stress leak-point pressure and maximum urethral closure pressure in patients with genuine stress incontinence. Obstet Gynecol 85:704–708

Swift S, Utrie J (1996) The need for standardization of the Valsalva leak-point pressure. Int Urogynecol J 7:227–230

Taylor E (ed) (1988) Dorland's illustrated medical dictionary. Saunders, Philadelphia

Theofrastous J, Bump R, Elser D, et al (1995) Correlation of urodynamic measure of urethral resistance with clinical measures of incontinence severity in women with pure genuine stress incontinence. The Continence Program for Women Research Group. Am J Obstet Gynecol 173:407–412

Urinary Incontinence Guideline Panel (1992) Urinary incontinence in adults: clinical practice guidelines (publication no. 92-0038). Agency for Health Care Policy and Research, Public Health Service, US Department of Health and Human Services, Rockville van Kerrebroeck P, Abrams P, Chaikin D, et al (2002) The standardisation terminology in nocturia: report from the Standardisation Sub-Committee of the International Continence Society. Neurourol Urodyn 21:179–183

van Waalwijk van Doorn E, Anders K, Khullar V, et al (2000) Standardisation of ambulatory urodynamic monitoring: report of the Standardisation Sub-Committee of the International Continence Society for Ambulatory Urodynamic Studies. Neurourol Urodyn 19:113–125

Wall L, Norton P, DeLancey J (1993) Practical urogynecology. Lippincott Williams and Wilkins, Baltimore, pp 83–124

Walters M, Shields L (1988) The diagnostic value of history, physical examination, and the Q-tip cotton swab test in women with urinary incontinence. Am J Obstet Gynecol 159:145–149

Wang S, McGuire E, Bloom D (1988) A bladder pressure management system for myelodysplasia – clinical outcome. J Urol 140:1499–1502

Weber A, Walters M (2000) Cost-effectiveness of urodynamic testing before surgery for women with pelvic organ prolapse and stress urinary incontinence. Am J Obstet Gynecol 183:1338–1347

Weidner A, Myers E, Visco A, et al (2001) Which women with stress incontinence require urodynamic evaluation? Am J Obstet Gynecol 184:20–27

4.6 Anorectal Physiology

A.V. Emmanuel

CONTENTS

4.6.1 Introduction *101*
4.6.2 Clinical Features *101*
4.6.3 Anorectal Manometry *101*
4.6.3.1 Vector Manometry *103*
4.6.3.2 Anal Electromyography *103*
4.6.3.3 Pudendal Nerve Latency Measurement *103*
4.6.4 Anal Sensation *104*
4.6.5 Rectal Sensation *104*
4.6.6 Colonic Transit *105*
4.6.7 Conclusion *105*
References *106*

4.6.1 Introduction

Understanding the physiology of defaecation and continence requires an appreciation of the interplay between the anal sphincter, rectum and pelvic floor, which although anatomically simple is physiologically complex. Gold standards to define function remain elusive. Nevertheless, there are in routine use a number of techniques for studying the motor and sensory elements of anorectal physiology. This chapter focuses primarily on the rationale for, and the clinical value of, performing these tests with only brief detail of the methodology.

4.6.2 Clinical Features

The interpretation of anorectal physiological must take into account the perceived impact of a patient's symptoms on the lifestyle of that patient. An accurate history, which also encompasses an enquiry into relevant aetiological factors, is the starting point of assessment. Symptom diaries and assessment questionnaires, com-

A.V. Emmanuel, MD, MRCP
Physiology Unit, St Mark's Hospital, Northwick Park, Watford Road, Harrow, Middlesex, HA1 3UJ, UK

pleted prior to clinical examination, greatly assist this process by quantifying the extent, timing and social context of symptoms. However, questionnaires are only an adjunct to history taking. There is no existing symptom questionnaire that on its own addresses anorectal dysfunction comprehensively (Jorge and Wexner 1993; Vaizey et al. 1999). Basic questioning in constipation should elicit a history of infrequent defaecation or evacuatory difficulty (or both).

In a patient with incontinence it is essential to differentiate between urge incontinence (loss of stool despite attempts to inhibit defaecation) and passive incontinence (loss of stool without patient awareness). Urge incontinence is usually associated with external anal sphincter dysfunction, whilst passive leakage reflects internal anal sphincter dysfunction (Engel et al. 1995). Nocturnal faecal incontinence suggests a neurological causation of symptoms. Anorectal physiology is much more valuable in incontinence compared to constipation, where it is important only with a lifelong history of constipation without faecal soiling, as this raises the possibility of Hirschsprung's disease.

Physical examination may reveal a clue as to aetiology, such as a neurological or connective tissue disorder. Perineal examination may demonstrate soiling, or erythema and excoriation from chronic incontinence. Digital assessment may give an indication of anal tone, though this correlates poorly with clinical, manometric or histological assessment (Hallan et al. 1989; Sultan et al. 1994). If a patient is suspected of having an external rectal prolapse, this needs to be evaluated while the patient strains seated on a toilet. Rigid sigmoidoscopy is mandatory when there is any suspicion of organic disease. In a constipated patient, digital examination is of value to detect faecal impaction.

4.6.3 Anorectal Manometry

Anal manometry determines the functional strength of the anal sphincter complex. The length of this complex is defined as the region where the resting pressure is >5 mmHg above rectal pressure. Traditionally a station pull-through method has been used to measure sphincter pressures, where a manometry catheter is inserted transanally into the rectum and pressure measurements recorded at 0.5 cm intervals as the catheter is withdrawn. The original manometry systems used air- or water-filled microballoons, and whilst they gave a pressure that equated to a summated "global" pressure there remained a major problem of poor reproducibility. Modern manometric methods use water-perfused systems or solid-state pressure transducers mounted on catheters. Such catheters typically carry between four to eight measuring ports (Fig. 4.6.1). Sphincter pressures are typically expressed as an average of the recordings from each transducer. The repeatability of this technique has been studied in small series with only moderate interobserver reproducibility demonstrated (HALLAN et al. 1989; ROGERS et al. 1989). A larger more recent study from St Mark's (NICHOLLS et al. 2002) has shown that clinically accurate and reproducible results are obtained in up to 92% of patients. The limitations of solid-state catheters are that the sheer size (and expense) of these transducers limit the number of measurement ports that can be arranged radially. The water-perfused systems, being smaller, allow multiple measurement ports to be arranged radially and longitudinally along a catheter.

There are two primary measurements made with anorectal manometry – the resting and voluntary contraction anal sphincter pressures. Resting pressure correlates predominantly with internal anal sphincter tone while contraction ("squeeze") pressure reflects predominantly external anal sphincter function (ENGEL et al. 1995). This implies that when making resting sphincter pressure measurements, the patient should be as relaxed as possible so as not to be contracting their external sphincter due to anxiety. Contraction pressure values are obtained by asking the patient to voluntarily squeeze their anal sphincter whilst the catheter is pulled through the anal canal. This can be assessed either as the average value obtained while the catheter is pulled rapidly through the canal or alternatively the average of multiple measurements made at discrete 0.5-cm "stations". Typical values for resting, internal sphincter pressure are between 50 and 65 mmHg, being slightly higher in men than women (READ et al. 1979; LOENING-BAUCKE and ANURAS 1984; MCHUGH and DIAMANT 1987; NICHOLLS et al. 2002). The range of normal values for contraction pressure is between 60 and 150 mmHg above resting sphincter pressure. Contraction pressures are consistently higher in men

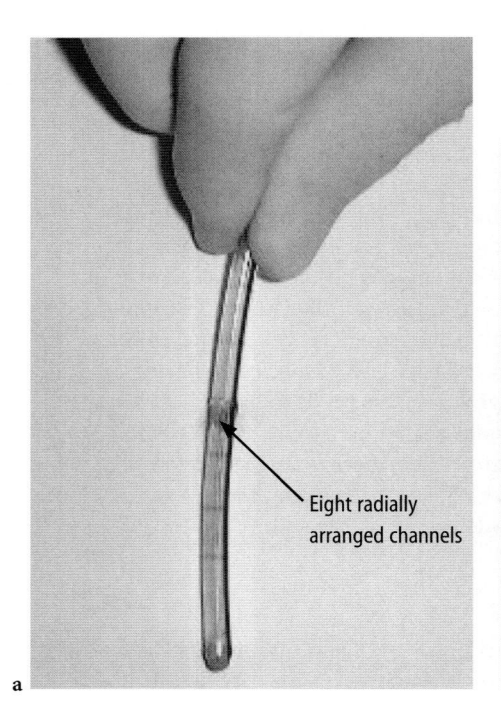

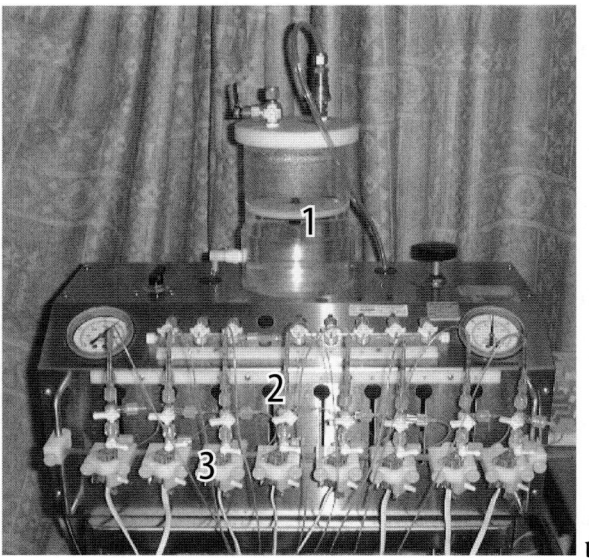

Fig. 4.6.1a, b. The eight radial catheter channels (a) are perfused with sterile water from (b) a pressurized reservoir (*1*) connected individually (*2*) to a capillary pressure transducer (*3*). Readings from each of these pressure transducers is sent to a PC for display and analysis

than women, and also tend to decline with age even in the absence of any pathology (READ et al. 1979; LOENING-BAUCKE and ANURAS 1984; MCHUGH and DIAMANT 1987; NICHOLLS et al. 2002).

Functional anal canal length is determined during the pull-through method, representing where anal sphincter pressure is greater than 5 mmHg above rectal pressure. There is seemingly a gender difference in this functional length, which in males is between 2.8 and 4.5 cm and in females is between 2.2 and 4.0 cm (LOENING-BAUCKE and ANURAS 1984; MCHUGH and DIAMANT 1987). An additional recording that is often made is of involuntary anal sphincter contraction pressure. The patient is asked to cough or in some other way to raise intraabdominal pressure whilst concurrently recording the reflex increase in external sphincter contraction that occurs. This involuntary measure is held to reflect the maximal potential strength of the external sphincter, and may be related to treatment outcome (NORTON and KAMM 2002). One other manometric measure that has been reported to reflect the fatigability of anal function is the duration of maximal squeeze pressure (READ et al. 1979; MARCELLO et al. 1998; NICHOLLS et al. 2002). These latter two measures, however, suffer from poor interobserver reproducibility, and their clinical value is as yet unproven.

One other clinically valuable manometric measure is confirming the presence of the rectoanal inhibitory reflex. This normal reflex is elicited by inflating a balloon in the rectum while simultaneously performing anal manometry. Absence of the reflex obviates the need for surgical histology in a patient with a history suggestive of Hirschsprung's disease (TOBON et al. 1968).

4.6.3.1
Vector Manometry

It is known that anal canal "pressures" are not radially symmetrical – in the proximal canal anterior quadrant pressures are lower, and in the distal canal posterior quadrant pressures are lower (TAYLOR et al. 1984). Vector manometry (vectometry) allows pressure profiling along the length of the anal canal to define this functional asymmetry. To date, however, there has been a disappointing absence of correlation between pressure asymmetry areas and defects on anal electromyography (see below) or endoanal ultrasound (PERRY et al. 1990; YANG and WEXNER 1994). Endoanal ultrasound remains the gold standard for identification of traumatic sphincter injury.

4.6.3.2
Anal Electromyography

Anal sphincter electromyography (EMG) provides information about the presence of sphincter defects and helps identify nerve injury. Measurement is performed by either needle electrode (concentric or single-fibre), surface EMG pads or anal plugs. Concentric EMG samples the action potentials from up to 25 motor units, identifying areas of absent electrical activity representing either scarring or a frank defect in the muscle. Single-fibre EMG can be used to further define these areas of absent electrical activity, identifying denervated or reinnervated areas of muscle based on the patterns of reinnervation potentials. To avoid the discomfort of needle insertion, in recent years EMG studies have been performed using anal plugs, although the reproducibility of such measurements is undetermined. Surface EMG may be of benefit as part of biofeedback treatment in patients with constipation and incontinence.

Patients with incontinence have higher single-fibre density than controls which is thought to reflect a neurogenic aetiology. However, there is no correlation between severity of symptoms and EMG changes (FELT-BERSMA et al. 1992), and furthermore there is no validation of EMG changes in relation to histological evidence of denervation. Overall, the advent of anal endosonography has vastly improved the accuracy of quantification of sphincter injury (SULTAN et al. 1994), and EMG is now of little value.

4.6.3.3
Pudendal Nerve Latency Measurement

KIFF and SWASH (1984) described a method to measure conduction in the pudendal nerve, using a stimulating and recording electrode which is worn on a gloved finger (Fig. 4.6.2). A stimulus is applied (at the finger tip) to the pudendal nerve and the latency until an external sphincter contraction occurs (recorded at the finger base) is measured. The normal value for this pudendal nerve terminal motor latency (PNTML) is 2 ± 0.5 ms, increasing with age. However the measurement technique is highly performer-related and the actual measure reflects only conduction of the fastest fibres. Thus, a damaged nerve with some conducting fibres will still produce a normal PNTML; typically the fastest fibres are the large ones which are the last to be damaged.

There does not seem to be a correlation between PNTML and either continence symptoms or anal electrosensation is 4.1±0.3 mA. The measure is an accurate reflection of denervation injury and has a role in predicting completeness of injury in spinal patients (EMMANUEL et al. 2002).

4.6.5
Rectal Sensation

Rectal sensitivity may be measured by either balloon distension or electrical stimulation. Balloon distension is performed by gradual inflation via a hand-held syringe of a balloon seated in the rectal ampulla. The patient is asked to report three separate feelings in succession: first ("threshold") sensation, feeling of urgency and finally maximal tolerable sensation. It is held that these sensations correlate to function of mucosal, muscular and serosal mechanoreceptors, respectively (LOENING-BAUCKE and ANURAS 1984; CARUANA et al. 1991). The volumes obtained for these sensations depend on the type of balloon and the protocol for distension used, and to minimize the variability that this generates between different centres it has been recommended that distension sensitivity is performed using a barostat. A barostat allows preset mechanical distension of an infinitely compliant balloon at fixed pressure, compensating for differences in rectal wall tension. Using a hand-held syringe and a party balloon, the normal range in St Mark's for threshold volume is 20–70 ml, for urge volume 35–120 ml and for maximum tolerated volume 100–260 ml (NICHOLLS et al. 2002). Heightened threshold volumes are found in patients with faecal incontinence, and these have been shown to normalize following successful biofeedback therapy (MINER et al. 1990).

Rectal electrical stimulation using a bipolar electrode as described for anal electrosensation is a more reproducible technique than balloon distension for measuring rectal sensation. The normal value for rectal electrosensation is 27.4±2.1 mA (KAMM and LENNARD-JONES 1990). This is a valuable technique for detecting hindgut denervation in patients with neurological disease (KAMM and LENNARD-JONES 1990; EMMANUEL et al. 2002).

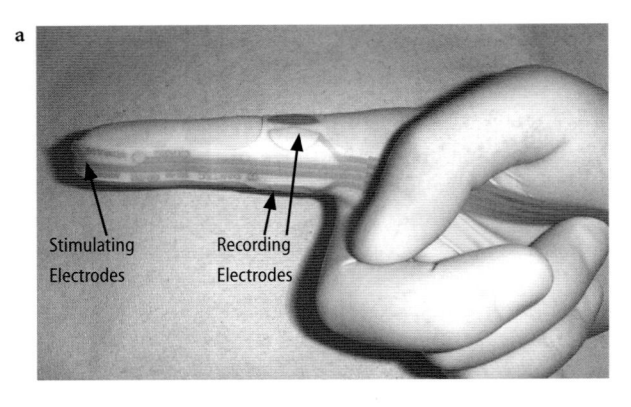

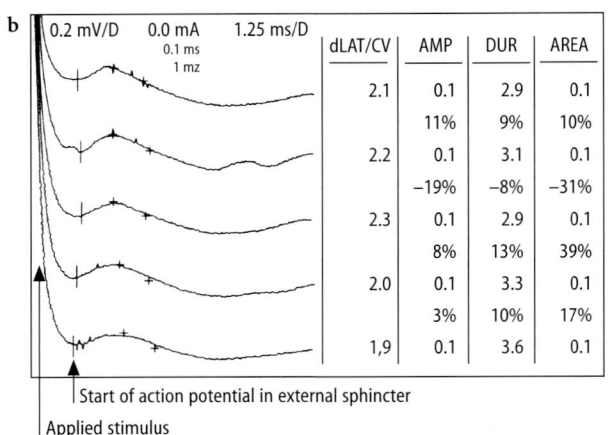

Fig. 4.6.2. a The St Mark's pudendal electrode for measuring pudendal nerve terminal motor latencies. The nerve is located by the tip of the ischial tuberosity. **b** The PNTML, measured in milliseconds, is the delay from the application of the stimulus to the onset of the external sphincter action potential

squeeze pressure (WEXNER et al. 1997; FYNES et al. 1999). Additionally, the balance of evidence does not support the idea that PNTML is predictive of surgical outcome, and the test can no longer be recommended in the assessment of the incontinent patient.

4.6.4
Anal Sensation

Anal sensation is served by specialized sensory endings in the anal mucosa, and is important in maintenance of continence mechanisms (MILLER et al. 1987; SUN et al. 1990). Reproducible thresholds for anal sensory perception can be obtained by passing a current between bipolar electrodes positioned in the anal canal (ROGERS et al. 1989; KAMM and LENNARD-JONES 1990). The normal value for anal

4.6.6
Colonic Transit

Radio-opaque marker studies provide a useful measure of whole gut transit. A well-validated technique involves the ingestion of three geometrically different marker sets of 20 markers each on days 1, 2 and 3 with a plain film of the abdomen on day 6 (i.e. 120 h after the first ingestion later) when the remaining markers are counted. This in effect gives three transit studies for the one film, and avoids the problem of clearing all the markers from a bowel motion early in the study if just one marker set was used (HINTON et al. 1969). The maximum number of markers that may be retained is less than four for the marker set given on day 1, less than six for the day-2 markers, and less than 12 for the day-3 markers (EVANS et al. 1992), and may be used to define slow colonic transit (Fig. 4.6.3). A modification of this is to give 20 markers for 3 days and then take a film on day 4. The number and distribution of markers may be used to calculate regional transit (METCALF et al. 1987), although the significance of the concept of regional transit is uncertain. Scintigraphic assessment of colonic transit is the most accurate, but also the most complex with no clear advantage over markers (VAN DER SIJP et al. 1993).

4.6.7
Conclusion

Anorectal physiological techniques are of value in diagnosis and assessment of patients with incon-

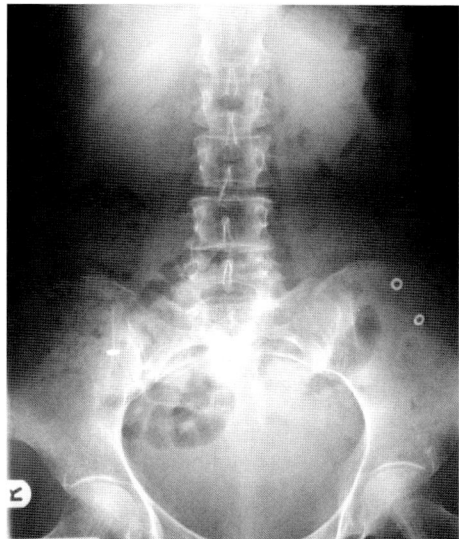

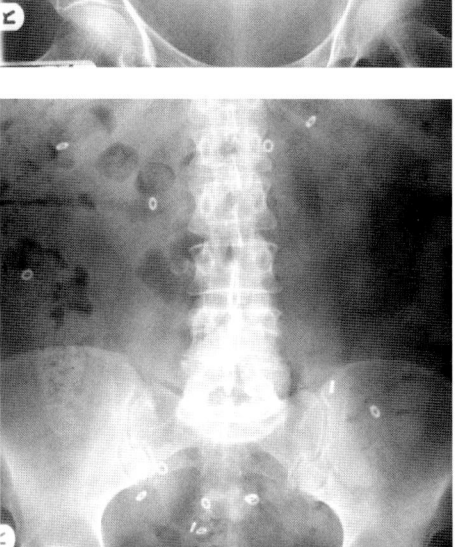

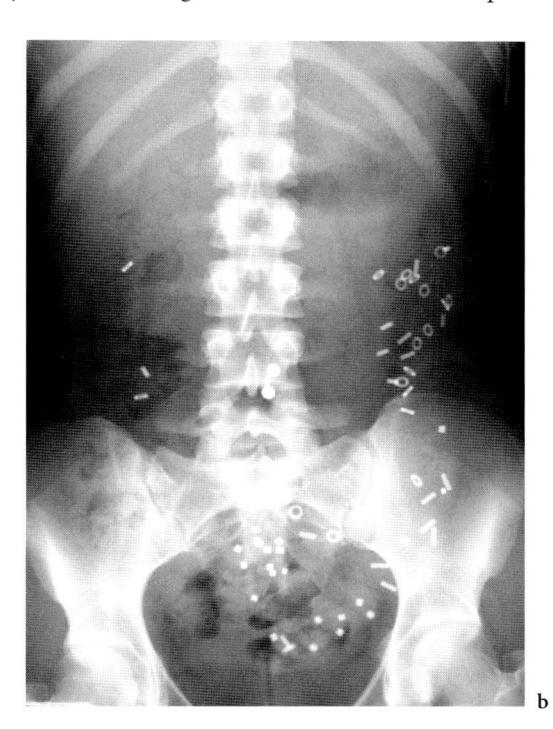

Fig. 4.6.3. a Normal transit with only 3 rings remaining (20 cubes given on day 1, 20 rods on day 2, 20 rings on day 3). **b** Slow colonic transit with 20 of each marker remaining. **c** Slow colonic transit on one of the marker sets only with all the cubes passed, 1 rod remaining, and 15 rings

tinence and constipation, but must be interpreted in the context of a comprehensive clinical history and appropriate imaging. Anal manometry is of unequivocal value in defining the functional integrity of the anal sphincter muscles and in excluding Hirschsprung's disease. Endoanal ultrasound remains superior to anal vector manometry or electromyography in defining traumatic sphincter injury. Pudendal nerve latency measurement is not of value in patients with faecal incontinence. Anorectal sensory testing is of value in defining patients with neurological damage.

References

Bersma RJF, van Baren R, Koorevar M, et al (1992) Anal endosonography: relationship with anal manometry and neurophysiologic tests. Dis Colon Rectum 35:944–949

Caruana BJ, Wald A, Hinds JP, et al (1991) Anorectal sensory and motor function in neurogenic faecal incontinence. Comparison between multiple sclerosis and diabetes mellitus. Gastroenterology 100:465–470

Emmanuel AV, Kamm MA, Middlever F, (2002) Gut specific autonomic testing and bowel dysfunction in spinal cord injury. Gastroenterology 122 Supp 1:M1535

Engel AF, Kamm MA, Bartram CI, et al (1995) Relationship of symptoms in faecal incontinence to specific sphincter abnormalities. Int J Colorectal Dis 10:152–155

Evans RC, Kamm MA, Hinton JM, et al (1992) The normal range and a simple diagram for recording whole gut transit time. Int J Colorect Dis 7:15–17

Fynes MM, Donelly V, Behan M, et al (1999) Effect of second vaginal delivery on anorectal physiology and faecal continence: a prospective study. Lancet 354:983–986

Hallan RI, Marzouk DE, Waldron DJ, et al (1989) Comparison of digital and manometric assessment of anal sphincter function. Br J Surg 76:973–975

Hinton JM, Lennard-Jones JE, Young AC (1969) A new method for studying gut transit times using radio-opapue markers. Gut 10:842–847

Jorge JM, Wexner SD (1993) Aetiology and management of faecal incontinence. Dis Colon Rectum 36:77–97

Kamm MA, Lennard-Jones JE (1990) Rectal mucosal electrosensory testing. Evidence for a sensory neuropathy in severe constipation. Dis Colon Rectum 33:419–423

Kiff ES, Swash M (1984) Slowed conduction in the pudendal nerves in idiopathic (neurogenic) faecal incontinence. Br J Surg 71:614–616

Loening-Baucke V, Anuras S (1984) Anorectal manometry in healthy elderly subjects. Am Geriatr Soc 32:636–639

Marcello PW, Barrett BS, Coller JA, et al (1998) Fatigue rate index as a new measurement of external sphincter function. Dis Colon Rectum 41:336–343

McHugh SM, Diamnt NE (1987) Effect of age, gender and parity on anal canal pressures: contribution of impaired anal sphincter function to faecal incontinence. Dig Dis Sci 32:726–736

Metcalf AM, Phillips SF, Zinsmeister AR, et al (1987) Simplified assessment of segmental colonic transit. Gastroenterology 92:40–47

Miller R, Bartolo DCC, Roe AE, et al (1988) Anal sensation and the continence mechanism. Dis Colon Rectum 31:433–438

Miner PB, Donnelly TC, Read NW (1990) Investigation of mode of action of action of biofeedback in treatment of faecal incontinence. Dig Dis Sci 35:1291–1298

Nicholls TJ, Solanki D, Emmanuel AV, et al (2002) Inter-examiner reproducibility of anorectal motor and sensory function test. Gut 51, Supp II:A60

Norton C, Chelvanayagam S, Kamm MA (2002) Randomised controlled trial of biofeedback for faecal incontinence. Gut 51, Supp II:A61

Perry RE, Blatchford GJ, Christensen MA, et al (1990) Manometric diagnosis of anal sphincter injuries. Am J Surg 159:112–117

Read NW, Harford WV, Schmulen AC, et al (1979) A clinical study of patients with faecal incontinence and diarrhoea. Gastroenterology 76:747–756

Rogers J, Laurberg S, Misiewicz JJ, et al (1989) Anorectal physiology validated: a repeatability study of the motor and sensory tests of anorectal function. Br J Surg 76:607–609

Sultan AH, Kamm MA, Talbot IC, et al (1994) Anal endosonography for identifying external sphincter defects confirmed histologically. Br J Surg 81:463–465

Sun WM, Read NW, Prior A, et al (1990) Sensory and motor responses to rectal distension vary according to rate and pattern of balloon inflation. Gastroenterology 99:1008–1015

Taylor BM, Beart RW Jr, Phillips SF (1984) Longitudinal and radial variations of pressure in the human anal sphincter. Gastroenterology 86:693–697

Tobon F, Reid NCRW, Talbert JL, et al (1968) Nonsurgical test for the diagnosis of Hirschsprung's disease. New Engl J Med 278:188–194

Vaizey CJ, Carapet E, Cahill JA, et al (1999) Prospective comparison of faecal incontinence grading systems. Gut 44:77–80

van der Sijp JR, Kamm MA, Nightingale JM, et al (1993) Radio-isotope determination of regional colonic transit in severe constipation: comparison with radio opaque markers. Gut 34:402–408

Wexner SD (1997) Re: manometric tests of anorectal function in the management of defecation disorders. Am J Gastroenterol 92:1400

Yang Y, Wexner SD (1994) Anal pressure vectography is of no apparent benefit for sphincter evaluation. Int J Colorectal Dis 9:989–996

5 Urogenital Dysfunction

D. S. Hale, F. M. Kelvin, K. Strohbehn

5.1 Surgery and Clinical Imaging for Pelvic Organ Prolapse

D. S. Hale

CONTENTS

5.1.1 Introduction 107
5.1.2 Anatomy of Support 107
5.1.3 Etiology of Prolapse 109
5.1.4 The Radiologist and the Clinician 110
5.1.5 Surgical Approach 113
5.1.6 The Anterior Vaginal Wall 113
5.1.6.1 Cystocele 114
5.1.6.2 Paravaginal Cystocele Repair 115
5.1.6.3 Graft Placement 115
5.1.6.4 Anterior Colporrhaphy 115
5.1.7 Surgery of the Vaginal Apex 116
5.1.7.1 Abdominal Sacral Colpoperineopexy 116
5.1.7.2 Sacrospinous Vault Suspension 117
5.1.7.3 Uterosacral Ligament Vault Suspension 118
5.1.7.4 Obliterative Surgery 118
5.1.7.5 Uterine Preservation Procedures 118
5.1.8 The Posterior Vaginal Wall 118
5.1.8.1 Rectocele 118
5.1.8.2 Posterior Colporrhaphy 119
5.1.8.3 Defect Repair 119
5.1.8.4 Graft Replacement 119
5.1.8.5 Imbrication 119
5.1.8.6 Transanal Repair 120
5.1.8.7 Enterocele 120
5.1.9 Conclusion 121
References 121

5.1.1 Introduction

The purpose of this chapter is to provide the radiologist interested in pelvic floor imaging with a surgical perspective of pelvic floor dysfunction. Although individual surgeons may have different reasons for requesting imaging studies, the basic question to be answered remains the same: the preoperative identification of all surgically treatable prolapse and pelvic floor dysfunction. It is estimated that 11.1% of women will undergo a single operation for pelvic floor dysfunction in their lifetime. Nearly 30% of these patients will require a second operation (Olsen et al. 1997).

Preoperative identification of these conditions is critical to appropriate intervention. In the past, division of the pelvic floor into an anterior, middle, and posterior compartment has lead to fragmentation of care. The anterior compartment with its urethra and bladder have been the realm of the urologist; the middle compartment containing the uterus and reproductive organs the domain of the gynecologist; the posterior compartment with the small and large bowel belonged to the colorectal surgeon. These artificial divisions of the pelvis did not recognize the symbiotic relationship of these "compartments". Treatment of one compartment influences the structure and function of the others. Radiological studies have helped clinicians recognize the interdependence of these compartments and the need to address them together in the treatment of pelvic disorders.

Advances in imaging techniques have evolved from studies involving single organs with their inherent limitations to more lengthy, but superior studies. Unfortunately, the best radiological techniques for evaluating these conditions are time consuming, as they require individual filling and emptying of the organs along with various dynamic maneuvers. However, by combining the patient history, physical examination, and radiological findings, the radiologist and the clinician can complement each other in the successful diagnosis and treatment of women with pelvic floor disorders.

5.1.2 Anatomy of Support

Care of women with these disorders begins with an understanding of the unique musculofascial system

D.S. Hale, MD, FACOG
Female Pelvic Medicine and Reconstructive Surgery, Methodist/Indiana University Hospital, 1633 N Capitol Avenue, Suite 436, Indianapolis, IN 46202, USA

that supports the pelvic organs. No single ligament or muscle is responsible for supporting the pelvic organs. Rather a unique musculofascial system is in place that must work together for proper organ support. The levator ani muscles (puborectalis, pubococcygeus, iliococcygeus) provide an active platform of support for the pelvic organs while a vast fascial connective tissue network suspend the organs on this platform. Damage to the levator ani muscles and pelvic nerves by childbirth, neurological disease or injury, disuse atrophy, or various other conditions affecting neuromuscular integrity, may lead to widening of the levator hiatus. As the hiatus widens, more stress is placed on the connective tissue network that holds the vaginal vault and pelvic organs in place. Eventually, this stress may lead to tearing or stretching of the supportive connective tissue. As the vaginal vault loses its support the surrounding organs will begin to prolapse through the levator hiatus.

In place of true ligamentous support, the connective tissue of the pelvis is made up of varying degrees of collagen, elastin, smooth muscle, neural tissue, and vascular channels (CAMPBELL 1950). The cardinal (Mackenrodt) ligament and uterosacral ligaments form a continuous complex of support for the upper vagina and uterus. These should not be thought of as distinct, separate structures. The cardinal ligaments fan out to blend laterally with the parietal fascia of the pelvic sidewall muscles. The uterosacral ligaments are the posteromedial continuation of this complex eventually joining the presacral fascia close to the sacroiliac joint. The importance of these structures for their role in support has been demonstrated in elegant yet simple cadaver studies (MENGERT 1936). Working with these upper supports, a distinct fascial layer enveloping the vagina and serving as an independent support to the bladder and rectum has been described. Anteriorly this layer has been called the pubovesicocervical fascia while posteriorly the term rectovaginal septum (Denonvillier's fascia in the male) has been used. Pubovesicocervical fascia is found on the anterior vaginal wall, but has not been identified histologically as a separate layer from the vaginal muscularis (WEBER and WALTERS 1997; FARRELL et al. 2001). This may be due to blending of the uterosacral-cardinal connective tissue with vaginal muscularis, so there is no defined plane of attachment (UHLENHUTH and NOLLEY 1957). It is, therefore, important for both surgeons and radiologists involved in pelvic floor dysfunction to appreciate that there is no distinct connective tissue layer that is separate from the anterior vaginal wall muscularis.

A similar controversy existed concerning the presence of a connective tissue layer supporting the posterior vaginal wall. Although there is a rectovaginal septum distinct from the posterior vaginal muscularis, problems arise in demonstrating the septum as a separate structure due to its fusion with the caudal half to one-third of the vagina and relatively short length (MILLEY and NICHOLS 1968). In a study of 44 women at laparoscopy, the mean length of the rectovaginal septum was found to be 2.1 cm while the rectovaginal pouch extended 5.3 cm below the posterior vaginal apex (KUHN and HOLLYOCK 1982). The short length of the rectovaginal septum has been confirmed histologically and on cadaveric dissection (DELANCEY 1999). Therefore, the superior edge of the rectovaginal septum fuses with the muscularis of the posterior vaginal wall approximately 3 cm above the perineal body. Laterally, the rectovaginal septum fuses with the fascia of the levator ani muscles (LEFFLER et al. 2001). The perineal body is indirectly suspended to the sacrum by a series of connective tissue links involving the rectovaginal septum, the midvaginal muscularis, and the uterosacral ligaments.

To summarize, three different levels of support are recognized for the vagina (DELANCEY 1992) (Fig. 5.1.1). The cardinal-uterosacral complex, which blends with the vaginal muscularis, supports the upper vagina and uterus. The mid vagina, level II support, is provided by the attachment of the vaginal muscularis to the arcus tendineus fascia pelvis and an intact vaginal muscularis. Level III support is the function of the rectovaginal septum and the perineal membrane. At all levels, the levator ani muscles have connective tissue extensions to aid with this support network (ZACCHARIN 1980). Not only do the well-recognized "ligamentous" supports of the urethra, vaginal vault, and lower uterine segment need to be intact but also it appears the musculofascial tissue enveloping the vaginal epithelium must remain unbroken. As in all aspects of anatomy, variations do exist between patients and this fact may help explain some of the pathogenesis of prolapse. Many surgeons correct breaks in the connective tissue support system at the time of surgery. MRI may have a role in identifying these connective tissue breaks that will then aid in the surgical planning. Understanding the anatomy and effectively communicating such imaging findings are paramount to the radiologist's interaction with the clinician.

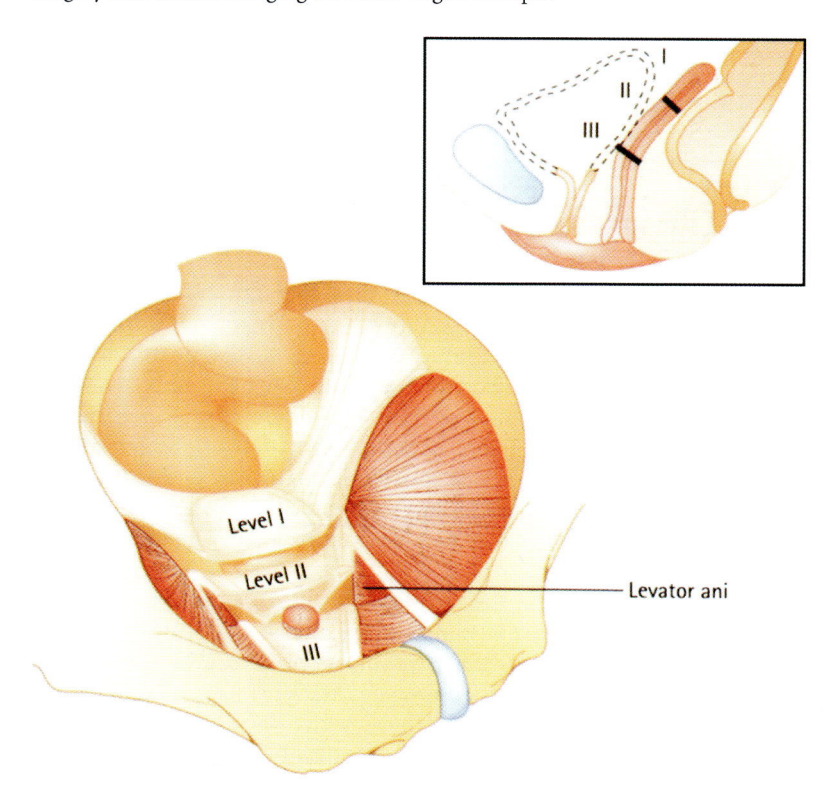

Fig. 5.1.1. Three levels of vaginal connective tissue support: level I uterosacral-cardinal complex, level II arcus tendineus fascia pelvis, level III perineal membrane and crura of levator muscles

5.1.3
Etiology of Prolapse

Pelvic organ prolapse has a multifactorial etiology. Vaginal parity, neuropathy, obesity, excessive Valsalva, connective tissue disorders, prior surgery, estrogen status, and advancing age are the most often cited risk factors (SMITH et al. 1989; GILPIN et al. 1989; NORTON et al. 1995; DAVIS 1996; SMITH et al. 1990). Of these, vaginal parity and its associated neuropathy are the most important.

Few epidemiological studies exist following the direct cause and progression of prolapse, although some are now being conducted. As noted above, dysfunction of the levator ani muscle, whether from childbirth, neuropathy, or other factors, leads to an increased area between the levator ani muscles, i.e. widening of the levator hiatus. Forces directed at the pelvic floor, namely Valsalva type maneuvers, further stress this situation by driving the organs through this hiatus. The connective tissue network begins to stretch and tear with resulting loss of support. Pelvic organ prolapse should not be thought of as the problem; rather it is the result of the problem, namely levator ani dysfunction.

Reconstructed three-dimensional MRI comparison of the levator ani muscles has shown a marked difference in levator volume, shape, and integrity between asymptomatic patients, those with genuine stress incontinence, and those with prolapse, providing indirect evidence that levator ani dysfunction is intimately involved in the different clinical manifestations of pelvic floor dysfunction (HOYTE et al. 2001). Histological studies have documented evidence of neurological damage in the levator ani of patients with prolapse (GILPIN et al. 1989; HEIT et al. 1996). Therefore, instead of focusing on a "dropped bladder" or "dropped bowel", physicians need to realize the role that the levator ani plays in the genesis of pelvic organ prolapse. The radiologist can help the clinician by differentiating between a global problem involving the levator ani, and one where there is a focal break in the connective tissue. If the levator hiatus is pathologically enlarged as a result of neuromuscular damage, fixing the connective tissue break alone will not suffice. Without the support of the levator ani, the same stresses will be placed on the connective tissue and prolapse will recur. Patients with a permanent, unrecoverable neuromuscular condition of the levator ani will often require graft placement to replace the damaged connective tissue. This graft material must be stronger than the native tissue and hold up better to the demands placed on the damaged pelvic floor. Such global levator dysfunction may be diagnosed on MRI by levator ani ballooning, an enlarged levator hiatal area, or abnormal levator ani position and movement. This added knowledge can have a major impact on the surgical procedure chosen.

5.1.4
The Radiologist and the Clinician

A standardized pelvic organ prolapse grading system accepted by both radiologists and surgeons is the single most important factor slowing collaboration between radiologists and surgeons in the area of pelvic organ prolapse. The International Continence Society (ICS) has agreed on such a system for clinicians (Bump et al. 1996b). Adopted in 1996, the Pelvic Organ Prolapse Quantification (POPQ) examination identifies nine points for measurement and prolapse staging (Fig. 5.1.2). This allows a standardized examination to be used for follow-up, for communication between clinicians, and in scientific papers. The examination has shown good inter- and intraobserver correlation (Hall et al. 1996). The hymeneal ring serves as the reference point for most of these measurements, an anatomic landmark not readily visible during radiological studies. Current radiological measurements for determining prolapse are based predominantly on bony landmarks, most commonly the pubococcygeal line. Other radiological grading systems have been employed but none is universally accepted. The pubococcygeal line is not only cephalad to the hymeneal ring, but it lies in an altogether different plane. Its more cephalad location may result in a tendency to exaggerate the degree of prolapse. Two studies have compared the ICS staging system to dynamic MRI (Hale and Kelvin 1998; Singh et al. 2001). The first used the pubococcygeal line while the second used the midpubic line to approximate the hymen. Although there was general agreement between the clinical and radiological studies, there were also discrepancies.

One problem is that the ICS system uses the hymen as a reference point. This is not a fixed anatomic structure, particularly at the posterior fourchette. Detachment of the perineal body from the rectovaginal septum cannot be appreciated by the current POPQ examination. Another problem is that the ICS system does not report on the highest level of support in cases where a hysterectomy has been performed. This information may influence surgical approach.

From the radiological side, failure to understand the normal range of findings has led to overstating the presence of prolapse. An example is the presence of an enterocele. Many radiologists diagnose an enterocele if there is any descent of small bowel posteriorly below the level of the vagina apex. However, the cul-de-sac depth in normal individuals may average over 5 cm, so that the radiological over-diagnosis of enteroceles becomes inevitable. Further limitations are evident when one looks at the paucity of data regarding "normals". An ICS stage II prolapse is a common finding in asymptomatic women on physical examination. In one study, nearly 50% of 497 women seen for routine gynecological care were asymptomatic and had ICS stage II prolapse (Swift 2000).

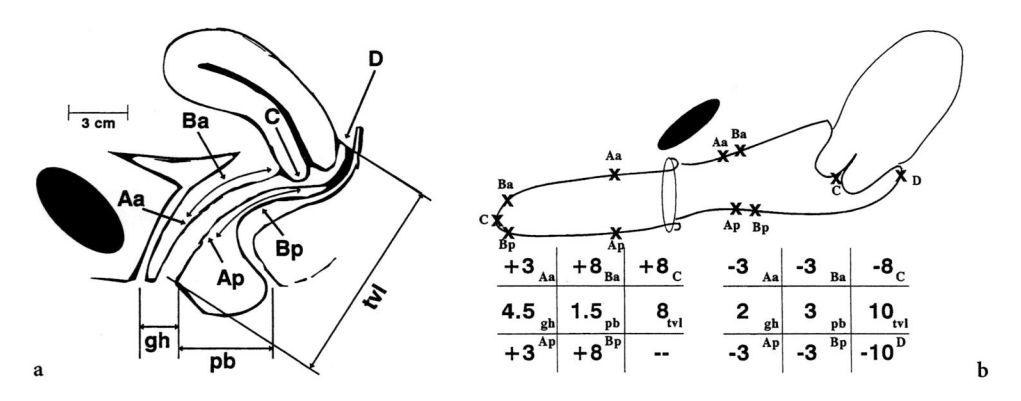

Fig. 5.1.2a, b. International Continence Society Pelvic Organ Prolapse grading system (Bump et al. 1996b). **a** Nine points are measured in centimeters and recorded. The hymeneal ring serves as the reference point for most measurements. This diagram illustrates the measurements of the anterior vaginal wall (Aa, Ba), cuff or cervix (C), posterior fornix (D), posterior vaginal wall (Ap, Bp), total vaginal length (TVL), genital hiatus (gh), and perineal body (pb). **b** A total uterovaginal vault eversion is juxtaposed with normal support. Where indicated, positive numbers represent tissue outside the hymeneal ring while negative numbers represent tissue above the hymen. Overall and individual site staging can then be assigned based on these measurements

Radiologically, very few studies on normals have been performed and most of these findings were obtained during an investigation of patients with prolapse. The overlap of normal subjects and symptomatic patients is considerable. Fig. 5.1.3 shows an asymptomatic 19-year-old subject who by radiographic criteria has a moderate, contrast-retaining rectocele. Clearly, she does not require surgery. However, the same conclusion might not have been reached in a 60-year-old patient complaining of an evacuation disorder with similar radiological findings. Rectoceles diagnosed radiologically may have no clinical symptoms. The complex, multifactorial etiology of bowel function makes reliance on one finding questionable. Nonetheless, a standardized staging system acceptable to both surgeons and radiologists is mandatory if further progress is to be made. If agreement cannot be reached on what constitutes prolapse and how it is measured, meaningful communication cannot take place.

Historically, a gold standard for the presence or absence of prolapse has not been established. In general, radiographic studies have shown a higher degree of prolapse when compared to physical examination. This has been attributed to the complete relaxation of the levator ani muscles achieved during defecation on imaging studies, a condition rarely achieved during a physical examination. This relaxation allows maximum distension of the urogenital hiatus, which in turn increases the extent of prolapse identified. As seen in Table 5.1.1, multiple comparative studies have shown that prolapse is more readily demonstrated on an imaging study than on physical examination. The discrepancy between the physical examination and imaging studies may lead to a change in surgical planning. One recent study found that 41% of initial surgical plans were changed on the basis of the results of the imaging study while a second earlier study showed that imaging changed the clinical diagnosis in 75% of subjects (KAUFMAN et al. 2001; ALTRINGER et al. 1995).

Competition for the limited space within the urogenital hiatus is a major concern during both physical examination and imaging studies of the pelvis. The first organ to descend into the urogenital hiatus may prevent the descent of other organs. An unemptied

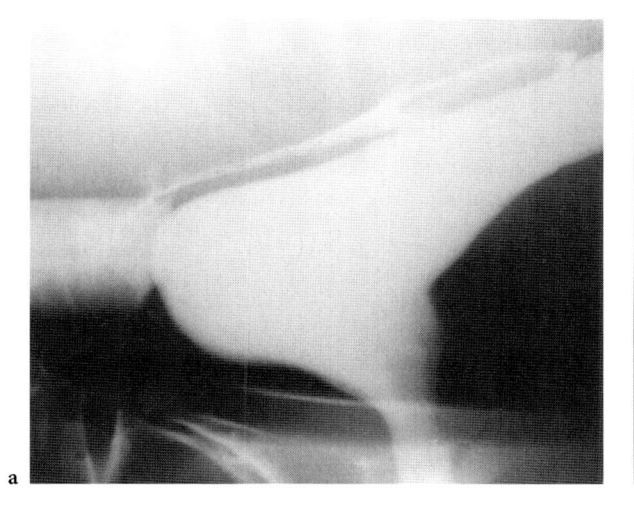

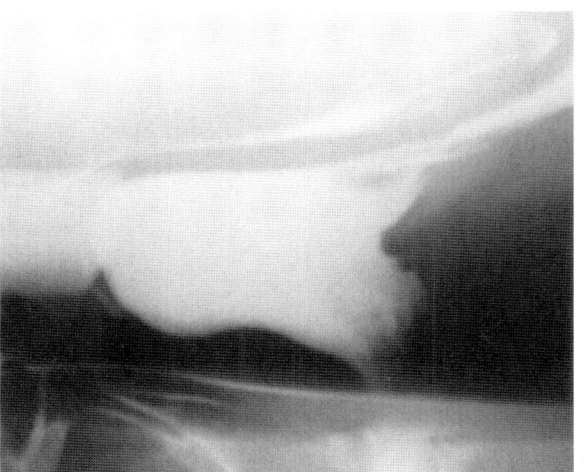

Fig. 5.1.3. a Moderate sized rectocele during evacuation in a 19-year-old asymptomatic control. **b** Following evacuation, contrast is retained in the same control. This demonstrates the difficulty in interpreting the clinical utility of these studies as an isolated finding

Table 5.1.1. Comparison of physical examination (PE) with fluoroscopic dynamic cystoproctography (DCP) in the detection of pelvic organ prolapse

Study	Rectocele			Enterocele			Cystocele		
	Found at DCP	Found at PE		Found at DCP	Found at PE		Found at DCP	Found at PE	
	n	n	%	n	n	%	n	n	%
Hock et al. (1993)	225	70	31	111	18	16	112	46	41
Altringer et al. (1995)	46	24	52	33	16	48	44	32	73
Kelvin et al. (1999)	155	119	77	47	24	51	159	132	83

cystocele may block descent of a rectocele or enterocele and therefore prevent its identification. Similarly, a large rectocele may prevent a cystocele or enterocele from being recognized (Fig. 5.1.4). Quickly performed imaging studies that do not systematically fill and empty the organs will miss the complete picture and add little to the physical examination. A triphasic technique has been proposed and seems to best address this issue. This systematic approach requires individual filling and emptying of the pelvic organs along with various dynamic maneuvers to help diagnose all organ prolapse (KELVIN et al. 2000).

Another example where imaging is helpful is the patient who may have an obvious posterior wall defect on physical examination that appears to be an enterocele, but imaging shows this to be a sigmoidocele (Fig. 5.1.5). Sigmoidoceles are virtually never diagnosed on physical examination, and may be present in up to 5% of patients with pelvic organ prolapse. Although some surgeons play down the distinction between a sigmoidocele and enterocele and do not change their surgical approach, others will. These surgical changes include a partial colectomy if a large sigmoidocele is associated with long-standing constipation (JORGE et al. 1994). In addition, detachment of the rectosigmoid from the presacral hollow with resulting prolapse may represent a different condition than a simple sigmoidocele alone, requiring rectopexy to re-establish rectosigmoid support rather than only a cul-de-sac correction. This represents a major change in surgical approach, and one that is made only with radiological help. Some surgeons argue that all prolapse may be identified at the time of surgery, so that little is gained by preoperative imaging. However, at the time of surgery the patient is asleep, unable to Valsalva, and usually in the dorsal lithotomy position, far from ideal conditions to identify prolapse and its extent.

For the clinician, different options exist when choosing an imaging study. Initial imaging studies of the pelvic floor were fluoroscopic. These have evolved into dynamic MRI studies and in some research centers, reconstructed three-dimensional imaging. The individual study ordered will depend on the experience of the radiologist and the equipment available.

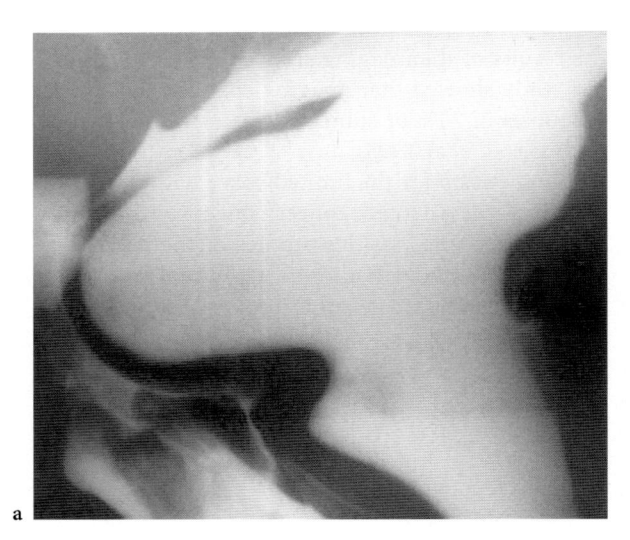

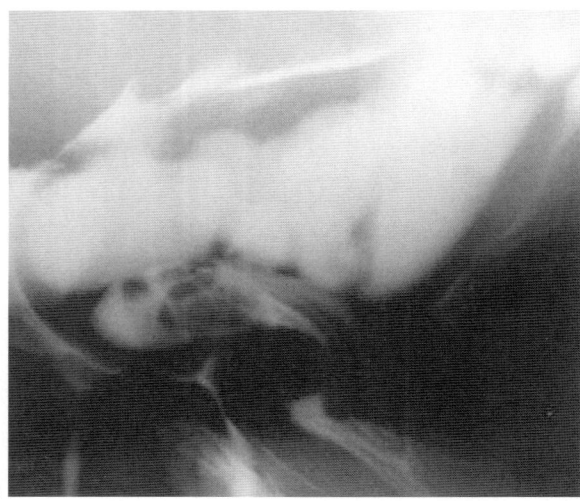

Fig. 5.1.4. a An unemptied rectocele obscuring a large enterocele prior to complete rectal emptying. **b** The same patient following complete contrast evacuation of the rectocele. A large enterocele is seen to descend into the urogenital hiatus demonstrating competition for this limited space. Single-phase studies miss these coexisting prolapses, demonstrating the need for multiphasic studies

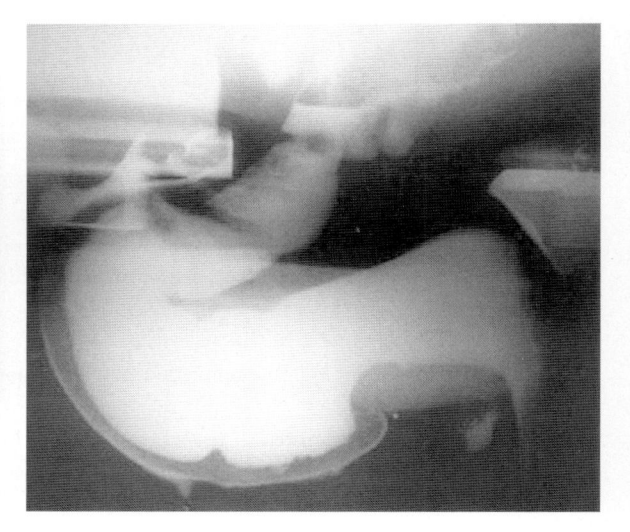

Fig. 5.1.5. Detachment of rectosigmoid from presacral hollow. A rectopexy is required to restore normal support in addition to appropriate vaginal support

The superior anatomic detail afforded by MRI would appear to make this the technique of choice. Other benefits of MRI are multiplanar views, detailed information about the levator ani muscle, patient comfort, and detection of other pelvic pathology as compared to fluoroscopic studies. Upright MRI, allowing a more physiological evacuation, is available in only a few centers. Cost may also be an issue. In a study of 22 patients having both MRI and fluoroscopy studies performed for constipation disorders, MRI was found to be ten times more expensive. In this small study there was no change in clinical management based on the results of one study compared to the other (Matsuoka et al. 2001).

Pelvic floor imaging is not needed in every case of pelvic floor dysfunction. When the physical examination and patient complaints correlate, little may be gained by the imaging study. In complicated patients where the physical examination and patient complaints disagree, an imaging study of the pelvic floor can be of diagnostic value and change surgical planning. As noted, the full extent of pelvic organ prolapse can only be appreciated when the levator ani completely relax. This relaxation happens only during evacuation, a condition not readily achieved during an office examination. As repeat surgery is invariably more difficult and exposes the patient to greater risk, care must be taken in planning the initial surgical repair. Although anatomic correction does not always lead to functional correction, the goal of pelvic surgery is to relieve patient symptoms and restore anatomy and function whenever possible.

5.1.5
Surgical Approach

Details of each surgical procedure are beyond the scope of this chapter. However, radiologists should have a basic understanding of the different surgeries available for prolapse. Many factors should be considered before selecting a route for reconstructive surgery. These include vaginal sexual function, concept of body image, a patient's medical condition, and possible fertility desires. Current surgical approaches include vaginal, abdominal, laparoscopic, or a combination of these routes. The experts who have published case series report a wide range of success rates with different techniques. Of course, the success rates of such experts may not apply universally. Only one prospective study has been published which randomized patients to either vaginal or abdominal routes. This attests to the difficulty in evaluating these important surgical issues. In this study, the vaginal route was found to have twice the failure rate when compared to abdominal surgery (Benson et al. 1996). A second, though retrospective, series found similar rates for recurrent prolapse when comparing the abdominal sacral colpopexy (19%) with sacrospinous fixation (33%) (Sze et al. 1999). This does not mean that vaginal surgery should be abandoned, but questions the overwhelming preponderance of the current vaginal surgery performed for pelvic organ prolapse.

Often, the connective tissue supports are so damaged that attempting to repair them alone makes little sense. If the levator ani is a healthy, robust muscle capable of supporting the vagina and pelvic organs, surgical correction of breaks in the connective tissue may be appropriate. If the levator muscle cannot be rehabilitated by physical therapy, surgical support limited to the connective tissues may lead to the historically documented high recurrence rates. In addition, there is also evidence that anterior vaginal wall dissection damages the nerve supply to the urethra and possibly also the bladder (Borirakchanyavat et al. 1997; Benson and McClellan 1993; Zivkovic et al. 1996; Ball et al. 1997). The most frequent offender is the anterior colporrhaphy, a procedure first described over 100 years ago (de Lamballe 1840) that has changed little since then. Although anterior colporrhaphy does have a place in the treatment of cystoceles, this role is limited.

Lastly, a laparoscopic approach may be useful in some patients. Long-term efficacy studies of such approaches are lacking. If they are chosen, laparoscopic procedures should be performed as described for open cases. At the present time, relatively few surgeons have the skills required to attempt these repairs with the laparoscope. As further studies are carried out, more of the "approach" questions will be answered.

5.1.6
The Anterior Vaginal Wall

A site-specific examination of the anterior vaginal wall focuses on the urethrovesical junction (UVJ), integrity of the lateral vaginal sulci, central vaginal wall defects, and lastly apical transverse defects (Richardson 1989) (Fig. 5.1.6). Patients with prolapse may also have coexisting or occult incontinence. A large prolapse may mask urinary incontinence by

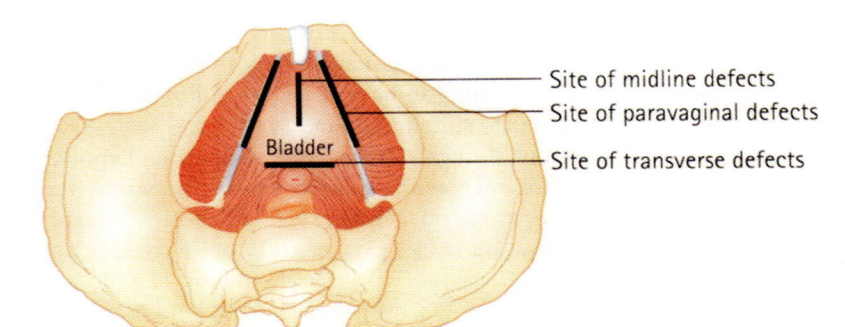

Fig. 5.1.6. Most common sites of anterior vaginal wall defects in the vaginal muscularis and connective tissue leading to cystocele: paravaginal, apical, central, and transverse

kinking of the urethra. In these cases, it has been suggested that the patients have the prolapse reduced and then have testing to uncover this occult incontinence. Occult incontinence is found with reduction testing in between 36–80% of patients with large prolapses (BUMP et al. 1988), though clinically the rate is lower, approximately 10% (BUMP et al. 1996a). Therefore, the decision as to whether to perform an anti-incontinence procedure in patients with occult incontinence is controversial. Selective support to the UVJ is encouraged in one form or another. This discussion needs to take place between the surgeon and the patient prior to surgery.

5.1.6.1
Cystocele

Historically, several terms have been used to describe cystoceles. Traction and displacement cystoceles are synonymous with paravaginal cystoceles, while pulsion or distension cystoceles are equivalent to central cystoceles (PILLAI and BENSON 1996). In a central cystocele, the apparent loss of contact between the vaginal epithelium and the muscularis presumably leads to a smooth cystocele with no rugae. The bladder can be visualized herniating through the defect, separating the epithelium from the muscularis (Fig. 5.1.7). This contrasts with a paravaginal cystocele where the central vaginal epithelium remains attached to the muscularis and rugae are maintained, but the lateral vaginal wall attachments to the arcus tendineus fascia pelvis are disrupted. Many surgeons feel that identification of the musculofascial defects is essential to select the correct surgical approach. Use of the posterior blade of a speculum to isolate the anterior vaginal wall allows these defects to be identified. "Urethrocele" is used to denote loss of support of the distal anterior vaginal wall that is fused with the urethra. It was previously thought that the urethra was supported by the pubourethral ligaments, making the diagnosis of an urethrocele relevant. However, these ligaments are really just the termination of the arcus tendineus levator ani, so that the differentiation of

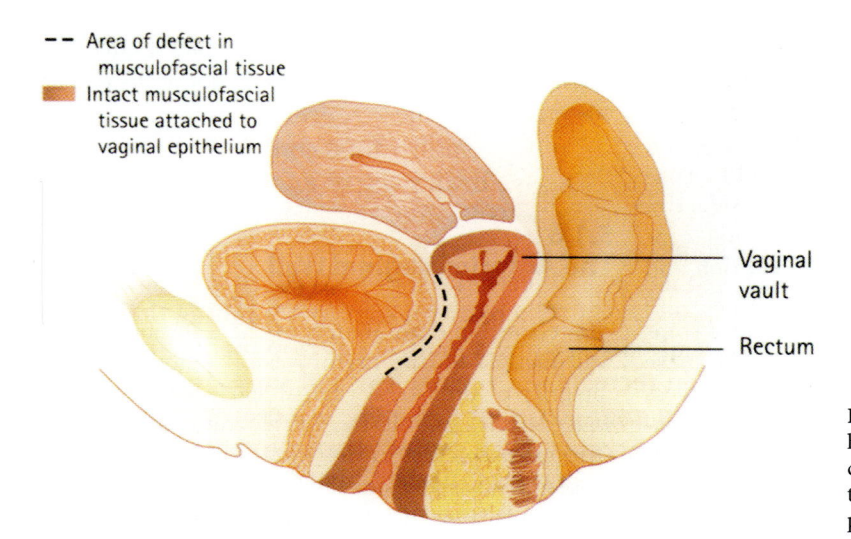

Fig. 5.1.7. Central cystocele: note the herniation of bladder through the muscularis separating the epithelium from the muscularis. No rugae will be seen on physical examination

a urethrocele and cystocele is merely the level at which anterior vaginal wall support is lost. The role of MRI in detecting these defects is evolving.

5.1.6.2
Paravaginal Cystocele Repair

The abdominal paravaginal cystocele repair (Fig. 5.1.8) is a popular and anatomically correct way to repair an anterior wall prolapse. Paravaginal cystoceles are reported to be the most commonly encountered (WHITE 1909; RICHARDSON et al. 1976). Two series ($n=149$, follow-up 6–48 months, and $n=213$, follow-up 2–8 years) (SHULL and BADEN 1989; RICHARDSON et al. 1981) found 95% success rates for abdominal paravaginal repairs. Success was defined with respect to anterior wall support only. A vaginal approach to repair of paravaginal cystoceles has been described in several case series. One series of 56 women (follow-up 0.1–5.6 years, mean 1.6 years) showed 15 women (27%) had recurrent bladder support defects after surgery with 4 (7%) being either to or through the hymen. No defects were worse postoperatively (SHULL et al. 1994). In another series of 100 women followed for a mean of 10.6 months, 22 had recurrent midline cystoceles while 22 had persistent paravaginal cystoceles (YOUNG et al. 2001).

5.1.6.3
Graft Placement

Experts may use an alternative to this procedure in a patient with multiple anterior wall defects. A vaginal paravaginal repair using synthetic mesh, an allograft, or a xenograft may be chosen. The graft is cut into a trapezoidal shape and strung like a hammock between the two arcus tendinei (Fig. 5.1.9). The superior edge of the graft is anchored to the apex of the vagina. The vaginal epithelium is then sutured to the graft repairing the anterior vaginal wall defects (WORD et al. 1992). One case series showed no recurrence in anterior wall prolapse when a permanent synthetic mesh was used for the graft material. However, 25% of patients had mesh-related complications (JULIAN 1996). Outcome analyses for these techniques are limited.

5.1.6.4
Anterior Colporrhaphy

An anterior colporrhaphy is indicated for repair of central defects. The basic technique typically involves a midline vaginal incision with dissection laterally until adequate vaginal muscularis is identified. The muscularis is then plicated in the midline with one or several layers elevating the prolapsed bladder. A

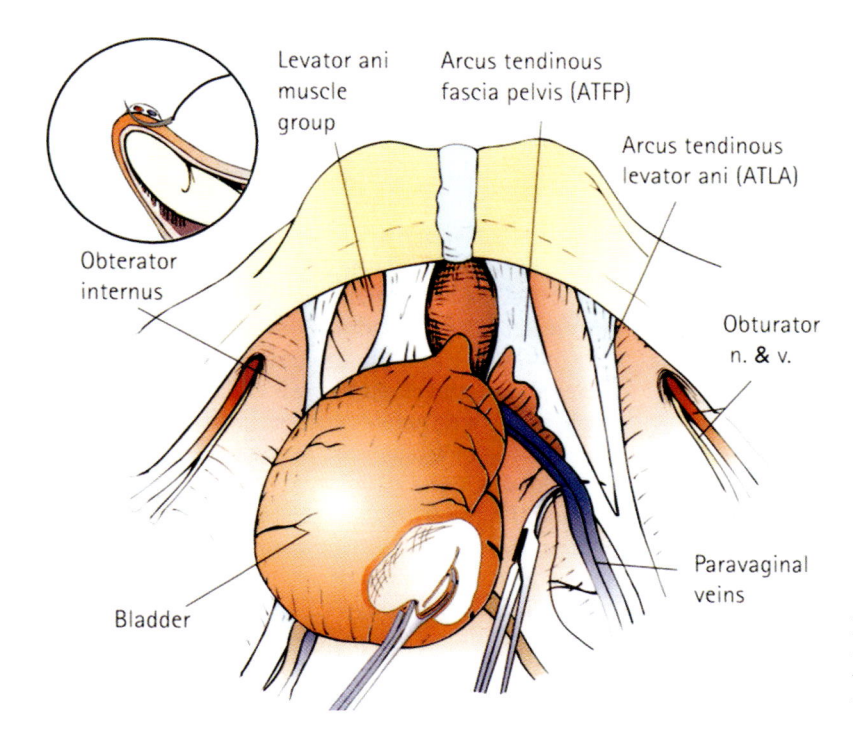

Fig. 5.1.8. Paravaginal cystocele repair: encircling the paravaginal veins with vaginal wall placement to the arcus tendineus fascia pelvis

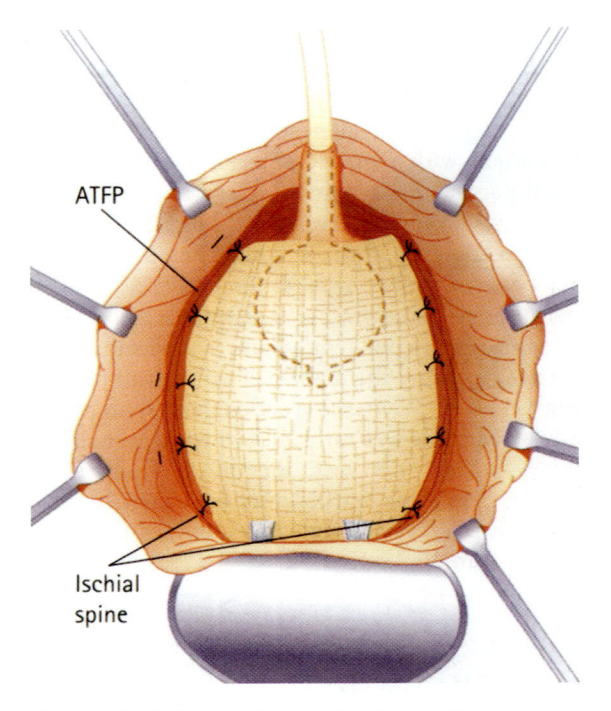

Fig. 5.1.9. Vaginal paravaginal repair using a graft to correct coexisting central and paravaginal defects. The superior edge of the fascia is sutured to the cuff and uterosacral ligaments. Bilaterally, the graft is anchored to the arcus tendineus

recent study randomized patients with anterior wall prolapse to one of three anterior colporrhaphy techniques: standard anterior colporrhaphy, standard repair plus polygalactin 910 mesh, or ultralateral anterior colporrhaphy. With a median follow-up of 23 months, there was no significant difference noted between the techniques. Satisfactory or optimal results were obtained in 30% of anterior colporrhaphy patients, 42% of those with the added absorbable mesh, and 46% of the ultralateral patients (WEBER et al. 2001). These numbers indicate the problem of using the patient's own tissue as the foundation of prolapse repair. The risk of damage to the urinary continence mechanism from nerve damage with anterior wall dissection must be considered before choosing this route of surgical correction.

5.1.7
Surgery of the Vaginal Apex

Uterine preservation is an option for some women who desire future fertility or have other reasons for avoiding hysterectomy, but for most women with uterovaginal prolapse, hysterectomy is added to the reconstruction. With lesser degrees of apical prolapse (ICS stage 0–II), the uterosacral-cardinal ligament complex can be used to provide vault support, either through an abdominal or a vaginal approach. Often these ligaments will need shortening prior to being used and ureteral location is essential before proceeding (BADEN and WALKER 1992a,b). After identifying these ligaments and possible shortening, the uterosacral complex is reattached to the musculofascial tissue of the anterior and posterior vaginal walls and a culdoplasty performed as needed. Consideration of these techniques should be given when performing any hysterectomy. For more severe apical prolapse, three surgical options exist: abdominal reconstruction, vaginal reconstruction, or obliterative surgery.

5.1.7.1
Abdominal Sacral Colpoperineopexy

Abdominal sacral colpopexy is a well-established, effective method for apical suspension. The first techniques of sacral colpopexy described supporting the vaginal apex with a graft, being either a synthetic mesh or autologous fascia (TIMMONS et al. 1992). Evolution of this technique has extended the support to the perineal body (CUNDIFF et al. 1997; FISCHER et al. 1997). This approach involves reinforcing the anterior and posterior vaginal wall with an allograft, xenograft, or synthetic mesh. The disadvantages of synthetic meshes include the potential of erosion in up to 9–11% of cases and an unnatural feel to the vaginal wall (IGLESIA et al. 1997). The advantages of synthetic meshes are their strength, longevity, and in some the propensity to stimulate scar tissue formation which may aid pelvic support. Autologous fascia is an option, but often impractical because such a large piece must be harvested. One series of ten patients had a 90% success rate (mean follow-up 26 months) with autologous fascia (MALONEY et al. 1990). Allografts may also be used, although long-term studies are not available for use in pelvic reconstructive surgery. Some of these materials have a well-documented record in orthopedic procedures (COOPER and BECK 1993). The advantages of most allografts are their pliability and natural feel without the apparent risk of erosion. Xenografts have been added to the pool of graft materials, but long-term studies are lacking.

The technique of abdominal sacral colpoperineopexy involves placement of a graft along the anterior and posterior vaginal walls. Posteriorly and distally, the graft is attached to the perineal body. Distally and laterally the posterior graft is attached to the fascia overlying the levator ani muscles. This initial graft attachment uses a vaginal approach. The remaining procedure is performed abdominally. Over the proximal two-thirds of the posterior wall, the graft is attached directly to the vaginal muscularis by spreading the graft as widely as possible. A Lucite stent within the vagina aids graft placement and dissection (Fig. 5.1.10). Anteriorly, a second graft leaf is placed after dissecting into the vesicovaginal space. This also is spread as widely as possible on the anterior vaginal wall and sutured in place. By enveloping the vaginal vault in a graft, the integrity of the connective tissue network can be restored. Appropriate tension is applied and the apices of the grafts are attached to the anterior longitudinal ligament of the spine over the S2-S3 levels. The grafts are usually placed retroperitoneally to minimize bowel adhesions. Symmetrical placement of the graft over the vaginal wall is important to allow for equal distribution of forces. If a rectocele is not present, the approach may be completely abdominal. This requires that there is good support of the rectovaginal septum to the perineal body, and that the upper edge of the rectovaginal septum is located high enough to be reached abdominally through the rectovaginal space. Often the perineal body is excessively mobile, and support should be extended to this level. Complications unique to this procedure include presacral hemorrhage and rarely osteomyelitis at the sacral site of graft attachment (SUTTON et al. 1981; WEIDNER et al. 1997).

5.1.7.2
Sacrospinous Vault Suspension

Over the last 25 years the most common procedure performed for vaginal vault prolapse has been the vaginal sacrospinous vault suspension. Introduced into this country in 1971 (RANDALL and NICHOLS 1971), there have been several clinical series citing its success in providing apical support. Modified techniques utilizing iliococcygeus fascia, pubococcygeus fascia, or multiple points of vaginal fixation over the levator plate have been described. In a meta-analysis of transvaginal repairs of vault prolapse, 1062 patients pooled from 18 studies undergoing sacrospinous vault suspension and 322 patients (four studies) treated with endopelvic vault suspension were reviewed. Recurrent prolapse occurred in 18% of the sacrospinous, and 11% of the endopelvic fascial suspensions (SZE and KARRAM 1997).

During sacrospinous vault suspension, the right sacrospinous ligament and overlying coccygeus muscle are reached after vaginal dissection. Frequently two permanent sutures are placed 4 cm medial to the ischial spine into the sacrospinous ligament-coccygeus complex. Important structures in this region include the pudendal neurovascular bundle, inferior gluteal neurovascular bundle, and superiorly located lumbosacral plexus. The support sutures are then placed into the apical vaginal muscularis. This technique deviates the vaginal axis to the right. Occasionally, a bilateral sacrospinous suspension is performed, but there are no data to support one technique over the other. Variations of this

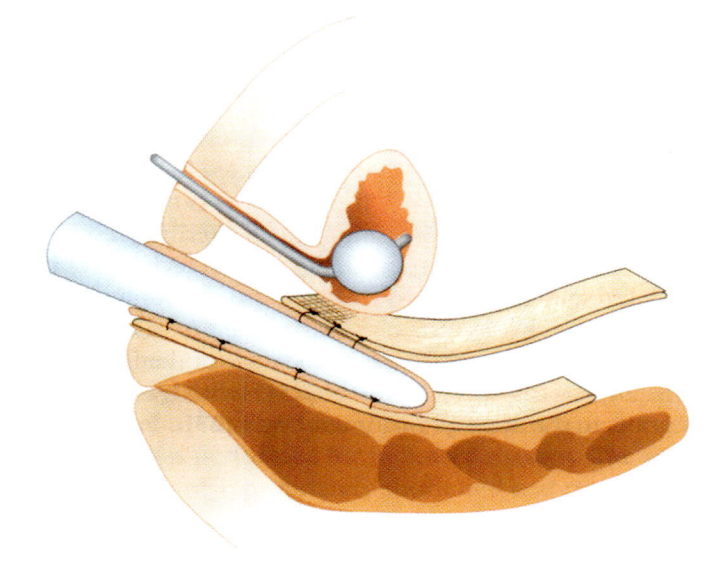

Fig. 5.1.10. Abdominal sacral colpoperineopexy, sagittal view. Anterior and posterior vaginal wall graft placement using a vaginal stent as a guide

procedure involve slightly different sites of suture placement, as well as using several points of vaginal fixation (PETERS and CHRISTENSON 1995; MORLEY and DELANCEY 1988).

5.1.7.3
Uterosacral Ligament Vault Suspension

Recently, a more extensive use of the uterosacral ligaments has been described for apical vault support via a vaginal approach. By placing sutures in the uterosacral ligaments, then successively through both the anterior and posterior vaginal walls, multiple points of fixation are used to obtain vaginal vault support. In several case series a success rate of nearly 90% using this more extensive vaginal repair has been reported (SHULL et al. 2000; BARBER et al. 2000; KARRAM et al. 2001).

5.1.7.4
Obliterative Surgery

Uterovaginal prolapse can be effectively treated with obliterative surgery. A LeFort colpocleisis that attaches rectangles of anterior and posterior vaginal walls that have been denuded of their epithelium below the cervix does not remove the uterus, and may be performed quickly although indications for this are becoming rare (THOMPSON 1992). It is usually reserved for a debilitated patient with minimal risk for endometrial cancer. In women who have had a hysterectomy, total colpocleisis can be performed. A single case series of 33 women reports a 97% cure ($n=33$, average follow-up 35 months) (DELANCEY and MORLEY 1997). This technique can also be done in conjunction with vaginal hysterectomy if the uterus is present.

Following vaginal hysterectomy if a uterus is present, the vaginal epithelium is removed close to the level of the hymen. The apex of the prolapsing mass is identified and successive purse string sutures are placed around the leading edge of the prolapse. As these sutures are tied, the enclosed tissue is reduced. The levator ani muscles are palpated and then approximated using a 0 or #1 permanent or delayed absorbable suture. Some support should be given to the UVJ, whether in the form of a Kelly plication, needle procedure, or pubovaginal sling to compensate for the downward traction that will be placed on the UVJ with the levator plication. The vaginal epithelium is then closed with a running suture, leaving a shortened vault, being at most 3 cm in length. A perineorrhaphy is performed to complete the procedure.

5.1.7.5
Uterine Preservation Procedures

Both vaginal and abdominal procedures exist to preserve the uterus in patients with symptomatic uterovaginal prolapse. These procedures are chosen for women who cannot tolerate the prolapse or pessary use and desire uterine preservation. In general, patients should be counseled to complete childbearing before reconstructive surgery is performed. If this is not acceptable, data from several small series exist. Pregnancy rates for potentially fertile patients ranged from 25–67% ($n=168$) in abdominally performed surgeries to 24–67% ($n=68$) in vaginally performed surgeries. Term deliveries were 9–50% and 5–67% respectively (JULIAN 1993; CHAUDHURI 1979; NASSAR 1967; DURFEE 1966; DASTUR et al. 1967; KOVAC and CRUIKSHANK 1993).

A wide range of operative techniques have been described, including the use of graft material, uterosacral ligament fixation to the sacrospinous ligament, uterosacral ligament plication, the Manchester procedure, and round ligament suspension of the uterus (NICHOLS 1991; SHAW 1933; THOMS et al. 1995; GILLIAM 1900). The lack of long-term studies makes these procedures speculative at best.

5.1.8
The Posterior Vaginal Wall

Defects of the posterior vaginal vault involve rectocele, enterocele, and sigmoidocele. Correction of the bulging may be attainable but often the patient's symptoms are not relieved and in fact may be worsened (KAHN and STANTON 1997). Techniques of rectocele repair include traditional posterior colporrhaphy, defect repair, fascial replacement, rectal wall imbrication, and transanal repair.

5.1.8.1
Rectocele

Controversy remains regarding the symptoms and diagnosis of rectoceles. Symptoms linked to, but not diagnostic of, rectocele include incomplete rectal emptying, manual assisted defecation, rectal pressure, bleeding, pain, and constipation. Fluoroscopic and MRI studies have had their greatest impact in the diagnosis of posterior wall defects. There are no clear criteria that predict successful rectocele repair. Unfortunately, anatomic repair does not always lead to functional correction.

5.1.8.2
Posterior Colporrhaphy

The posterior colporrhaphy has its roots in the repair of perineal lacerations, dating back to the 16th century. Many modifications to this procedure have been made, but the basic procedure remains unchanged. In the traditional posterior colporrhaphy the musculofascial tissue (rectovaginal septum and vaginal muscularis) is plicated in the midline.

The posterior vaginal epithelium is opened in the midline and dissected laterally and superiorly. The thickened musculofascial tissue is plicated in the midline. Epithelial trimming is done only to remove redundant epithelium. Some experts recommend plication of the levator muscles between the vagina and rectum while other experts avoid this as it may result in dyspareunia. Apareunia or severe dyspareunia have been reported in 30% of patients undergoing posterior repair where the levator muscles are exposed and sutured (Jeffcoate 1959). In one study evaluating both subjective and objective outcomes, representative results for traditional rectocele repair were seen (Mellgren et al. 1995). Patients ($n=25$) were evaluated with preoperative and postoperative questionnaires, physical examination, and defecography. Preoperatively, 96% suffered from constipation while 48% used digital support for evacuation. All patients showed a rectocele on defecography, while 88% had a rectocele on physical examination. Surgical repair consisted of a posterior colporrhaphy with levator plication. Mean follow-up was 1 year. Constipation was eliminated in 52% of patients, an occasional complaint persisted in 32%, and complaint was frequent in 16%. No patient required digital maneuvers to aid defecation following surgical correction. Defecography showed that rectoceles were eliminated in 79% of patients. Physical examination detected rectoceles in only 4% of patients postoperatively. Following repair, 19% of patients suffered from dyspareunia. Subjective and objective improvement was achieved in approximately 80% of patients.

5.1.8.3
Defect Repair

An alternative technique can be performed if a clear break in the rectovaginal septum is identified (Richardson 1993). The defect repair is approached as in a traditional repair with a posterior midline incision just beneath the vaginal epithelium and continued with lateral dissection. With a finger placed rectally, the operator palpates the borders of the defect that is repaired using deep bites into the musculofascial tissue and rectovaginal septum with a long-lasting absorbable suture. Although sound in theory, one small study ($n=16$) showed a decrease in rectocele size in only 50% of patients. The rectocele was unchanged in 25% of patients and larger in 25% by physical examination. Of these women, 75% reported a decrease in straining, 44% improved with regard to rectal emptying, and no change was observed in digital maneuvers to aid in emptying (Pillai 1994). Larger studies with objective measures are needed.

5.1.8.4
Graft Replacement

Replacement of fascia along the posterior wall has been described as part of sacral colpoperineopexy. In the unusual event that an isolated rectocele exists with poor musculofascial tissue, donor fascia may be attached to the perineal body, anchored to the levator ani muscles bilaterally, and lastly placed to the uterosacral ligaments superiorly (Fig. 5.1.11). Typically a 4×12-cm graft will be more than adequate. The graft is individualized according to each patient's anatomy. Care is taken not to bridge the fascia too tightly across the rectum. There is no case series describing this technique, so no outcome detail is available.

5.1.8.5
Imbrication

Rectal wall imbrication can be approached either transvaginally or transrectally. In the transvaginal approach a midline posterior vaginal wall incision extending into the rectovaginal space is used (Benson 1992). Running interlocking sutures are placed in the rectal muscularis for the length of the rectocele. This results in the imbrication of the rectal wall narrowing the lumen. No long-term outcome study for this technique has been published. With the transrectal approach, the running interlocking suture

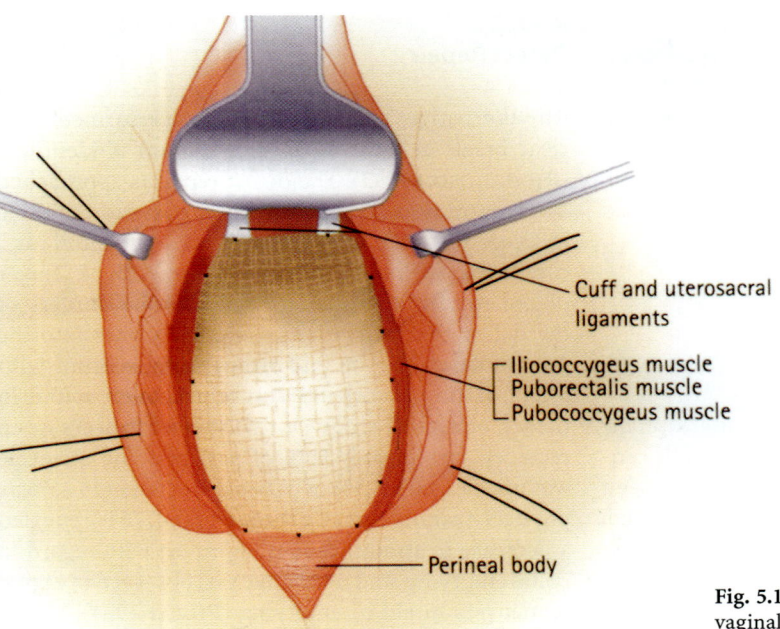

Fig. 5.1.11. Repair of rectocele using a posterior vaginal wall allograft or xenograft. Superiorly the graft is attached to the uterosacral ligament, laterally to the fascia of levator ani muscles, and inferiorly to the perineal body

is placed through the mucosa and submucosa. The incorporated tissue will undergo necrosis purportedly narrowing the rectal lumen and strengthening the muscularis layer. Outcome studies are also lacking for this technique.

5.1.8.6
Transanal Repair

Transanal rectocele repair has been reported only rarely in the gynecological literature, although its use by colorectal surgeons is well documented (Sullivan et al. 1968; Sehapayak 1985; Khubchandani et al. 1997; Karlbom et al. 1996; Janssen and van Dijke 1994). Rectal dilators are used to access the rectum; long slightly curved clamps are placed along the rectal mucosa and redundant mucosa is pulled into the clamp. This mucosal excision is performed in one to three areas depending on the degree of redundancy. The musculofascial tissue and rectal muscularis are then reinforced with horizontal suturing. Several series of transanal repair with minor variations have been published with subjective improvement/cure rates ranging from 82% to 98% (Sehapayak 1985; Khubchandani et al. 1997). Postoperatively a fluoroscopic decrease in rectocele size, a decrease in rectal area at rest, and increased rectal evacuation in 25/31 patients (81%) has been reported (Karlbom et al. 1996). In this study, a large rectal area at rest and use of enemas or bowel stimulants preoperatively was related to poor outcome. A second study using postoperative fluoroscopy also evaluated manometric measurements (Janssen and van Dijke 1994). Rectocele was eliminated objectively in 62% and reduced in the remaining 38% ($n=39$). Subjectively at 1 year, an 87% improvement or cure rate was noted ($n=76$). No predictive defecographic parameter was identified, but on manometry a large first urge to defecate volume was a predictor of good clinical outcome. It makes inherent sense that some rectoceles will not respond to vaginal wall operations alone, as the rectal side of the rectocele may be intimately involved (Marks 1967).

5.1.8.7
Enterocele

The cul-de-sac depth may have little bearing on the finding of an enterocele (Zaccharin 1977). The belief that a defect in the musculofascial layer of the posterior vaginal wall is responsible for an enterocele has been challenged (Tulikangas et al. 2001), and although still debated, an enterocele seems most likely to be the result of small bowel herniation through the posterior levator hiatus. In any repair to correct enterocele, the upper vaginal axis needs to be restored over the levator plate as part of the repair. The vaginal axis can be restored using an appropriate apical support technique. An alternative approach involves suturing the posterior vaginal vault to the levator plate. Using this technique, the urogenital hiatus is shortened by a levator plication posterior to the rectum followed by vaginal fixation to the levator plate (ZACCHARIN 1985). No outcome measure is available for this technique.

More traditionally a Halban, Moschcowitz, or McCall type culdoplasty may be performed. The Halban or Moschcowitz approach requires sutures being placed only through peritoneal or serosal surfaces. Using the Halban technique, successive vertical sutures are placed down the serosal surface of the sigmoid colon, across the cul-de-sac and along the posterior vaginal wall (NICHOLS et al. 1996). The sutures are placed 1 cm apart and no further laterally than 1 cm medial to the ureters to avoid small bowel herniating between the sutures and kinking of the ureters. A Moschcowitz culdoplasty uses successive purse-string sutures to occlude the cul-de-sac (MOSCHCOWITZ 1912). The ureters must be identified to avoid being pulled medially when the sutures are tied. These procedures do not rely upon the strength of this tissue, but rather provide apposition of peritoneal surfaces for scarification.

With a vaginal approach, a McCall type culdoplasty can be used (MCCALL 1957). This requires the uterosacral ligaments to be identified, shortened and then reattached to the vaginal apex. Certain patients with apparent enteroceles may have sigmoidoceles. Of patients undergoing defecography for pelvic floor defects, 4% ($n=234$) were found to have sigmoidoceles. None was diagnosed by physical examination (FENNER 1996). Rarely, sigmoid resection may be indicated (JORGE et al. 1994).

Many patients with POP will have an enlarged vaginal introitus and reduced perineal body. Although experts agree that this procedure is frequently needed for a comprehensive reconstruction, the specific indications for this remain vague. With significant perineal body descent, sacral fixation using abdominal sacral colpoperineopexy may be considered.

5.1.9
Conclusion

The relationship between the radiologist and surgeon in the area of pelvic floor dysfunction continues to actively evolve. A unified language for grading dysfunction is missing. Radiologists need a thorough understanding of the supportive anatomy of the pelvis to aid in this communication. Clinicians need to recognize the value of imaging studies in helping to understand pelvic floor disorders. Physicians must also acknowledge the limitations of imaging remembering the multifactorial nature of pelvic floor disorders. Radiographic findings do not always correlate with patient symptoms. However, pelvic floor imaging can represent an unbiased high-quality assessment tool in the study of the pelvic floor and in surgical outcome studies. Working together, care for patients with these problems will continue to improve.

References

Altringer WE, Saclarides TJ, Dominguez JM, et al (1995) Four-contrast defecography: pelvic "floor-oscopy". Dis Colon Rectum 38:695–699

Baden WF, Walker T (1992a) Abdominal approach to superior vaginal defects. In: Baden WF, Walker T (eds) Surgical repair of vaginal defects. Lippincott, Philadelphia, p 119

Baden WF, Walker T (1992b) Vaginal approach to superior vaginal defects. In: Baden WF, Walker T (eds) Surgical repair of vaginal defects. Lippincott, Philadelphia, p 161

Ball TP Jr, Teichman MH, Sharkey FE, et al (1997) Terminal nerve distribution to the urethra and bladder neck: consideration in the management of stress urinary incontinence. J Urol 158:827–829

Barber MD, Visco AG, Weidner C, et al (2000) Bilateral uterosacral ligament vault suspension with site-specific endopelvic fascia defect repair for treatment of pelvic organ prolapse. Am J Obstet Gynecol 183:1402–1410

Benson JT (1992) Rectocele, descending perineal syndrome, enterocele. In: Benson JT (ed) Female pelvic floor disorders: investigation and management. Norton, New York, p 384

Benson JT, McClellan E (1993) The effect of vaginal dissection on the pudendal nerve. Obstet Gynecol 82:387–389

Benson JT, Lucente V, McClellan E (1996) Vaginal versus abdominal reconstructive surgery for the treatment of pelvic support defects: a prospective randomized study with long-term outcome evaluation. Am J Obstet Gynecol 175:1418–1422

Borirakchanyavat S, Aboseif SR, Carroll PR, et al (1997) Continence mechanism of the isolated female urethra: an anatomical study of the intrapelvic somatic nerves. J Urol 158:822–826

Bump RC, Fantyl JA, Hurt WG (1988) The mechanism of urinary continence in women with severe uterovaginal prolapse: results of barrier studies. Obstet Gynecol 72:291

Bump RC, Hurt WG, Theofrastus JP, et al (1996a) Randomized prospective comparison of needle colposuspension versus endopelvic fascia plication for potential stress incontinence prophylaxis in women undergoing vaginal reconstruction for stage III or IV pelvic organ prolapse. Am J Obstet Gynecol 175:326

Bump RC, Mattiasson A, Bo K, et al (1996b) The standardization of terminology of female pelvic organ prolapse and pelvic floor dysfunction. Am J Obstet Gynecol 175: 1467–1471

Campbell RM (1950) The anatomy and histology of the sacrouterine ligaments. Am J Obstet Gynecol 59:1–12

Chaudhuri SK (1979) The place of sling operations in treating genital prolapse in young women. Int J Gynaecol Obstet 16:314–320

Cooper JL, Beck CL (1993) History of soft-tissue allografts in orthopedics. Sports Med Arthrosc Rev 1:2–16

Cundiff GW, Harris RL, Coates K, et al (1997) Abdominal sacral colpoperineopexy: a new approach for correction of posterior compartment defects and perineal descent associated with vaginal prolapse. Am J Obstet Gynecol 177:1345–1355

Dastur B, Gurubaxani G, Palnitkar SS (1967) Shirodkar sling operation in the treatment of genital prolapse. Obstet Gynaecol Br Commonw 74:125–128

Davis GD (1996) Uterine prolapse after laparoscopic uterosacral transection in nulliparous airborne trainees. A report of 3 cases. J Reprod Med 41:279–282

De Lamballe J (1840) Mem de l'Acad Roy De Med VIII:697

DeLancey JOL (1992) Anatomic aspects of vaginal eversion after hysterectomy. Am J Obstet Gynecol 166:1717–1728

DeLancey JOL (1999) Structural anatomy of the posterior compartment as it relates to rectocele. Am J Obstet Gynecol 180:815–823

DeLancey JOL, Morley GW (1997) Total colpocleisis for vaginal eversion. Am J Obstet Gynecol 176:1228–1235

Durfee RB (1966) Suspension operations for treatment of pelvic organ prolapse. Clin Obstet Gynecol 9:1047–1061

Farrell SA, Dempsey T, Geldenhuys L (2001) Histologic examination of "fascia" used in colporrhaphy. Obstet Gynecol 98: 794–798

Fenner D (1996) Diagnosis and assessment of sigmoidoceles. Am J Obstet Gynecol 175:1438–1441

Fischer JR, Hale DS, Benson JT, et al (1997) Combined rectocele repair and abdominal sacral colpopexy. A new method for repair of Denonvillier's fascia. Presented at the AUGS 18th Annual Scientific Meeting, Tucson, Arizona

Gilliam DT (1900) Round-ligament ventrosuspension of the uterus: a new method. Am J Obstet 52:1028

Gilpin SA, Gosling JA, Smith ARB, et al (1989) The pathogenesis of genitourinary prolapse and stress incontinence of urine. A histological and histochemical study. Br J Obstet Gynaecol 96:15–23

Hale DS, Kelvin FM (1998) Dynamic cystoproctography vs. dynamic MRI vs. physical exam in patients with pelvic organ prolapse. Presented at the 20th Annual AUGS Scientific Meeting, Washington DC

Hall AF, Theofrastus JP, Cundiff GW, et al (1996) Interobserver and intraobserver reliability of the proposed International Continence Society, Society of Gynecologic Surgeons and American Urogynecologic Society pelvic organ prolapse classification system. Am J Obstet Gynecol 175:1467–1471

Heit M, Benson JT, Russell B, et al (1996) Levator ani muscle in women with genitourinary prolapse: indirect assessment of muscle by histopathology. Neurol Urodyn 15:17–29

Hock D, Lombard R, Jehaes C, et al (1993) Colpocystodefecography. Dis Colon Rectum 36:1015–1021

Hoyte L, Schierlitz L, Zou K, et al (2001) Two- and 3-dimensional MRI comparison of levator ani structure, volume and integrity in women with stress incontinence and prolapse. Am J Obstet Gynecol 185:11–19

Iglesia CB, Fenner D, Brubaker L (1997) The use of mesh in gynecologic surgery. Int Urogynecol J 8:105–115

Janssen LWM, van Dijke CF (1994) Selection criteria for anterior rectal wall repair in symptomatic rectocele and anterior rectal wall prolapse. Dis Colon Rectum 37: 1100–1107

Jeffcoate TNA (1959) Posterior colpoperineorrhaphy. Am J Obstet Gynecol 77:490–502

Jorge JM, Yang YK, Wexner SD (1994) Incidence and clinical significance of sigmoidoceles as determined by a new classification system. Dis Colon Rectum 37:1112–1117

Julian TM (1993) Response to Kovac SR, Cruikshank SH Successful pregnancies and vaginal deliveries after sacrospinous uterosacral fixation in five of nineteen patients. Am J Obstet Gynecol 168:1778–1786

Julian TM (1996) The efficacy of Marlex mesh in the repair of severe, recurrent vaginal prolapse of the anterior vaginal wall. Am J Obstet Gynecol 175:1472–1475

Kahn MA, Stanton SI (1997) Posterior colporrhaphy: its effects on bowel and sexual function. Br J Obstet Gynecol 104:82–86

Karlbom U, Wilhelm G, Nilsson S, et al (1996) Does surgical repair of a rectocele improve rectal emptying? Dis Colon Rectum 39:1296–1302

Karram M, Goldwasser S, Kleeman S, et al (2001) High uterosacral vault suspension with fascial reconstruction for vaginal repair of enterocele and vaginal vault prolapse. Am J Obstet Gynecol 185:1339–1343

Kaufman HS, Buller JL, Thompson JR, et al (2001) Dynamic pelvic magnetic resonance imaging and cystocolpoproctography after surgical management of pelvic floor disorders. Dis Colon Rectum 44:1575–1584

Kelvin FM, Hale DS, Maglinte DDT, et al (1999) Female pelvic organ prolapse: diagnostic contribution of dynamic cystoproctography and comparison with physical exam. AJR Am J Roentgenol 173:31–37

Kelvin FM, Maglinte DDT, Hale DS, et al (2000) Female pelvic organ prolapse: a comparison of triphasic dynamic MR imaging and triphasic fluoroscopic cystocolpoproctography. AJR Am J Roentgenol 174:81–88

Khubchandani IT, Clancy JP, Riether RD, et al (1997) Endorectal repair of rectocele revisited. Br J Surg 84:88–91

Kovac SR, Cruikshank SH (1993) Successful pregnancies and vaginal deliveries after sacrospinous uterosacral fixation in five of nineteen patients. Am J Obstet Gynecol 168: 1778–1786

Kuhn RJP, Hollyock VE (1982) Observations on the anatomy of the rectovaginal pouch and septum. Obstet Gynecol 59: 445–447

Leffler KS, Thompson JR, Cundiff GW, et al (2001) Attachment of the rectovaginal septum to the pelvic sidewall. Am J Obstet Gynecol 185:41–43

Maloney JC, Dunton CJ, Smith K (1990) Repair of vaginal vault prolapse with abdominal sacropexy. J Reprod Med 35:6–10

Marks MM (1967) The rectal side of the rectocele. Dis Colon Rectum 10:387–388

Matsuoka H, Wexner S, Desia MB, et al (2001) A comparison between pelvic magnetic resonance imaging and videoproctography in patients with constipation. Dis Colon Rectum 44:571–576

McCall ML (1957) Posterior culdoplasty: surgical correction of enterocele during vaginal hysterectomy: a preliminary report. Obstet Gynecol 10:595

Mellgren A, Anzen B, Nilsson BY, et al (1995) Results of rectocele repair. A prospective study. Dis Colon Rectum 38:7–13

Mengert WF (1936) Mechanics of uterine support and position. Am J Obstet Gynecol 31:775–782

Milley PS, Nichols DH (1968) A correlative investigation of the human rectovaginal septum. Anat Rec 163:443–452

Morley GW, DeLancey JO (1988) Sacrospinous ligament fixation for eversion of the vagina. Am J Obstet Gynecol 158:872–881

Moschcowitz AV (1912) The pathogenesis, anatomy and cure of prolapse of the rectum. Surg Gynecol Obstet 15:7

Nassar GF (1967) Modified Williams-Richardson operation for uterine prolapse. Obstet Gynecol 30:233–237

Nichols DH (1991) Fertility retention in the patient with genital prolapse. Am J Obstet Gynecol 164:1155–1158

Nichols DH, Randall CL (1996) Enterocele. In: Nichols DH, Randall CL (eds) Vaginal surgery, 4th edn. Williams and Wilkins, Baltimore, p 348

Norton PA, Baker JE, Sharp HC, et al (1995) Genitourinary prolapse and joint hypermobility in women. Obstet Gynecol 85:225–228

Olsen A, Smith VJ, Bergstrom JO, et al (1997) Epidemiology of surgically managed pelvic organ prolapse and urinary incontinence. Obstet Gynecol 89:501–506

Peters WA, Christenson ML (1995) Fixation of the vaginal apex to the coccygeus fascia during repair of vaginal vault eversion with enterocele. Am J Obstet Gynecol 172:1894–1902

Pillai A (1994) Rectocele repair: defect approach, an early review. Proceedings of the 5th Annual Scientific Meeting of the American Urogynecologic Society, Toronto, Ontario, Canada

Pillai A, Benson JT (1996) Cystocele. In: Brubaker LT, Saclarides TJ (eds) The female pelvic floor: disorders of function and support. Davis, Philadelphia, p 269

Randall CL, Nichols DH (1971) Surgical treatment of vaginal inversion. J Obstet Gynecol 38:327–332

Richardson AC (1989) Pelvic support defects in women (urethrocele, cystocele, uterine prolapse, enterocele and rectocele). In: Skandalakis J, Gray S, Mansberger A Jr, Colborn G, Skandalakis L (eds) Hernia: surgical anatomy and technique. McGraw-Hill, New York, pp 238–263

Richardson AC (1993) The rectovaginal septum revisited: its relationship to rectocele and its importance in rectocele repair. In: Pitkin RM, Scot JR, DeLancey JOL (eds) Clinical obstetrics and gynecology, vol 36/4. Lippincott, Philadelphia, p 977

Richardson AC, Lyon JB, Williams NL (1976) A new look at pelvic relaxation. Am J Obstet Gynecol 126:568

Richardson AC, Edmonds PB, Williams NL (1981) Treatment of stress urinary incontinence due to paravaginal fascial defect. Obstet Gynecol 57:357–362

Sehapayak S (1985) Transrectal repair of rectocele: an extended armamentarium of colorectal surgeons, a report of 355 cases. Dis Colon Rectum 28:422–433

Shaw WF (1933) The treatment of prolapses uteri, with special reference to the Manchester operation of colporrhaphy. Am J Obstet Gynecol 26:667

Shull BL, Baden WF (1989) A six-year experience with paravaginal defect repair for stress urinary incontinence. Am J Obstet Gynecol 160:1432–1440

Shull BL, Benn SJ, Kuehl TJ (1994) Surgical management of prolapse of the anterior vaginal segment: an analysis of support defects, operative morbidity, and anatomic outcome. Am J Obstet Gynecol 171:1429–1439

Shull BL, Bachofen C, Coates KW, et al (2000) A transvaginal approach to repair of apical and other associated sites of pelvic organ prolapse with uterosacral ligaments. Am J Obstet Gynecol 183:1365–1373

Singh K, Reid WM, Berger LA (2001) Assessment and grading of pelvic organ prolapse by use of dynamic magnetic resonance imaging. Am J Obstet Gynecol 185:71–77

Smith ARB, Hosker GL, Warrell DW (1989) The role of partial denervation of the pelvic floor in the aetiology of genitourinary prolapse and stress incontinence of urine. A neurophysiologic study. Br J Obstet Gynaecol 96:24–28

Smith P, Heimer G, Norgen A, et al (1990) Steroid hormone receptors in pelvic muscles and ligament in women. Gynecol Obstet Invest 30:27–30

Sullivan ES, Leaverton GH, Hardwick CE (1968) Transrectal perineal repair: an adjunct to improved function after anorectal surgery. Dis Colon Rectum 11:106–114

Sutton GP, Addison WA, Livengood CH III, et al (1981) Life-threatening hemorrhage complicating sacral colpopexy. Am J Obstet Gynecol 140:836–837

Swift SE (2000) The distribution of pelvic organ support in a population of female subjects seen for routine gynecologic care. Am J Obstet Gynecol 183:277–285

Sze EHM, Karram MM (1997) Transvaginal repair of vault prolapse: a review. Obstet Gynecol 89:466–475

Sze EHM, Kohli N, Miklos J, et al (1999) A retrospective comparison of abdominal sacrocolpopexy with Burch colposuspension versus sacrospinous fixation with transvaginal needle suspension for the management of vault prolapse and coexisting stress incontinence. Int Urogynecol J 10:390–393

Thompson JD (1992) Malposition of the uterus. In: Thompson JD, Rock JA (eds) TeLinde's operative gynecology, 7th edn. Lippincott, Philadelphia, pp 846–849

Thoms AG, Brodman ML, Dottino PR, et al (1995) Manchester procedure vs. vaginal hysterectomy for uterine prolapse: a comparison. J Reprod Med 40:299–304

Timmons MC, Addison WA, Addison SB, et al (1992) Abdominal sacral colpopexy in 163 women with post hysterectomy vaginal vault prolapse and enterocele: evolution of operative techniques. J Reprod Med 37:323–327

Tulikangas PK, Walters MD, Brainard JA, et al (2001) Enterocele: is there a histologic defect? Obstet Gynecol 98:634–637

Uhlenhuth E, Nolley GW (1957) Vaginal fascia, a myth? J Obstet Gynecol 10:349–358

Weber AM, Walters MD (1997) Anterior vaginal prolapse: review of anatomy and techniques of surgical repair. Obstet Gynecol 89:311–318

Weber AM, Walters MD, Piedmonte MR, et al (2001) Anterior colporrhaphy: a randomized trial of three surgical techniques. Am J Obstet Gynecol 185:1299–1306

Weidner AC, Cundiff GW, Harris RL, et al (1997) Sacral osteomyelitis: an unusual complication of abdominal sacral colpopexy. Obstet Gynecol 90:689–691

White GR (1909) Cystocele. A radical cure by suturing lateral sulci of vagina to white line of pelvic fascia. JAMA 21:1701–1710

Word BH, Montgomery HA, Baden WF, et al (1992) Vaginal approach to anterior paravaginal repair: alternative techniques. In: Baden WF, Walker T (eds) Surgical repair of vaginal defects. Lippincott, Philadelphia, p 201

Young SB, Daman JJ, Bony LG (2001) Vaginal paravaginal repair. One-year outcomes. Am J Obstet Gynecol 185:1360–1367

Zaccharin RF (1977) A Chinese anatomy – the supporting tissues of the Chinese and Occidental female compared and contrasted. Aust NZ J Obstet Gynaecol 17:1–11

Zaccharin RF (1980) Pulsion enterocele: review of functional anatomy of the pelvic floor. Obstet Gynecol 55:135–140

Zaccharin RF (1985) Abdomino-perineal repair of large pulsion enterocele. In: Zaccharin RF (ed) Pelvic floor anatomy and the surgery of pulsion enterocele. Springer, Vienna New York, pp 135–155

Zivkovic F. Famussino K, Ralph G, et al (1996) Long-term effects of vaginal dissection on the innervation of the striated urethral sphincter. Obstet Gynecol 87:257–260

5.2 Urinary Incontinence: Clinical and Surgical Considerations

K. Strohbehn

CONTENTS

5.2.1 Introduction 125
5.2.1.1 Definition 125
5.2.1.2 Epidemiology 126
5.2.2 Types of Urinary Incontinence 127
5.2.2.1 Disorders of the Urethral/Bladder Neck 128
5.2.2.2 Disorders of the Bladder 128
5.2.2.3 Mixed Urinary Incontinence 128
5.2.2.4 Overflow Incontinence 128
5.2.2.5 Functional/Cognitive Incontinence 129
5.2.2.6 Extraurethral Incontinence 129
5.2.3 Clinical Evaluation 129
5.2.3.1 History 130
5.2.3.2 Physical Examination 130
5.2.4 Further Testing 131
5.2.5 Treatment Options 131
5.2.5.1 Behavioral Treatment 132
5.2.5.2 Pharmacologic Treatment 132
5.2.5.3 Surgical Treatment 133
5.2.5.4 Other Management Options 138
5.2.6 Summary 138
References 139

5.2.1 Introduction

Urinary incontinence is a prevalent disorder that occurs more commonly in subjects with pelvic support disorders. As reviewed briefly in Chapter 4.5 on urodynamic testing, conditions affecting bladder control can be divided into problems affecting proper storage of urine and those of normal bladder emptying. This chapter primarily focuses on problems of bladder storage that result in loss of urinary control. The epidemiology, clinical evaluation and treatment options for urinary incontinence are discussed.

K. Strohbehn, MD, FACOG, FACS
Associate Professor, Dartmouth Medical School, Department of Obstetrics and Gynecology; Director, Division of Urogynecology/Reconstructive Pelvic Surgery, Dartmouth-Hitchcock Medical Center, One Medical Center Drive, Lebanon, NH 03756, USA

5.2.1.1 Definition

Urinary incontinence has been defined by the International Continence Society (ICS): "urinary incontinence is involuntary loss of urine which is objectively demonstrable and a social or hygienic problem" (Abrams et al. 1988a, 1988b). The definition is similar to the that of the consensus panel of the US Agency for Healthcare Policy and Research (Urinary Incontinence Guideline Panel 1992): "involuntary loss of urine which is sufficient to be a problem." The ICS definition includes three separate and important concepts:
1. The loss of urine is not voluntary.
2. Urine loss must be demonstrable on objective testing, such as cystometry or cough testing.
3. The incontinence must be perceived by the patient (or the patient's care provider) as a social or hygienic problem.

The definitions of urinary incontinence are important to consider, as the studies regarding outcomes often use different definitions for urinary incontinence. Variation in definitions occurs because there are differences in amounts of urine lost, frequency of these events and how the incontinent events impact the individual. In addition to the ICS definition of urinary incontinence, an important concept is that the term urinary incontinence denotes three different meanings (Blaivas et al. 1997):
- A *symptom*: subjective involuntary urine loss
- A *sign*: objective demonstration of urine loss
- A *condition*: the pathophysiology underlying incontinence by clinical or urodynamic techniques.

To illustrate the importance of delineating the different meanings of the term urinary incontinence, let us consider a paradigm paraphrased from Drs. John DeLancey and Lewis Wall (DeLancey and Wall, personal communication):

Consider a set of multiparous identical twin mothers who are both 35 years old and who are similar build, weight, height and appearance. The sisters had similar childbirth experience, similar vaginal parity and both had babies of equal birthweights, similar labor and pushing times. Consider, however, that one mother is very active. She teaches physical education, she plays tennis, jogs, and routinely practices aerobic exercise. She now experiences urinary incontinence with these activities and impacts her lifestyle greatly since this is her employment. Her sister, on the other hand, is a librarian who lives a fairly sedentary lifestyle. She does not note urinary incontinence and never uses pads for incontinence.

Let us suppose that a physical examination, including a pelvic examination is performed, as well as urodynamic testing. It is conceivable that the testing would show exactly the same mobility of the bladder neck and the similar urodynamic parameters (bladder capacity, sensitivity, urethral closure pressures, leak point pressures). By objective testing, both of these women are found to have urinary incontinence as a *sign*. By subjective evaluation, only the more active twin has urinary incontinence, as a *symptom*.

Herein lies the dilemma: Do both of the women have urinary incontinence as a *condition*? ... How best to study outcome measurements for urinary incontinence when the objective measurement tools do not correlate with subjective measurements?

Based, on this paradigm, it is clear that we must be precise in defining whether we are discussing patient symptoms, objective findings or the overall condition of urinary incontinence when we utilize this term. In their review of the epidemiology of urinary incontinence, Hunskaar et al. note "The absence of a unifying definition for urinary incontinence is a fundamental problem which has not been resolved" (Hunskaar et al. 2000).

5.2.1.2
Epidemiology

5.2.1.2.1
Prevalence

While not a life-threatening condition, urinary incontinence is exceptionally common. Two excellent recent reviews summarize the epidemiology of urinary incontinence (Bump and Norton 1998; Hunskaar et al. 2000). It is estimated that 30–40% of older Americans suffer from the symptom of urinary incontinence (Burgio et al. 1991; Diokno et al. 1986; Teasdale et al. 1988). Prevalence estimates increase with increasing age (Brown et al. 1999; Malmsten et al. 1997). However, in two studies of nulliparous women aged under 25 years, the prevalence of some degree of urinary incontinence was 50%, but it was recognized as a severe or unacceptable problem in only 5–6% (Nemir and Middleton 1954; Wolin 1969). Women are generally twice as likely to experience incontinence as men, but this ratio is actually much higher in the age range 25–64 years (Fig. 5.2.1) (Bump and Norton 1998; Thom 1998).

Among women, increasing parity is associated with increasing rates of urinary incontinence (Schulman et al. 1997). Estimates from other countries have shown similar ranges in prevalence rates of urinary incontinence (Lee et al. 1998; Schulman et al. 1997; Temml et al. 2000; Ushiroyama et al. 1999). There is also a marked increase in the rate of urinary incontinence among individuals who are institutionalized, reaching as high as 72.0% (Toba et al. 1996).

The epidemiologic studies are limited by the lack of consistent definitions regarding urinary incontinence (Hampel et al. 1997; Hunskaar et al. 2000). As mentioned above, there is variation in the definitions regarding frequency of urine loss, volume of urine loss as well as bothersome symptoms resulting from the loss (Thom 1998). Several studies show that high prevalence rates for symptoms of urinary incontinence, but much lower rates if the subject is asked if the leakage is bothersome to them, or if they would seek help to improve their symptoms (Hunskaar et al. 2000; Ushiroyama et al. 1999). In one study, men were more likely to seek care for symptoms than women (29% vs 13%), despite having a lower overall prevalence rate (24% vs 49%) (Robertson et al. 1998).

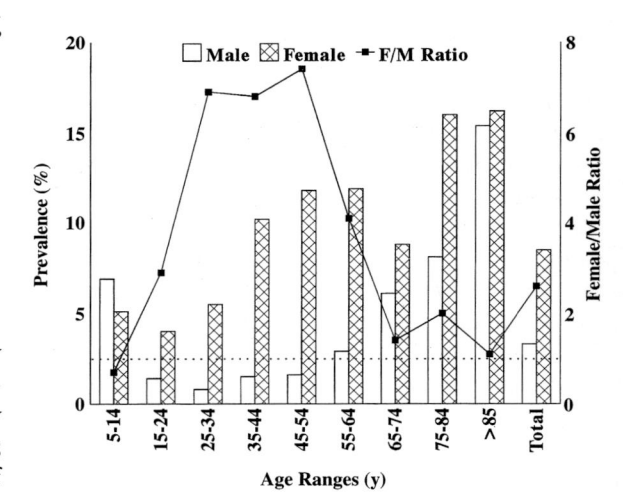

Fig. 5.2.1. Male-to-female ratios of urinary incontinence prevalence versus age, demonstrating larger female prevalence in younger age ranges (data from Thomas et al. 1980) (with permission, Bump and Norton 1998, p. 724)

Racial differences have also been described in the prevalence of urinary incontinence. The prevalence of stress incontinence is higher among white women than black women (BROWN et al. 1999).

Prevalence rates for surgical treatment of stress urinary incontinence provides another way to look at the concept of how bothersome the problem is to the individual. If it were bothersome enough that the subject opts for surgical treatment, one would assume that it is a considerable burden for them. OLSEN and colleagues investigated the prevalence of surgical treatment for women with incontinence or pelvic organ prolapse (OLSEN et al. 1997). Of 149, 554 women in a health maintenance organization from the northwestern United States, 395 women were identified as having undergone surgical repair in 1995. Based on this, they estimated that the risk of a woman undergoing a single operation for prolapse or urinary incontinence by age 80 years was 11.1%. Furthermore, 29.2% of the patients required more than one surgical repair for prolapse or urinary incontinence.

5.2.1.2.2
Incidence/Remission Rates

Interestingly, there are several reports identifying that urinary incontinence is a dynamic process that waxes and wanes (MOLLER et al. 2000; NYGAARD and LEMKE 1996; SAMUELSSON et al. 2000). Using serial surveys over a 6-year study period, as part of a larger epidemiologic study, NYGAARD and LEMKE (1996) studied a group of 2025 women aged 65 years or older living in a rural community setting. They found a 36.3% prevalence rate for urge incontinence and 40.3% for stress incontinence. Subjects were resurveyed between at the 3rd and 6th year and they found that remission and incidence rates for urge incontinence were 22.1% and 28.5%. For stress incontinence, the remission and incidence rates were 25.1% and 28.6%.

5.2.1.2.3
Risk Factors

Most studies of risk factors are limited in that they do not provide longitudinal data, but cross-sectional data, so that correlates can be identified, but cause and effect cannot. Risk factors associated with all types of urinary incontinence in women include (HUNSKAAR et al. 2000):
- Increasing age
- Current pregnancy
- Increased parity
- Menopause
- Hysterectomy
- Obesity
- Functional impairment
- Cognitive impairment
- Occupational risks
- Other

Other reported correlations include: history of childhood bedwetting, urinary tract infections, prior gynecologic surgery, constipation, diuretic use, perineal suturing, exercise, cystocele, uterine prolapse, history of radiation, poor levator ani function, current and former tobacco use, neurologic disease (Parkinson's, dementia, stroke), depression and congestive heart failure (HUNSKAAR et al. 2000). Dietary caffeine intake has also been correlated with urge incontinence (ARYA et al. 2000) and alpha-adrenergic agents used for treatment of hypertension have been linked to stress urinary incontinence (MARSHALL and BEEVERS 1996).

The epidemiology of male incontinence is less well studied, but reported risk factors include the following (HUNSKAAR et al. 2000):
- Age
- Lower urinary tract symptoms
- Functional and cognitive impairment
- Neurologic disorders
- Prostatectomy
- Other factors

The incidence of urinary incontinence after a transurethral resection of the prostate (TURP) is about 1%, whereas the rate is higher (5–34%) after radical prostatectomy (Hunskaar et al. 2000).

5.2.2
Types of Urinary Incontinence

In general, storage disorders that result in urinary incontinence are due to a problem where urethral resistance is overcome by the bladder pressures, leading to transient loss of urine. Therefore, urinary incontinence includes problems associated with: (1) a poorly functioning urethra due to loss or support or a weak sphincter muscle; (2) problems that cause increased internal bladder pressures, such as from contraction of the bladder detrusor muscle; or (3) external pressures generated from increased abdominal pressure that is transmitted to the bladder in excess of urethral resistance. Disorders of bladder emptying can also result in urinary incontinence: when the bladder becomes overfilled due to poor emptying, small increases in abdominal pressure or small bladder contractions can result in overflow incontinence. In the following sections the different types of incontinence are briefly discussed and defined. Further testing and treatment of the less common types of incontinence are discussed with definitions of these conditions. More extensive discussion follows in subsequent sections on the more common conditions of stress urinary incontinence and urge incontinence (overactive bladder).

5.2.2.1
Disorders of the Urethral/Bladder Neck

The outlet of the bladder is important in the normal control of urine storage. The control of bladder storage of urine relies on an intact neuromuscular control of the bladder. Neuromuscular control must regulate relaxation of the bladder detrusor muscle, while the bladder outlet provides resistance through contraction of the urethral sphincter muscle. In addition, support mechanisms maintain the urethrovesical neck in a stable position, including passive ligamentous support and active muscular support of the bladder neck (STROHBEHN and DELANCEY 1997).

5.2.2.1.1
Stress Urinary Incontinence

Stress urinary incontinence is the loss of urine from the urethra synchronous with coughing, sneezing or physical exertion (BLAIVAS et al. 1997). Stress urinary incontinence can be due to a poorly functioning urethral sphincter muscle, termed "intrinsic sphincter deficiency" (ISD) or due to hypermobility of the bladder neck, implying loss of the active supports (neurologic innervation and pelvic floor muscles) and/or connective tissue supports (passive supports) (STROHBEHN 1998; STROHBEHN and DELANCEY 1997). While it is common to artificially categorize the two conditions into separate entities there is a continuum, as is noted in Chapter 4.5. Many subjects who have urinary incontinence have elements of both a urethral sphincter problem and a bladder neck mobility problem. Additionally, some women have loss of urethral support, but are able to maintain continence due to a normally functioning urethra.

Subjects who have low urethral resistance are more likely to leak easily. This is the premise on which leak point pressures (Chapter 4.5) are established. Subjects who leak almost continuously or who leak with stress events at very low volumes (MCLENNAN and BENT 1998) are more likely to have intrinsic sphincter deficiency.

5.2.2.2
Disorders of the Bladder

Bladder abnormalities that can result in urinary incontinence are generally disorders of the bladder detrusor muscle, and/or its innervation. There is a move to simplify the definitions of different types of detrusor dysfunction and the term "overactive bladder" has been used over the past several years to simplify the problems of a bladder that contracts involuntarily (ABRAMS and WEIN 1999). BLAIVAS et al. (1997) has previously reviewed definitions of the following overactive bladder abnormalities that lead to urinary incontinence and subsequently has emphasized the importance of maintaining precise definitions (BLAIVAS 1999):

- *Detrusor overactivity:* a generic term to describe involuntary bladder contractions.
- *Detrusor instability:* involuntary contractions that are not due to a neurologic disorder.
- *Detrusor hyperreflexia:* involuntary contractions that are due to a neurologic condition.

5.2.2.3
Mixed Urinary Incontinence

It is foolhardy to believe that we can codify incontinence into distinct categories without overlap, and many subjects have both stress urinary incontinence and urge incontinence. Epidemiologic studies suggest that by symptoms, 48% of subjects have stress incontinence, 17% have urge incontinence and 34% have mixed incontinence (HUNSKAAR et al. 2000). SANDVIK et al. (1995) validated questions in a survey with urodynamic testing and found that stress incontinence in their population increased from 51% to 77%, urge incontinence increased from 10% to 12% and mixed incontinence was reduced from 39% to 11%.

5.2.2.4
Overflow Incontinence

Overflow incontinence refers to incontinence due to an overdistended bladder that usually has a relatively atonic detrusor muscle. In this circumstance, the patient may leak because of increased abdominal pressure forcing urine out of the over-distended bladder, or because of small detrusor contractions that cause continued small amounts of leakage, even at rest (detrusor hyperreflexia with impaired contractility, or DHIC). In general, overflow incontinence is due to neuropathologic conditions that result in loss of normal detrusor contractility and the term "neurogenic bladder" is often used synonymously. However, overflow incontinence can also be the result of obstruction at the outlet. Obstruction is most commonly from an enlarged prostate in men, or as a complication of incontinence surgery in women. In women, prolapse of the anterior vaginal wall can cause kinking of the bladder neck, resulting in relative obstruction. The mainstay of treatment for overflow incontinence due to a poorly functioning detrusor muscle is catheterization. If a patient is considered suitable, clean intermittent self-catheterization is taught. For women, if there is obstruction at the bladder neck from a prior anti-incontinence procedure, the obstruction can be successfully released with resumption of normal voiding in about 60% (BENT and McLENNAN 1998). Others have reported successful resumption of voiding in up to 93.5% (AMUNDSEN et al. 2000). For non-obstructive urinary retention, a new therapeutic option is sacral neuromodulation (JONAS et al. 2001; SIEGEL et al. 2000), which is described below.

5.2.2.5
Functional/Cognitive Incontinence

Functional incontinence refers to incontinence that is due to other medical problems that limit the patient's ability to get to the bathroom in a timely manner. Medical problems such as arthritis or other neurologic conditions can lead to urinary incontinence, simply due to decreased mobility. This is an important consideration, because these individuals would be expected to have normal bladder function on urodynamic testing. The diagnosis is usually established by history and physical evaluation. Treatment may be as simple as prescribing a bedside commode and focusing on ameliorating symptoms that limit the patient's mobility.

Cognitive incontinence is common among patients with dementia who simply forget to go to the bathroom and are not aware of their bladder fullness. Again, the diagnosis can frequently be established by history and examination. Treatment is primarily prompted voiding and special attention by caregivers to maintain hygiene.

5.2.2.6
Extraurethral Incontinence

Extraurethral urinary incontinence refers to urine loss other than from the urethra meatus. Examples include vesicovaginal, uterovaginal, ureterovaginal and urethrovaginal fistulae, as well as ectopic ureter. Presenting symptoms usually include continuous leakage throughout the day and night without correlation to stress or urge symptoms. The incontinence is often a result of a surgical complication and this is established by history. The other common source of fistulae is from obstetric trauma, although this is a much more significant problem in underdeveloped countries (DANSO et al. 1996).

The diagnosis is usually confirmed with examination of the vagina. Vesicovaginal fistulae may be diagnosed with a tampon placed in the vagina and retrograde instillation of methylene blue or indigo-carmine into the bladder via a catheter. The patient ambulates for 30 min and if blue dye stains the upper tampon, a vesicovaginal fistula is suspected. If the test is negative, a similar test can be performed, but with administration of oral pyridium or intravenous indigocarmine to look for staining of the tampon with orange or blue, respectively. In the setting of a negative bladder test for a fistula, staining with the second test is consistent with a ureterovaginal fistula. Diagnosis can be supplemented with cystoscopy, retrograde cystography, voiding cystourethrography and intravenous pyelography. Hysterosalpingography is useful to establish the diagnosis of a vesicouterine fistula (HURT 2000), which most commonly might occur after cesarean section or rarely after vaginal birth following cesarean section.

Treatment of fistulae is usually surgical, with reported successful repair rates in the range 67–100% (BLAIVAS et al. 1995).

5.2.3
Clinical Evaluation

As mentioned in Chapter 4.5, the evaluation of the incontinent subject relies on accurate history taking, a focused physical examination, and consideration of adjunctive testing, such as urodynamics.

5.2.3.1
History

The history for evaluation of urinary incontinence focuses on whether the individual's primary concern is due to insufficient urethral resistance or due to an overactive detrusor muscle or both, as these are the most common two types of incontinence. It is especially important to establish the chronicity of the incontinent episodes in relationship to other activities. Establishing the timing and frequency of these episodes is often best determined with a voiding diary, as described in Chapter 4.5. Patients who leak at night are more likely to have a detrusor-related problem, whereas those who leak only while ambulatory are more likely to have stress incontinence. It is also important to assess the impact of the problem on the patient's quality of life. Questions about pad usage, restriction of exercise or other activities, including coitus, help determine the impact of incontinence on the patient. As mentioned above, individuals surveyed in a general survey are more likely to volunteer symptoms of urinary incontinence but when asked if they are bothersome, many indicate these symptoms do not impact their lifestyle greatly. In comparing a survey of subjects seen in a general practice to a subspecialty practice where the individuals have been referred specifically for the evaluation of urinary incontinence, it is also more likely that the general practice patients will not indicate that their symptoms are severe or bothersome.

Questions about incontinence of stool or flatus should be addressed, as the prevalence of dual incontinence of anal incontinence among women with urinary incontinence has been reported to be as high as 31% (Jackson et al. 1997). Questions about prolapse symptoms should also be addressed.

The past medical history should be explored, especially conditions that limit mobility, neurologic function and normal comprehension. Prior bladder problems such as recurrent urinary tract infections, stones or malignancy are addressed. Coexistent conditions such as congestive heart failure, diabetes or back problems are noted. Congestive heart failure and resultant dependent peripheral edema can lead to nocturia as the third-spaced fluids return to circulation when the individual is recumbent at night. Prior pelvic surgeries including hysterectomy, bladder and bowel surgeries are reviewed. Obstetrical events are also reviewed to determine vaginal parity, the largest birthweight and whether or not forceps were utilized during delivery.

In one series, clinical diagnosis of urinary incontinence with history and physical examination alone was accurate in only 65% of cases when compared to a urodynamic diagnosis (Jarvis et al. 1980). As mentioned above, when the treatment plan is conservative, it is unlikely that harm could be inflicted when empiric therapy is based on history if the postvoid residual and urinalysis are negative.

There are also several validated questionnaires for determining the life quality and symptom distress of women with urinary incontinence. The Incontinence Impact Questionnaire (IIQ) includes 30 questions that assess the effects on life quality, including effects on emotional health, physical activity, travel, daily living activities, sexual activity and sleep (Wyman et al. 1987). The Urogenital Distress Inventory (UDI) uses 19 questions to assess the types of symptoms that the subject is experiencing (Wyman et al. 1987). Short forms of both the IIQ and UDI have been developed and validated that include only seven and six questions, respectively (Ubersax et al. 1995). While these questionnaires do not correlate well with urodynamic diagnoses (Fitzgerald and Brubaker 2002; Lemack and Zimmern 1999), the twin paradigm above (DeLancey and Wall 1995) illustrates how important the subjective aspects of urinary incontinence are in measuring outcomes.

5.2.3.2
Physical Examination

A targeted clinical examination includes an examination of the back, abdomen, pelvis, rectum and distal extremities. In the back examination evidence of paraspinal tenderness, costovertebral angle tenderness, asymmetry or surgical scars are investigated. The abdominal examination focuses on whether there are masses, suprapubic tenderness or surgical scars. On pelvic examination, the urethral meatus is inspected for irritation or prolapse of the mucosa. The bladder neck is assessed to determine if there is excessive mobility. A cotton swab test can help identify if hypermobility is present. A sterile swab is lubricated with sterile gel or, preferably, a topical anesthetic gel and inserted into the urethra after sterile preparation of the urethral meatus. It is then withdrawn until resistance is met at the bladder neck. The mobility is determined by looking at the resting angle and straining angle of the swab. Greater than 30 degree excursion is consistent with hypermobility, but it is important to remember that this does not confirm that the patient's incontinence is due solely to a mobility problem. Many women have hypermobility of the bladder neck without incontinence.

Other important aspects of the pelvic examination are whether or not there is concomitant prolapse of other vaginal tissues or the uterus, and how strong the levator ani are.

Rectal examination is performed to assess normal sphincter tone and integrity. A normal sphincter tone and ability to contract the levator ani suggest an intact innervation to the pelvic floor through sacral roots S2–4. Distal extremity examination focuses on normal innervation and sensory dermatomes for the sacral nerve roots, and to rule out peripheral edema.

5.2.4
Further Testing

The decision of what additional testing is required is, in part, determined by what recommendations are considered for treatment. If the patient has a strong history of stress urinary incontinence and an examination consistent with hypermobility of the bladder neck, but the patient desires to try conservative treatments such as pelvic floor exercises, then urodynamic testing is less likely to be of value. As discussed in Chapter 4.5, many advocate urodynamic testing if surgical treatment for stress incontinence is considered, but the cost of testing is high and simple testing may provide enough information to make a decision on treatment, especially for uncomplicated cases (WEBER and WALTERS 2000). The Agency for Health Care Policy and Research incontinence guidelines suggest the following criteria for establishing when to proceed with further evaluation (FANTL et al. 1996):

- Uncertain diagnosis and inability to develop a reasonable treatment plan based on the diagnostic evaluation. Uncertainty in diagnosis may occur when there is lack of correlation between symptoms and clinical findings.
- Failure to respond to the patient's satisfaction to an adequate therapeutic trial, and the patient is interested in pursuing further therapy.
- Consideration of surgical intervention, particularly if previous surgery failed or the patient is a high surgical risk.
- Hematuria without infection.
- The presence of comorbid conditions:
  - Incontinence associated with recurrent symptomatic urinary tract infections
  - Persistent symptoms or difficult bladder emptying
  - History of previous anti-incontinence surgery or radical pelvic surgery
  - Beyond hymen and symptomatic pelvic prolapse
  - Prostate nodule, asymmetry, or other suspicion of prostate cancer
  - Abnormal postvoid residual (PVR) urine
  - Neurologic condition, such as multiple sclerosis and spinal cord lesions or injury.

Determination of the postvoid residual and a urinalysis are a requirement for evaluation of all patients with incontinence. Overflow incontinence can mimic either stress incontinence or urge incontinence and empiric treatment of stress or urge incontinence without first ruling out overflow incontinence could worsen the condition.

5.2.5
Treatment Options

In general, approach to the incontinent patient should progress from conservative treatment to more aggressive treatment. Scheduled follow-up evaluation is crucial to prevent the patient from thinking they have been abandoned or that all treatment options have been exhausted (URINARY INCONTINENCE GUIDELINE PANEL 1992).

Therapy should focus on ameliorating the subject's most bothersome symptoms. A patient with mixed urinary incontinence may describe leaking related to a sudden urge and loss of control, but also leakage with coughing and exercise. If surgery is performed to treat the stress incontinence on a patient in whom the urge symptoms predominate, the patient will obviously be distressed if, as is often the case, the urge symptoms worsen after the surgery. A discussion of treatment options follows.

Where possible, the outcome data from studies available from multicenter trials with evidence-based medicine are cited, including the Cochrane Database of Systematic Reviews. Ideally, outcome studies should address the different measures of urinary incontinence available (LOSE et al. 2001):
- Patient observations (symptoms)
- Quantification of symptoms (bladder diary, pad-weighing tests)
- Clinician's observations (examination, urodynamics)
- Quality of life measures (SF-36, IIQ, UDS questionnaires)
- Socioeconomic costs (cost-effectiveness)

5.2.5.1
Behavioral Treatment

Behavioral therapy is the term for several different therapeutic interventions that are available to treat both stress and urge urinary incontinence. Treatment options that are included under behavioral treatment of stress urinary incontinence include all forms of pelvic floor muscle training (PFMT), including unsupervised exercises, supervised exercises, biofeedback, vaginal weights, and electrical stimulation. Behavioral treatment options to treat urge urinary incontinence include: PFMT (including biofeedback, vaginal weights, electrical stimulation), and habit training. The Cochrane Database of Systemic Reviews currently includes 43 studies which were randomized trials using PFMT (Hay-Smith et al. 2002).

5.2.5.1.1
Pelvic Floor Muscle Training

For the treatment of urinary incontinence, the mainstay of behavioral treatment is pelvic floor rehabilitation. Pelvic floor muscle exercises, also called "Kegel's exercises" (Kegel 1948, 1951), are performed repetitively during the day to improve the muscle tone of the pelvic floor and provide improved support to the bladder neck. The optimal frequency and duration of contractions that are optimal for improved outcome has not been determined (Hay-Smith et al. 2002). There is one randomized study that suggests there is no difference in outcome when urodynamic testing is used to establish the diagnosis before initiation of pelvic muscle exercises (Ramsay et al. 1996). Analyzing the combined studies included in the Cochrane Database of Systemic Reviews, pelvic floor muscle exercises are found to subjectively cure or improve urinary incontinence when compared to placebo (relative risk 23.04, 95% confidence interval 7.56–70.22) (Hay-Smith et al. 2002).

There are several innovative ways to improve PFMT. These include the use of vaginal weighted cones, biofeedback with vaginal or anal probes to assess strength, electrical stimulation of the levator ani muscles, also using vaginal or anal probes, and magnetic coil stimulation of the muscles. The Cochrane Database indicates that neither weighted vaginal cones nor electrical stimulation improve the outcome of PFMT exercises considerably. "PFMT appeared to be consistently better than no treatment and placebo treatments for women with both stress and/or mixed incontinence. Few side effects of PFMT were noted and all were minor and easily reversible.

There is some evidence to support the widespread recommendation that PFMT should be offered as first line conservative management to women with stress and/or mixed incontinence" (Hay-Smith et al. 2002).

5.2.5.1.1.1
Stress Incontinence

The majority of the trials in the Cochrane Database of Systemic Reviews for PFMT were for treatment of stress urinary incontinence or mixed urinary incontinence. There are currently 31 trials in the Cochrane Database that compared pelvic floor muscle training in subjects with stress urinary incontinence (Hay-Smith et al. 2002). As noted above, PFMT was felt to be of benefit when compared to placebo. In addition, one study identified that teaching the "knack" of precontracting the pelvic floor in anticipation of a cough substantially reduced the incontinence in a short period of time (Miller et al. 1998). The trials comparing pelvic floor exercises to surgery were limited, but there were improved self-reported cures among those undergoing surgery (Hay-Smith et al. 2002; Klarsov et al. 1991).

5.2.5.1.1.2
Urge Incontinence

Only a few trials in the Cochrane Database of Systemic Reviews for PFMT compared treatment of isolated urge incontinence or detrusor instability (Burgio et al. 1998; Nygaard et al. 1996; Wyman et al. 1988). There were not enough subjects to conclude the efficacy of PFMT for the treatment of detrusor instability (Hay-Smith et al. 2002).

5.2.5.1.1.3
Mixed Incontinence

Mixed incontinence is usually included with stress urinary incontinence in the Cochrane Database of Systemic Reviews for PFMT. The conclusions reached are the same as those noted for stress urinary incontinence (Hay-Smith et al. 2002).

5.2.5.1.2
Bladder Training

Bladder training, often called behavioral training, involves reeducating voluntary control of the bladder. "Bladder training aims to increase the time interval between voiding, either by a mandatory or self adjusted schedule, so that incontinence is ultimately avoided and continence regained" (Roe et al. 2002). Each week the patient is instructed to increase the time between voids by 15 minutes. The interval goal between voids may differ for different individuals, but would ideally be to void every 3–4 hours without loss of control. Other terms for bladder training include "bladder retraining" or "bladder drills". In general, bladder training is used to treat subjects with urge incontinence or mixed incontinence. The Cochrane Database of Systemic Reviews for bladder training identified seven trials that were acceptable for review and were last reviewed in 1999. There is a trend towards improvement of symptoms with bladder training, but the authors caution that the outcome measurements and definitions differed greatly amongst the studies. Addition of pharmacologic agents did not improve the treatment of urge incontinence when bladder training was the primary treatment.

5.2.5.1.3
Habit Retraining

Habit retraining is prescribed to assess an individual's normal voiding pattern. It is generally used for institutionalized subjects who have cognitive or functional impairments contributing to their incontinence (Hadley 1986). "It involves identification of an incontinent person's individualized toileting pattern and development of a toileting schedule which pre-empts involuntary bladder emptying by decreasing voiding intervals, while aiming to keep intervals as long as possible without incontinence" (Ostaszkiewicz et al. 2002). In one randomized controlled study of nursing home patients, improvement in urinary incontinence was seen in 86% of subjects (Colling et al. 1992). Prompted voiding is a similar technique, in which the caregiver reminds the individual when to void, with good results in terms of reduction of incontinent events (Eustice et al. 2002; Fantl et al. 1996). Timed voiding is the same as prompted voiding, but the individual is asked to void whether or not they have the sensation of fullness (Anders 2000).

5.2.5.2
Pharmacologic Treatment

Pharmacologic management of urinary incontinence relies on the neurophysiology of continence. To treat bladder overactivity, antimuscarinic drugs, alpha-adrenoceptor antagonists, beta-adrenoceptor agonists, and prostaglandin synthesis inhibitors are used (Andersson 2000). In addition, several other agents are under investigation, including serotonin reuptake inhibitors, as well as intravesical agents (Fowler 2000). In general, pharmacologic interventions for the management of urge incontinence focus on peripheral or central nervous system-mediated relaxation of the detrusor muscle. The most common drug used is an anticholinergic agent. Newer anticholinergic agents such as extended-release oxybutynin (Gleason et al. 1999) and tolterodine extended release have improved side effect profiles, with less common dry mouth and constipation than oxybutynin. Reductions in incontinent episodes by up to 77% have been described in a randomized placebo-controlled study with tolterodine extended release (Van Kerrebroeck et al. 2001).

For the treatment of stress urinary incontinence, alpha-adrenergic agents increase the tone of the urethral sphincter and may help with mild stress urinary incontinence. For mixed urinary incontinence, imipramine has properties of both an anticholinergic agent and an alpha-adrenergic agent and thus may allow simultaneous detrusor relaxation and increased urethral sphincter tone.

There are seven proposed Cochrane Databases proposed for reviewing anticholinergic agents, alpha-adrenergic agents and estrogens in the management of urinary incontinence. At present, all seven database protocols are in the development stage.

5.2.5.3
Surgical Treatment

Surgical treatment should be considered when conservative measures fail. In general, surgery is reserved for the treatment of stress urinary incontinence, but a few surgical options for treatment of urge incontinence are mentioned below. For the management of stress urinary incontinence, hundreds of operations have been described (Bent and McLennan 1998), but they essentially fall into five categories (Table 5.2.1) Over the past one or two decades, it has been the trend that the surgical approach should depend upon the urodynamic diagnosis. A decision tree is shown in Fig. 5.2.2, which summarizes different approaches to the management of urinary incontinence. As noted in Chapter 4.5, subjects with evidence of intrinsic sphincter deficiency on urodynamic testing have higher failure rates when treated with a support operation (Bowen et al. 1989; McGuire 1981; Sand et al. 1987).

Table 5.2.1. Surgical approaches to treat stress urinary incontinence

Anatomic deficiency	Surgical approach	Procedure name
Bladder neck hypermobility	Vaginal	Kelly plication (suburethral plication, pubourethral ligament suspension)
	Vaginal needle	Needle urethropexy (Stamey, Raz, Pereyra procedures)
		Tension-free vaginal tape
	Abdominal	Retropubic urethropexy (colposuspension)
		Burch procedure
		Marshall-Marchetti-Krantz procedure
		Paravaginal defect repair
Intrinsic sphincter deficiency	Transurethral/periurethral injections	Bulking agent injectables (bovine collagen, polytetrafluoroethylene, pyrolytic carbon beads, autologous fat or chondrocytes)
	Abdominal/vaginal	Autologous pubovaginal sling procedures (rectus abdominis fascia, fascia lata)
		Allograft slings (cadaveric)
		Synthetic slings
		Mesh
		Tension-free vaginal tape

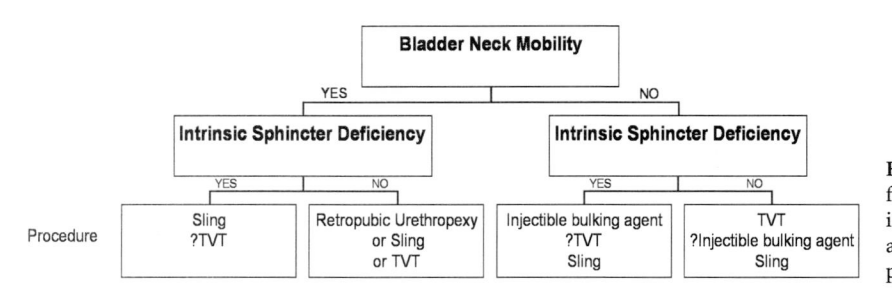

Fig. 5.2.2. Decision analysis tree for surgical treatment of stress incontinence (adapted from BENT and MCLELLAN 1998, p. 884, with permission)

5.2.5.3.1
Anterior Colporrhaphy

Anterior colporrhaphy is not considered an effective treatment of stress urinary incontinence. A Cochrane Database of Systematic Reviews identified eight randomized studies comparing anterior vaginal repair to open abdominal retropubic suspension. The authors found both short-term and long-term failure rates to be significantly higher with anterior colporrhaphy (Table 5.2.2) (GLAZENER and COOPER 2002).

Table 5.2.2. Summary of eight studies comparing subjective outcomes of anterior colporrhaphy with open retropubic urethropexy (data from Glazener and Cooper 2002)

	Failure rate (%)		Relative risk	95% confidence interval
	Anterior colporrhaphy	Open retropubic suspension		
First year	29	14	1.89	1.39–2.59
After first year	41	17	2.50	1.92–3.26

Anterior colporrhaphy is an appropriate procedure to treat midline defects of the anterior vaginal wall resulting in a cystocele.

5.2.5.3.2
Needle Urethropexy

Needle urethropexies have previously been a common procedure to treat stress urinary incontinence. There are several named modifications as noted in Table 5.2.1. A needle is passed bilaterally alongside the bladder neck from the abdominal approach, through the Space of Retzius. Sutures at the bladder neck are brought back through the Space of Retzius and attached to the abdominal wall. Poor long-term success rates (BERGMAN and ELIA 1995) have led to this procedure being performed rarely.

5.2.5.3.3
Abdominal Retropubic Urethropexy (Colposuspension)

For hypermobility of the bladder neck with a normally functioning urethra, an open retropubic urethropexy has been considered the standard of care over the past several decades. There are two common approaches: the Burch colposuspension (BURCH 1961, 1968) and the Marshall-Marchetti-Krantz procedure (MARSHALL et al. 1949). Both operations rely on placing sutures abdominally at the bladder neck after dissection of the Space of Retzius. For the Burch operation, two permanent sutures are placed at each side of the bladder neck. The sutures are all anchored to Cooper's ligament, with each passed through the ipsilateral side (Fig. 5.2.3). For the Marshall-Marchetti-Krantz procedure, on to three pairs of nonabsorbable sutures are placed at the bladder neck which is then sutured to the cartilage at the symphysis pubis.

Open retropubic suspensions have had success rates of 85–90% at 1 year, and a 10-year objective cure rate of over 70% (BENT and MCLENNAN 1998). The 5-year cure rates for surgical treatment of stress urinary incontinence have been compared in a randomized trial, comparing anterior colporrhaphy, needle suspensions and the Burch procedure (BERGMANN and ELIA 1995). The objective urodynamic success rates among patients who received these procedures at 5 years was 37%, 43%, and 82%, respectively and the decline in the success rate after the first year was 26%, 22%, and 7%, respectively, in 4 years.

Complications for retropubic suspensions are summarized in Table 5.2.3 (BENT and MCLENNAN 1998). Radiologic imaging can assist in ruling out complications of a hematoma, abscess, or ureteral or bladder injury. Additionally, imaging can assist

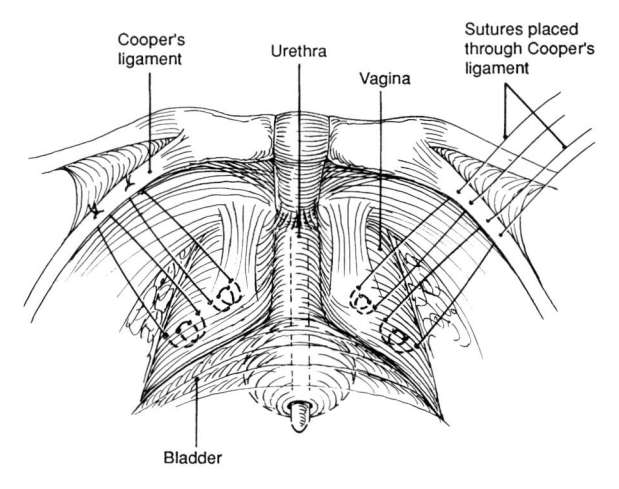

Fig. 5.2.3. Burch retropubic urethropexy. Bilateral pairs of permanent sutures are placed in the paravaginal fascia to support the anterior vaginal wall at the level of the bladder neck. Each suture is anchored to Cooper's ligament on the ipsilateral side (with permission, CHEN and HORBACH 1997)

in ruling out osteitis pubis or osteomyelitis as a complication from the Marshall-Marchetti-Krantz procedure (LENTZ 1995).

5.2.5.3.4
Suburethral Sling

The suburethral sling has traditionally been the operation of choice for the treatment of intrinsic sphincter deficiency and recurrent stress incontinence after a primary operation. There has been a trend towards the use of slings for the primary treatment of stress urinary incontinence, regardless of whether there is hypermobility or intrinsic sphincter deficiency (BEZERRA and BRUSCHINI 2002; GROUTZ et al. 2001). There are vari-

Table 5.2.3. Complications of retropubic suspension (adapted from BENT and MCLELLAN 1998, p. 887, with permission)

Intraoperative	Acute postoperative	Chronic postoperative
Hemorrhage	Fever	Urinary retention
Injury to adjacent structures	Infection	Voiding dysfunction
Ureter	Anemia	De novo detrusor instability
Bladder	Hematoma	Chronic urinary tract infections
Obturator nerve	Urinary tract infection	
Obturator vessels	Urinoma	Pelvic organ prolapse
Femoral nerve	Ileus	Persistent urinary incontinence
Femoral vessels	Catheter obstruction	
	Deep venous thrombosis	Abscess
	Pulmonary	Pain
	Cardiac	

ous sling materials that have been utilized, including autologous fascial grafts from the rectus abdominis muscle or the fascia lata. Cadaveric fascia lata allograft has been also been utilized. Several reports have indicated cure rates as low as 33.3–72.2% with cadaveric allografts (HUANG et al. 2001; SOERGEL et al. 2001), whereas others have noted success rates similar to that of autologous fascia (BROWN and GOVIER 2000), but with less postoperative pain (FLYNN and YAP 2002). Synthetic materials have also been used for slings, with some reports of erosion of the material into the vagina, bladder or urethra (BARBALIAS et al. 1997; CLEMENS et al. 2000; YOUNG et al. 2001). The slings can be secured to the rectus abdominis fascia, Cooper's ligament, or the pubic bone itself with bone anchors (BENT and MCLENNAN 1998).

Complications from slings include many of the complications listed in Table 5.2.3 for the retropubic suspensions. Urinary retention, voiding complications and de novo detrusor instability have been reported as higher than with retropubic suspensions in the older literature (BENT and MCLENNAN 1998; BEZERRA and BRUSCHINI 2002), but in newer literature, these complication rates are comparable to the retropubic suspension (CHAIKIN et al. 1998). Other complications include erosions of sling material into the urethra, bladder and vagina. The erosion rates are higher with synthetic materials than with autologous materials.

5.2.5.3.5
Tension-Free Vaginal Tape

A variant of the sling procedure, the tension-free vaginal tape, or TVT, has become very popular in the treatment of stress urinary incontinence for women. A synthetic polypropylene mesh is positioned at the mid urethra rather than at the bladder neck for the pubovaginal sling procedures. The polypropylene tape is then directed under the symphysis pubis via a large curved needle to a small incision in the abdominal wall on each side of the urethra. The tape is adjusted with the subject awake and does not require suturing as the mesh stays in place once a protective plastic sleeve is removed. The tension is adjusted prior to moving these sleeves with a full bladder and the patient coughing. Tension is tightened just to the point where leakage stops.

In one multicenter, randomized study, the success of the TVT was similar to the open retropubic urethropexy (WARD et al. 2000). In that series, quite varying success rates, which were dependent upon subjective reporting (no stress incontinence, reporting of cure) or objective testing (negative 1-hour pad testing, cystometrogram) were reported. The cure rates ranged from 38% to 89% depending upon which outcome measure was used to determine success. Another series of 49 women with intrinsic sphincter deficiency reported a 74% cure rate for complete cure of any incontinence, with 90% reporting improved quality of life (REZAPOUR et al. 2001).

Advantages of TVT are that it is usually performed under regional or local anesthesia with short operating times and quicker recovery time. Complications are similar to those reported for slings and retropubic suspensions, including voiding dysfunction and urinary retention at a lower rate. Bladder injury occurs in 2–24% of TVT procedures, usually during placement of the needles into the Space of Retzius (LEBRET et al. 2001; NIEMCZYK et al. 2001; REZAPOUR et al. 2001). Injuries are usually not a problem if recognized intraoperatively with replacement of the needle and temporary drainage of the bladder and lessen with experience of the surgeon (LEBRET et al. 2001). There have been reports of bowel injury (TAMUSSINO et al. 2001), vascular injury and/or retropubic hematomas, obturator nerve injury (MESCHIA et al. 2001), and mesh erosion into the bladder or urethra (MADJAR et al. 2002; PITS 2002). One of the largest series of patients is from the Austrian registry, which reported a reoperation rate of 68/2795 women (2.4%) who underwent the TVT procedure.

5.2.5.3.6
Urethral Bulking Agents

In the presence of intrinsic sphincter deficiency without urethral hypermobility, the surgical treatment of choice has traditionally been periurethral injection of a bulking agent (BENT and MCLENNAN 1998; HORBACH 1997). Bulking agents have also been used with moderate success in subjects with urethral hypermobility who want to avoid major surgery (BENT et al. 2001b). More recently, success with the use of TVT for treatment of intrinsic sphincter deficiency has been reported (REZAPOUR et al. 2001).

A urethral injection is performed at the submucosa of the bladder neck and can be performed as a transurethral injection via a cystourethroscope (Fig. 5.2.4) or as a periurethral injection using a needle adjacent to the urethra (Fig. 5.2.5). Several agents have been used, including bovine collagen (Contigen Implant; C.R. Bard, Covington, Ga.), polytetrafluoroethylene (Teflon; Dupont Co., Wilmington, De.), silicone, pyrolytic carbon-coated zirconium oxide beads (Durasphere; Advanced Uroscience, St. Paul, Minn.), and autologous fat or chondrocytes (BENT

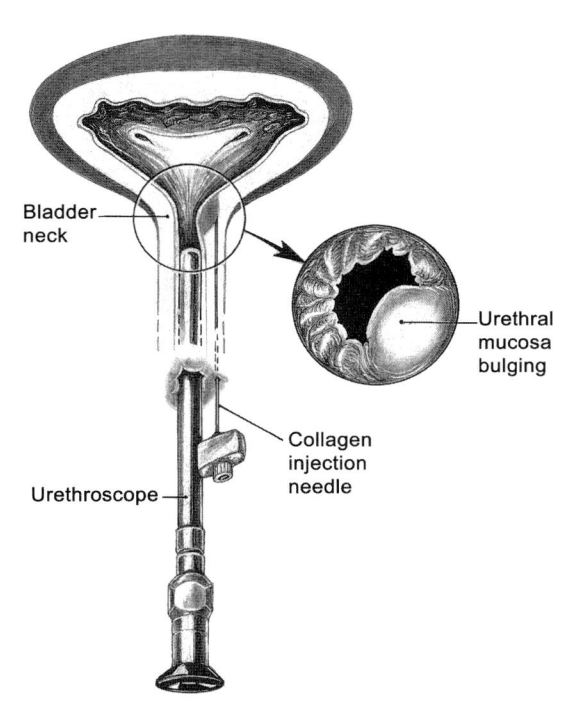

Fig. 5.2.4. Transurethral collagen injection. Collagen is injected through a port on the cystourethroscope at the level of the bladder neck. Injection is shown at 2 o'clock and would continue at other sites until the mucosa coapts from each side (with permission BENT 1997, p. 54)

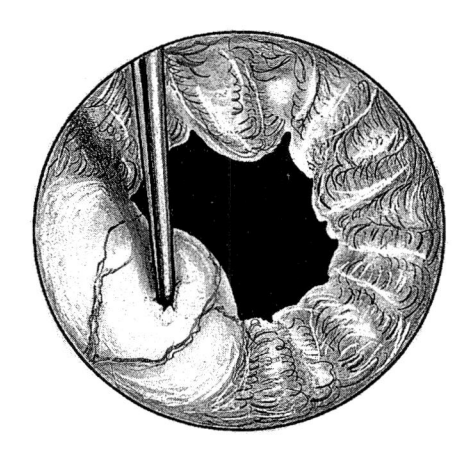

Fig. 5.2.5. Periurethral collagen injection (with permission, BENT 1997, p. 52)

et al. 2001a). Currently, silicone and Teflon are not FDA-approved in the United States, due to concerns about migration of the material to other organs. Autologous fat has a high initial reported success rate, but the effect diminishes over time, probably due to reabsorption of the fat (BENT and McLENNAN 1998). The risks of urinary retention are minimal with bulking agents, but the success rates are also lower than with many of the other procedures with an overall cure rate reported at 20–30%, but with another 50–60% of subjects noting marked improvement (BENT and McLENNAN 1998). Repeat injections are often performed over time with similar results to the primary injection if the bulking agent seems to have lost effectiveness. Periurethral bulking agents have been reported to have some success in treating male subjects with post-prostatectomy urinary incontinence.

5.2.5.3.7
Artificial Urethral Sphincter

Artificial urethral sphincters have been utilized to treat women with no hypermobility and intrinsic sphincter deficiency who fail periurethral injectable bulking agents and sling procedures (BENT and McLENNAN 1998). The procedure has been used to treat men with post-prostatectomy urinary incontinence. An artificial sphincter is placed around the urethra and a reservoir allows the sphincter to be inflated to maintain continence, and then deflated to allow emptying. Success rates for the treatment of post-prostatectomy subjects are approximately 80%, but reoperation rates approach 50% for the treatment of complications including infection and malfunction (CLEMENS et al. 2001). A recent review of 207 women treated with an artificial sphincter for intrinsic sphincter deficiency without mobility showed success in 88.7% with a reoperation rate of 5.9% (COSTA et al. 2001).

5.2.5.3.8
Surgical Approaches for Detrusor Instability

As mentioned above, surgical treatment of detrusor instability is limited to rare cases where the symptoms persist despite traditional pharmacologic and behavioral interventions. Over the past decade, sacral neuromodulation has been used to treat subjects resistant to traditional pharmacologic and behavioral approaches. Sacral neuromodulation involves implantation of a wire lead to the sacral nerve roots that innervate the bladder (SIEGEL et al. 2000). The subjects who have improvement with a test wire have implantation of a permanent wire and pack, similar to a pacemaker, but applied at the sacral nerve roots. Almost 60% of subjects have been shown to have a greater than 50% reduction in leaking episodes.

Other surgical procedures for the treatment of detrusor instability include an augmentation cystoplasty, also called clam cystoplasty, where a segment of gut is interposed in the bladder. This causes the detrusor muscle to be ineffective during contraction and as a result, many subjects will need to use intermittent self-catheterization to empty afterwards. Other long-term complications with this procedure include fluid/electrolyte disturbances, bladder stones, tumors and diarrhea (VENN and MUNDY 2000). Other approaches have included continent urinary reservoirs from a neobladder, usually constructed from gut and with a stoma through the abdominal skin. One other procedure described by INGELMAN-SUNBERG involves denervation of the bladder detrusor muscle (INGELMAN-SUNDBERG 1975) or phenol injection to destroy the innervation at the trigone. The latter procedure has only a 14% cure rate in longer term follow-up and vesicovaginal fistulas have been reported, so this procedure has been essentially abandoned (RAMSAY et al. 1992).

5.2.5.4
Other Management Options

5.2.5.4.1
Absorbent Products

While bothersome, many subjects with urinary incontinence elect to manage their symptoms with the use of absorbent pads. The data concerning the use of absorbent products are limited despite the high prevalence of use. A series of Swedish women who were using home delivery and free provision of incontinence pads were surveyed regarding their incontinence pad use. Of the women surveyed, 24% used pads as the primary solution to their problem of incontinence and did not desire further evaluation by a health-care provider or consideration of a trial of curative treatments (KINN and ZAAR 1998). Menstrual pads are more commonly used to manage incontinence and less expensive than incontinence pads (MCCLISH et al. 1999). However, despite their higher cost, superabsorbent disposable urinary pads have been shown to perform better than other products, including nondisposable products (BRAZZELLI et al. 2002).

5.2.5.4.2
Mechanical Devices

Mechanical devices have also been used to treat urinary incontinence and can be divided into three categories:
1. Intraurethral devices
2. Vaginal support devices
3, Extraurethral covering shields

The intraurethral devices have a median corrected cured/improved rate of 43%, with a high rate of urinary tract infections (VIERHOUT and LOSE 1997). These are primarily devices that are inserted into the urethra and secured in place with a balloon, similar to a Foley catheter balloon. They are disposable and after each void, a new one is inserted. Hematuria and migration of the device into the bladder are also reported complications. Vaginal devices include tampons, contraceptive diaphragms, bladder neck prosthetic devices and pessaries. Mean corrected cured/improved rates are 63% for several different devices (VIERHOUT and LOSE 1997). Side effects include vaginal discharge, pelvic pressure and sexual problems. The last category includes urethral occlusive devices for women that are applied by the patient. One type uses a suction cap that is squeezed and fitted over the urethral meatus. Silicone gel helps maintain the seal and it is removed for voiding (MOORE et al. 1999). Another device is a pad applied over the urethral meatus that seals the urethra.

5.2.6
Summary

There are many treatment options available for the treatment of urinary incontinence, both conservative and surgical. Surgical cure rates are higher for the treatment of stress urinary incontinence than conservative options, but the complication rates are also higher. Treatment planning requires investigation into whether the incontinence is primarily related to urgency and detrusor overactivity versus insufficient resistance at the urethra to be able to compensate for increased intravesical and abdominal pressures. Evaluation of coexistent problems of anal incontinence and/or pelvic organ prolapse is also important. For incontinence among women, there is a continuum between hypermobility of the bladder neck and intrinsic sphincter deficiency. Therefore, surgical therapy for stress incontinence must be directed at what is felt to be the primary cause of the incontinence. The TVT has shown promising results that may be applicable to patients with either hypermobility or intrinsic sphincter deficiency.

References

Abrams P, Wein A (1999) The overactive bladder and incontinence: definitions and a plea for discussion. Neurourol Urodyn 18:413–416

Abrams P, Blaivas J, Stanton S, et al (1988a) The standardisation of terminology of lower urinary tract function. Neurourol Urodyn 7:403–406

Abrams P, Blaivas J, Stanton S, et al (1988b) The standardisation of lower urinary tract function. Scand J Urol Nephrol [Suppl] 114:5–19

Amundsen C, Guralnick M, Webster G (2000) Variations in strategy for the treatment of urethral obstruction after a pubovaginal sling procedure. J Urol 164:434–437

Anders K (2000) Bladder retraining. In: Stanton S, Monga A (eds) Clinical urogynaecology. Churchill Livingstone, London, pp 575–581

Andersson KE (2000) Drug therapy for urinary incontinence. Baillieres Best Pract Res Clin Obstet Gynaecol 14:291–313

Arya L, Myers D, Jackson N (2000) Dietary caffeine intake and the risk for detrusor instability: a case-control study. Obstet Gynecol 96:85–89

Barbalias G, Liatsikos E, Barbalias D (1997) Use of slings made of indigenous and allogenic material (GoreTex) in type III urinary incontinence and comparison between them. Urology 31:394–400

Bent AE (1997) Periurethral collagen injections. Oper Tech Gynecol Surg 2:54

Bent A, McLennan M (1998) Surgical management of urinary incontinence. Obstet Gynecol Clin North Am 25:883–906

Bent A, Tutrone R, McLennan M, et al (2001a) Treatment of intrinsic sphincter deficiency using autologous ear chondrocytes as a bulking agent. Neurourol Urodyn 20:157–165

Bent A, Foote J, Siegel S, et al (2001b) Collagen implant for treating stress incontinence in women with urethral hypermobility. J Urol 166:1354–1357

Bergman A, Elia G (1995) Three surgical procedures for genuine stress urinary incontinence: five year follow-up of a prospective randomized study. Am J Obstet Gynecol 173:66–71

Bezerra C, Bruschini H (2002) Suburethral sling operations for urinary incontinence in women (Cochrane Review). The Cochrane Library, Issue 3. Update Software, Oxford

Blaivas J (1999) Defining words: overactive bladder (editorial). Neurourol Urodyn 18:417–418

Blaivas J, Heritz D, Romanzi L (1995) Early versus late repair of vesicovaginal fistulas: vaginal and abdominal approaches. J Urol 153:1110–1112

Blaivas J, Appell R, Fantl J, et al (1997) Definition and classification of urinary incontinence: recommendations of the Urodynamic Society. Neurourol Urodyn 16:149–151

Bowen L, Sand P, Ostergard D, et al (1989) Unsuccessful Burch retropubic urethropexy: a case-controlled urodynamic study. Am J Obstet Gynecol 160:452–458

Brazzelli M, Shirran E, Vale L (2002) Absorbent products for containing urinary and/or fecal incontinence in adults. J Wound Ostomy Continence Nurs 29:45–54

Brown J, Grady D, Ouslander J, et al (1999) Prevalence of urinary incontinence and associated risk factors in postmenopausal women. Heart and Estrogen/Progestin Replacement Study (HERS) Research Group. Obstet Gynecol 94:66–70

Brown S, Govier F (2000) Cadaveric versus autologous fascia lata for the pubovaginal sling: surgical outcome and patient satisfaction. J Urol 164:1633–1637

Bump R, Norton P (1998) Epidemiology and natural history of pelvic floor dysfunction. Obstet Gynecol Clin North Am 25:723–746

Burch J (1961) Urethrovaginal fixation to Cooper's ligament for correction of stress incontinence, cystocele, and prolapse. Am J Obstet Gynecol 81:281–290

Burch J (1968) Cooper's ligament urethrovesical suspension for stress incontinence. Nine years' experience – results, complications, technique. Am J Obstet Gynecol 100:764–774

Burgio K, Matthews K, Engel B (1991) Prevalence, incidence and correlates of urinary incontinence in healthy, middle-aged women. J Urol 146:1255–1259

Burgio K, Locher J, Goode P, et al (1998) Behavioral vs drug treatment for urge urinary incontinence in older women: a randomized controlled trial. JAMA 280:1995–2000

Chaikin D, Rosenthal J, Blaivas J (1998) Pubovaginal fascial sling for all types of stress incontinence: long-term analysis. J Urol 160:1312–1316

Chen AH, Horbach NS (1997) Abdominal retropubic urethropexy procedures. Oper Tech Gynecol Surg 2:26

Clemens J, DeLancey J, Faerber G, et al (2000) Urinary tract erosions after synthetic pubovaginal slings: diagnosis and management strategy. Urology 56:589–594

Clemens J, Schuster T, Konnak J, et al (2001) Revision rates after artificial urinary sphincter implantation for incontinence after radical prostatectomy: actuarial analysis. J Urol 166:1372–1375

Colling J, Ouslander J, Hadley B, et al (1992) The effects of patterned urge-response toileting (PURT) on urinary incontinence among nursing home residents. J Am Geriatr Soc 40:135–141

Costa P, Mottet N, Rabut B, et al (2001) The use of an artificial urinary sphincter in women with type III urinary incontinence and a negative Marshall test. J Urol 165:1172–1176

Danso K, Martey J, Wall L, et al (1996) The epidemiology of genitourinary fistulae in Kumasi, Ghana, 1977–1992. Int Urogynecol J 7:117–120

Diokno A, Brock B, Brown M, et al (1986) Prevalence of urinary incontinence and other urological symptoms in the noninstitutionalized elderly. J Urol 136:1022–1025

Eustice S, Roe B, Paterson J (2002) Prompted voiding for the management of urinary incontinence in adults (Cochrane Review). The Cochrane Library, Issue 3. Update Software, Oxford

Fantl J, Newman D, Colling J, et al (1996) Urinary incontinence in adults: acute and chronic management. Clinical practice guideline. US Department of Health and Human Services. Public Health Service, Agency for Health Care Policy and Research, Rockville, pp 1–154

Fitzgerald M, Brubaker L (2002) Urinary incontinence symptoms scores and urodynamic diagnoses. Neurourol Urodyn 21:30–35

Flynn B, Yap W (2002) Pubovaginal sling using allograft fascia lata versus autograft fascia for all types of stress urinary incontinence: 2-year minimum followup. J Urol 167:608–612

Fowler C (2000) Intravesical treatment of overactive bladder. Urology 55:60–64

Glazener C, Cooper K (2002) Anterior vaginal repair for urinary incontinence in women (Cochrane Review). The Cochrane Library, Issue 3. Update Software, Oxford

Gleason D, Susset J, White C, et al (1999) Evaluation of a new once-daily formulation of oxybutynin for the treatment of urinary urge incontinence. Ditropan XL Study Group. Urology 54:420–423

Groutz A, Blaivas J, Hyman M, et al (2001) Pubovaginal sling surgery for simple stress urinary incontinence: an analysis by outcome score. J Urol 165:1597–2000

Hadley E (1986) Bladder training and related therapies for urinary incontinence in older people. JAMA 256:372–379

Hampel C, Weinhold D, Benken N, et al (1997) Prevalence and natural history of urinary incontinence. Eur Urol 32 [Suppl 2]:3–12

Hay-Smith E, Bo K, Berghmans L, et al (2002) Pelvic floor muscle training for urinary incontinence in women (Cochrane Review). The Cochrane Library, Issue 3. Update Software, Oxford

Horbach N (1997) Choosing the appropriate surgery for genuine stress urinary incontinence. Oper Tech Gynecol Surg 2:1–4

Huang Y, Lin A, Chen K, et al (2001) High failure rate using allograft fascia lata in pubovaginal sling surgery for female stress urinary incontinence. Urology 58:943–946

Hunskaar S, Arnold E, Burgio K, et al (2000) Epidemiology and natural history of urinary incontinence. Int Urogynecol J 11:301–319

Hurt W (2000) Genitourinary fistulae. In: Monga A (eds) Clinical urogynaecology. Churchill Livingstone, London, pp 247–257

Ingelman-Sundberg A (1975) Urge incontinence in women. Acta Obstet Gynecol Scand 54:153–156

Jackson S, Weber A, Hull T, et al (1997) Fecal incontinence in women with urinary incontinence and pelvic organ prolapse. Obstet Gynecol 89:423–427

Jarvis G, Hall S, Stamp S, et al (1980) An assessment of urodynamic examination in the incontinent woman. Br J Obstet Gynaecol 87:893–896

Jonas U, Fowler C, Chancellor M, et al (2001) Efficacy of sacral nerve stimulation for urinary retention: results 18 months after implantation. J Urol 165:15–19

Kegel A (1948) Progressive resistance exercise in the functional restoration of the perineal muscles. Am J Obstet Gynecol 56:238–248

Kegel A (1951) Physiologic therapy for urinary stress incontinence. JAMA 1951:915

Kinn A, Zaar A (1998) Quality of life and urinary incontinence pad use in women. Int Urogynecol J 9:83–87

Klarsov P, Kroyer K, Kromann B, et al (1991) Long-term results for female genuine stress floor training and surgery for female genuine stress incontinence. Int Urogynecol J 12:132–135

Lebret T, Lugagne P, Herve J, et al (2001) Evaluation of tension-free vaginal tape procedures. Its safety and efficacy in the treatment of female stress incontinence during the learning phase. Eur Urol 40:543–547

Lee E, Yoo K, Kim Y, et al (1998) Prevalence of lower urinary tract symptoms in Korean men in a community-based study. Eur Urol 33:17–21

Lemack G, Zimmern P (1999) Predictability of urodynamic findings based on the Urogenital Distress Inventory-6 questionnaire. Urology 54:461–466

Lentz S (1995) Osteitis pubis: a review. Obstet Gynecol Surv 50:310–315

Lose G, Fantl J, Victor A, et al (2001) Outcome measures for research in adult women with symptoms of lower urinary tract dysfunction. Standardization Committee of the International Continence Society. Acta Obstet Gynecol Scand 80:981–985

Madjar S, Tchetgen M, van Antwerp A, et al (2002) Urethral erosion of tension-free vaginal tape. Urology 59:601

Malmsten U, Milsom I, Molander U, et al (1997) Urinary incontinence and lower urinary tract symptoms: an epidemiologic study of men aged 45 to 99 years. J Urol 158:1733–1737

Marshall H, Beevers D (1996) Alpha-adrenergic blocking drugs and female urinary incontinence: prevalence and reversibility. Br J Clin Pharmacol 42:507–509

Marshall V, Marchetti A, Krantz K (1949) The correction of stress incontinence by simple vesicourethral suspension. Surg Gynecol Obstet 88:509–518

McClish D, Wyman J, Sale P, et al (1999) Use and costs of incontinence pads in female study volunteers. Continence Program for Women Research Group. J Wound Ostomy Continence Nurs 26:210–213

McGuire E (1981) Urodynamic findings in patients after failure of stress incontinence operations. Prog Clin Biol Res 78:351–360

McLennan M, Bent A (1998) Supine empty stress test as a predictor of low Valsalva leak point pressure. Neurourol Urodyn 17:121–127

Meschia M, Pifarotti P, Bernasconi F, et al (2001) Tension-free Vaginal Tape: analysis of outcomes and complications in 404 stress incontinent women. Int Urogynecol J 12:S24–S27

Miller J, Ashton-Miller J, DeLancey J (1998) A pelvic muscle precontraction can reduce cough-related urine loss in selected women with mild SUI. J Am Geriatr Soc 46:870–874

Moller L, Lose G, Jorgensen T (2000) Incidence and remission rates of lower urinary tract symptoms at one year in women aged 40-60: longitudinal study. BMJ 320:1429–1432

Moore K, Simons A, Dowell C, et al (1999) Efficacy and user acceptability of the urethral occlusive device in women with urinary incontinence. J Urol 162:464–468

Nemir A, Middleton R (1954) Stress incontinence in young nulliparous women. Am J Obstet Gynecol 68:1166–1168

Niemczyk P, Klutke J, Carlin B, et al (2001) United States experience with tension-free vaginal tape procedure for urinary stress incontinence: assessment of safety and tolerability. Tech Urol 7:261–265

Nygaard I, Lemke J (1996) Urinary incontinence in rural older women: prevalence, incidence and remission. J Am Geriatr Soc 44:1049–1054

Nygaard I, Kreder K, Lepic M, et al (1996) Efficacy of pelvic floor muscle exercises in women with stress, urge, and mixed urinary incontinence. Am J Obstet Gynecol 174:120–125

Olsen A, Smith V, Bergstrom J, et al (1997) Epidemiology of surgically managed pelvic organ prolapse and urinary incontinence. Obstet Gynecol 89:501–506

Ostaszkiewicz J, Johnston L, Roe B (2002) Habit retraining for the management of urinary incontinence in adults (Cochrane Review). The Cochrane Library, Issue 1. Update Software, Oxford

Pits M (2002) Rare complications of tension-free vaginal tape procedure: late intraurethral displacement and early misplacement of the tape. J Urol 167:647

Ramsay I, Clancy S, Hilton P (1992) Subtrigonal phenol injections in the treatment of idiopathic detrusor instability in the female – a long-term urodynamic follow-up. Br J Urol 69:363–365

Ramsay I, Ali H, Hunter M, et al (1996) A prospective, randomized controlled trial of inpatient versus outpatient continence programs in the treatment of urinary incontinence in the female. Int Urogynecol J 7:260–263

Rezapour M, Falconer C, Ulmsten U (2001) Tension-free vaginal tape (TVT) in stress incontinent women with intrinsic sphincter deficiency (ISD) – a long-term follow-up. Int Urogynecol J 12:S12–S14

Robertson R, Jacobsen S, Rhodes T, et al (1998) Urinary incontinence in a community-based cohort: prevalence and healthcare-seeking. J Am Geriatr Soc 46:467–472

Roe B, Williams K, Palmer M (2002) Bladder training for urinary incontinence in adults (Cochrane Review). The Cochrane Library, Issue 3. Update Software, Oxford

Samuelsson E, Victor F, Svardsudd K (2000) Five-year incidence and remission rates of female urinary incontinence in a Swedish population less than 65 years old. Am J Obstet Gynecol 183:568–574

Sand P, Bowen L, Panganiban R, et al (1987) The low pressure urethra as a factor in failed retropubic urethropexy. Obstet Gynecol 69:399–402

Sandvik H, Hunskaar S, Vanvik A (1995) Diagnostic classification of female urinary incontinence: an epidemiologic survey corrected for validity. J Clin Epidemiol 48:339–343

Schulman C, Claes H, Matthijs J (1997) Urinary incontinence in Belgium: a population-based epidemiologic survey. Eur Urol 32:315–320

Siegel S, Catanzaro F, Dijkema H, et al (2000) Long-term results of a multicenter study on sacral nerve stimulation for treatment of urinary urge incontinence, urinary frequency, and retention. Urology 56:87–91

Soergel T, Shott S, Heit M (2001) Poor surgical outcomes after fascia lata allograft slings. Int Urogynecol J 12:247–253

Strohbehn K (1998) Normal pelvic floor anatomy. Obstet Gynecol Clin North Am 25:683–705

Strohbehn K, DeLancey J (1997) The anatomy of stress incontinence. Oper Tech Gynecol Surg 2:5–16

Tamussino K, Hanzal E, Kolle D, et al (2001) Tension-free vaginal tape operation: results of the Austrian registry. Obstet Gynecol 98:732–736

Teasdale T, Taffet G, Luchi R, et al (1988) Urinary incontinence in a community-residing elderly population. J Am Geriatr Soc 36:600–606

Temml C, Haidinger G, Schmidbauer J, et al (2000) Urinary incontinence in both sexes: prevalence rates and impact on quality of life and sexual life. Neurourol Urodyn 19:259–271

Thom D (1998) Variation in estimates of urinary incontinence prevalence in the community: effects of differences in definition, population characteristics, and study type. J Am Geriatr Soc 46:473–480

Thomas TM, Plymat KR, Blannin J, et al (1980) Prevalence of urinary incontinence. BMJ 281:1243–1245

Toba K, Ouchi Y, Orimo H, et al (1996) Urinary incontinence in elderly inpatients in Japan: a comparison between general and geriatric hospitals. Aging (Milano) 8:47–54

Ubersax J, Wyman J, Shumaker S, et al (1995) Short forms to assess life quality and symptom distress for urinary incontinence in women: the incontinence impact questionnaire and the urogenital distress inventory. Neurourol Urodyn 14:131–139

Urinary Incontinence Guideline Panel (1992) Urinary incontinence in adults: clinical practice guidelines. Agency for Health Care Policy and Research publication no. 92-0038. Public Health Service, US Department of Health and Human Services. Rockville

Ushiroyama T, Ikeda A, Ueki M (1999) Prevalence, incidence, and awareness in the treatment of menopausal urinary incontinence. Maturitas 33:127–132

van Kerrebroeck P, Kreder K, Jonas U, et al (2001) Tolteridine once-daily: superior efficacy and tolerability in the treatment of overactive bladder. Urology 57:414–421

Venn S, Mundy T (2000) Detrusor instability. In: Stanton S, Monga A (eds) Clinical urogynaecology. Churchill Livingstone, London, pp 219–226

Vierhout M, Lose G (1997) Preventative vaginal and intra-urethral devices in the treatment of female urinary stress incontinence. Curr Opin Obstet Gynecol 9:325–328

Ward K, Hilton P, Browning J (2000) A randomised trial of colposuspension and Tension-free Vaginal Tape for primary stress genuine stress incontinence. Neurourol Urodyn 19:386–388

Weber A, Walters M (2000) Cost-effectiveness of urodynamic testing before surgery for women with pelvic organ prolapse and stress urinary incontinence. Am J Obstet Gynecol 183:1338–1347

Wolin L (1969) Stress incontinence in young, healthy nulliparous female subjects. J Urol 101:545–549

Wyman J, Harkins S, Choi S, et al (1987) Psychosocial impact of urinary incontinence in women. Obstet Gynecol 70:378–381

Wyman J, Fantl J, McClish D, et al (1988) Comparative efficacy of behavioral interventions in the management of female urinary incontinence. Continence Program for Women Research Group. Am J Obstet Gynecol 179:999–1007

Young S, Howard A, Baker S (2001) Mersilene mesh sling: short- and long-term clinical and urodynamic outcomes. Am J Obstet Gynecol 185:32–40

6. Coloproctological Dysfunction

S. Halligan, C. J. Vaizey, C. I. Bartram

6.1 Constipation and Prolapse

S. Halligan

CONTENTS

6.1.1 Introduction 143
6.1.2 Constipation 143
6.1.3 Investigation 144
6.1.4 Evacuation Proctography and Constipation 146
6.1.4.1 Rectal Prolapse 146
6.1.4.2 Pelvic Floor Descent 149
6.1.4.3 Rectocele 150
6.1.4.4 Functional Disorder 151
6.1.5 Summary 153
References 154

6.1.1 Introduction

Constipation is something of which we all have experience to one degree or another. The radiological investigation of severely affected patients has attracted considerable attention over recent years, in tandem with the parallel development of physiological techniques for assessment and a greater understanding of pathophysiology. Ultimately, the role of imaging remains controversial despite a wealth of research. This chapter defines the role of evacuation proctography in the constipated patient and details both structural and functional findings in these individuals, stressing the importance of a balanced interpretation.

6.1.2 Constipation

Constipation is the "disease of diseases" (Whorton 2000). The belief that constipation predisposes to "internal putrefaction" has been widely held since

S. Halligan, MD, MRCP, FRCR
Intestinal Imaging Centre, Level 4V, St. Mark's Hospital, Watford Road, Northwick Park, Harrow, Middlesex, HA1 3UJ, UK

at least the 16th century BC (Ebbell 1937). By the beginning of the 19th century, there was a general medical consensus that constipation was the foremost disease of civilization, a universal affliction of the industrialized societies. This concept was buttressed by the discovery that bacteria cause infection, so proving that "the colon was a sewage pit teeming with bacteria, a cesspit that, in patients with constipation, was not being regularly emptied" (Whorton 2000). This led directly to the concept of "autointoxication". The constipated patient, Charles Bouchard declared, "is always working towards his own destruction; he makes continual attempts at suicide by intoxication" (Bouchard 1906). The logical culmination of this theory is perhaps best expressed by Arbuthnot Lane, who advocated colectomy as the cure-all for "civilisation's curse" (Lane 1913). Even in the 21st century, the notion of autointoxication remains alive and well; witness the mantra of the colonic irrigationists.

What is constipation? Whilst all of us are familiar with the term, it should be borne in mind that this merely describes a symptom, an expression of a sensation, and so means different things to different people. Furthermore, because of the private nature of the act, what passes for normal bowel habit is particularly subjective. For example, there is considerable variation in response when people are asked to define constipation (Sandler and Drossman 1987). Some will concentrate on bowel frequency whilst others will be more concerned with ease of defaecation and stool size and consistency. Indeed, most people have more than one definition. However, it is generally accepted that a satisfactory definition of constipation must include concepts of both infrequent defaecation and difficult evacuation. Whilst a globally valid definition of constipation probably remains elusive, the following is broadly applicable: infrequent stools defined as fewer than three per week and/or difficult evacuation defined as forceful straining for more than 25% of the total time spent in the lavatory (Drossman 1994).

Chronic constipation is very common. It has been estimated that one in five apparently healthy middle-aged adults have symptoms suggesting functional constipation (TALLEY et al. 1993). There are approximately 2.5 million physician consultations for constipation per year in the USA (JOHANSON et al. 1989). The economic impact is also considerable: a 1987 study estimated that cathartics were prescribed for 3 million people yearly in the USA, with over 200 million dollars spent on laxatives (SANDLER and DROSSMAN 1987). Furthermore, a study of severely constipated patients found that three-quarters had taken time off work because of their affliction, with one-fifth losing their job (PRESTON and LENNARD-JONES 1986). It is also worth noting that the vast majority of people with constipation never visit a doctor for help and population-based studies have revealed a high prevalence amongst those not seeking health care. Nevertheless, as a group those individuals who do consult a doctor tend to have worse symptoms and, as a consequence, probably real cause for complaint (HEATON et al. 1991).

A physical sign can be elicited, but a subjective experience or symptom is much more difficult to prove. Interestingly, doctors usually accept patients' claims that they are constipated but patients are notoriously inaccurate when asked to define their own bowel frequency (CHAUSSADE et al. 1989). Indeed, some patients will deny the passage of stool even when there is objective evidence, via transit studies, that this has occurred (HINTON et al. 1969)! Supporting this diagnostic uncertainty, a study of 224 patients referred with severe constipation documented normal investigations in 49 (22%), with daily stools in 24 (11%) (REX et al. 1992). Infrequent defaecation and small hard stools both imply slow colonic transit, and documented objective criteria such as slow transit are a more objective way with which to determine symptom severity than merely relying on the patient's historical account and subjective experience (PROBERT et al. 1994). It is clearly inappropriate to investigate all patients presenting with constipation, even if this were economically feasible. The physician's role is to determine those whose symptoms are considered severe enough to warrant further investigation. Generally, severe constipation is three times more frequent in women, who comprise practically all those with severe symptoms; in one series, all of the patients being considered for colectomy were women (KAMM et al. 1988).

It should be remembered that the primary aim of investigation is to guide therapy by sorting patients into treatment-defined groups. Presently the treatment options for severe constipation are limited, and investigation may achieve little other than to confirm symptom severity. It must be appreciated that this is not a field where there is any final histological arbiter. Functional disorders are difficult to analyse. Interpretation must be cautious, and referenced to developments in related fields of diagnosis.

6.1.3 Investigation

Causes of constipation are myriad (Table 6.1.1). Indeed, the possibilities range from rare congenital abnormalities to carcinoma of the colon. Because the vast majority of cases are merely lifestyle- and diet-related, a sensible approach to investigation must be adopted. As stated above, further investigation is only warranted in those with severe symptoms or those in whom a sinister underlying cause could be responsible. "Change in bowel habit" is a common reason for referral in older patients. Carcinoma, however, usually results in a change from constipation to diarrhoea rather than vice versa, and sinister symptoms such as anaemia and rectal bleeding may also be present. These patients require total large bowel investigation in the first instance, usually via barium enema or colonoscopy.

The majority who consult a doctor will respond to simple dietary measures once an underlying cause has been excluded. This leaves a group of patients who are severely affected, and in whom simple measures have

Table 6.1.1. Causes of constipation

Simple constipation	
Dietary	Inadequate fibre
Lifestyle	Repressed defaecatory urge
Secondary constipation	
Congenital	Hirschsprung's disease, idiopathic megarectum/megacolon
Mechanical	Carcinoma
Drugs	e.g. Analgesics, antidepressants
Metabolic	e.g. Diabetic neuropathy, chronic renal failure
Endocrine	e.g. Hypothyroidism, hypercalcaemia
Neurological	Multiple sclerosis, spinal trauma, autonomic neuropathy, Parkinson's disease
Psychological	e.g. Depression, anorexia
Idiopathic slow colonic transit	
Evacuation disorders	
Functional	Anismus, ineffective straining, solitary rectal ulcer syndrome
Structural	Rectocele, descending perineum
Constipation-predominant irritable bowel syndrome	

not been effective. Buried within these will be a small but significant number of younger patients who have been markedly constipated all of their lives; this raises the possibility of a congenital disorder. Abdominal palpation may reveal a hugely loaded colon, often with abdominal distension. In these instances, a simple water-soluble enema is all that is required to diagnose or exclude a congenital abnormality, with the emphasis on a lateral view of the contrast-filled rectum. There are three possibilities: Hirschsprung's disease, idiopathic megarectum, or congenital megacolon. All three are defined by gross rectal dilatation, but there will be a short distal aganglionic segment of variable length in patients with Hirschsprung's (Fig. 6.1.1), whereas dilatation extends right down to the level of the pelvic floor in megarectum/megacolon. Distinction between the latter two depends on the sigmoid colon, which is of normal calibre in congenital megarectum (Fig. 6.1.2) but also dilated in those with congenital megacolon (Gattuso and Kamm 1997). Studies of colonic transit and rectal evacuation are unwarranted in any of these patients since the diagnosis is made by contrast studies. It should be noted that imaging is superior to physiological testing for diagnosis because the rectoanal inhibitory reflex, the absence of which is used to diagnose Hirschsprung's, may be impossible to elicit in those with megarectum simply because the balloon used is often insufficiently large to distend the rectum and elicit a reflex.

However, the majority of patients presenting with severe constipation have no readily identifiable "organic" cause and it seems reasonable to classify these on the basis of functional disturbance. This is achieved by a combination of anorectal physiology testing, transit studies and evacuation proctography. There are then a variety of possibilities: patients will be found to have slow colonic transit, abnormalities of rectal evacuation, or a combination of both. Transit studies and their interpretation are detailed in Chapter 4.6. Patients who solely exhibit slow colonic transit are likely to be suffering from "idiopathic slow transit constipation" (Preston and Lennard-Jones 1986). These individuals are almost exclusively young women and additionally suffer constitutional symptoms and abdominal bloating together with a dramatically reduced stool frequency. There is some evidence that the underlying abnormality is not merely confined to the colon but is more generalized. For example, many exhibit abnormal antroduodenal manometry (Glia and Lindberg 1998). The underlying disorder remains obscure but is likely to be related to a generalized sensory and autonomic neuropathy (Knowles et al. 1999), which might explain why colectomy so often fails to ameliorate symptoms (Bernini et al. 1998).

In other patients, the defined abnormality will be predominantly characterized by difficult defaecation, i.e. the patient cannot empty the rectum or may have to strain forcefully and for prolonged periods in order to do so, or experiences feelings of incomplete evacuation after stool passage. Most constipated patients with predominantly rectal symptoms probably experience a combination of all of these,

Fig. 6.1.1. Water-soluble enema in a 46-year-old man reveals a dilated proximal rectum with distal short segment, diagnosing Hirschsprung's disease

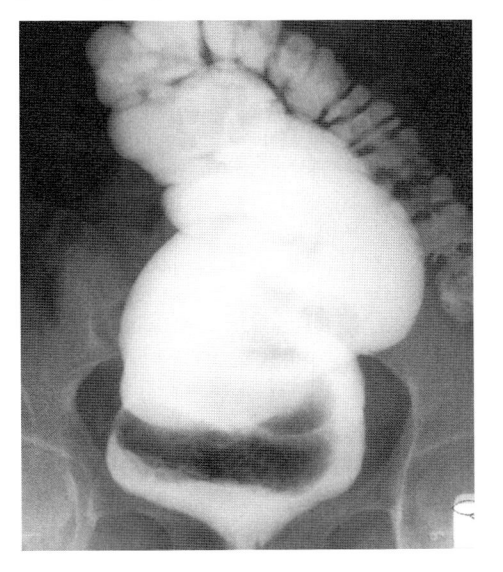

Fig. 6.1.2. Water-soluble enema in a 20-year-old man reveals a hugely dilated rectum that extends right down to the pelvic floor. There is no short segment and the sigmoid colon is of normal calibre, suggesting the diagnosis is idiopathic megarectum

a symptom complex termed "outlet obstruction" or "obstructed defaecation".

Whilst classification into those with colonic inertia and those with rectal outlet obstruction is now considered simplistic, it is clinically convenient and for this reason transit studies and evacuation proctography are frequently requested together. To further complicate matters, slow colonic transit and abnormal rectal evacuation frequently coexist. A study of 14 women suffering from idiopathic slow transit constipation found that they also had decreased rectal sensory perception when compared to controls and few were able to pass a simulated stool (READ et al. 1986). Perhaps this interrelationship should not be surprising since, intuitively, transit and rectal evacuation ought to be related; if they were not then stool delivered to the rectum at a normal rate in patients with isolated obstructed defaecation would cause a megarectum within days! An interrelationship has been proved in a study of normal volunteers who were asked to suppress the urge to defaecate; proximal colonic transit slowed dramatically within 1 week of suppression (KLAUSER et al. 1990). The situation is analogous to the "ileocaecal brake", in which increased delivery of intestinal contents to the caecum slows proximal small bowel transit. Furthermore, this relationship implies that treatment should be directed at normalizing rectal evacuation in any patient who demonstrates both slow transit and impaired voiding, since the former could merely be a normal physiological response to the latter. Moreover, this approach also suggests that an assessment of rectal evacuation is probably the single most important test in severely constipated patients since it most precisely characterizes the primary abnormality (READ 1989).

Alternatively, investigations will be entirely normal and the possibility of the irritable bowel syndrome should be considered. Although irritable bowel is defined by the Rome criteria (THOMPSON et al. 1989), which centre on abdominal pain and change in bowel habit, there are constipation predominant subgroups (PRIOR et al. 1990). Interestingly, many have heightened sensitivity to rectal distension, which might explain sensations of incomplete evacuation in those complaining of constipation (PRIOR et al. 1990).

6.1.4
Evacuation Proctography and Constipation

Constipation is the commonest reason to request evacuation proctography, although pelvic pain, prolapse (either rectal or otherwise) and anal incontinence may occasionally be other indications. For the reasons described above, the main aim of evacuation proctography is to characterize rectal evacuation, normal or not. The test will be of most use in those individuals in whom "obstructed defaecation" is clinically suspected.

Generally, proctographic findings may be broadly divided into two groups: abnormalities of rectal and pelvic floor configuration, and functional abnormalities of rectal emptying. Any proctographic report should incorporate an assessment of both of these. The overall picture is complicated by the fact that structural and functional rectal abnormalities usually coexist and it is therefore difficult to determine which is the primary cause of the patient's symptoms, if either. Luckily, there are only a few possibilities: structural rectal abnormalities may be broadly grouped into prolapse, rectocele, and pelvic floor descent, and functional abnormality generally means an inability to empty the rectum rapidly and completely, whatever its configuration.

6.1.4.1
Rectal Prolapse

Rectal prolapse may be external or internal. External rectal prolapse is circumferential and tends to be "complete" (i.e. all of the rectal wall layers are involved). Circumferential prolapse which remains confined to the rectal ampulla, or which only enters the anal canal, is termed intussusception (intrarectal and intraanal intussusception, respectively). Intussusception may involve all rectal wall layers or be confined to the mucosa and immediate subjacent layers. Additionally, intussusception implies a circumferential process. However, intussusception may be confined to the anterior rectal wall, where it is more correctly termed "anterior mucosal prolapse".

Complete rectal prolapse clearly needs surgical treatment. Diagnosis is usually not difficult although evacuation proctography is occasionally necessary if the prolapse cannot be demonstrated on the examination couch. Evacuation proctography facilitates the diagnosis of rectal prolapse and, because of the dynamic nature of the examination, its introduction enabled the mechanism of rectal prolapse to be studied directly for the first time. Cineradiographic studies have revealed that rectal prolapse develops from a circumferential intussusception 6 to 8 cm from the anal verge (BRODEN and SNELLMAN 1968) and it rapidly became clear that prolapse is frequently retained within the rectum, lending support to the concept of internal intussusception, first described in 1903 (TUTTLE 1903). Whilst clinical diagnosis of intussusception relies on direct proctoscopy during straining, the introduction of evacuation proctography meant that accurate diagnosis of intussusception, including subtle forms, was now possible.

Proctographic intussusception has been divided into a seven-point scale (SHORVON et al. 1989) but there is probably no practical need for such a detailed scoring system. It is easier to divide intussusception merely into high and low grades, which is an attempt to define whether it is abnormal or not since intussusception is known to occur in normal individuals. Low-grade intussusception is defined by a thin circumferential ampullary ring that originates in the rectal ampulla when emptying commences and travels towards the anorectal junction as voiding continues (Fig. 6.1.3). It remains confined to the rectum. High-grade intussusception also develops in the same way and also remains confined within the rectum but in this case the prolapsing folds are much thicker, bulkier, and capacious (Fig. 6.1.4).

Although it is possible to measure the thickness of prolapsing folds in order to differentiate between high- and low-grade intussusception, with 3 mm being the usually quoted figure, this is rarely clinically necessary; with experience, an accurate diagnosis can be simply made by inspection. It is worth remembering that the rectum has to empty for intussusception to be revealed – it is commonly believed that intussusception obstructs evacuation but this phenomenon is rarely seen proctographically (HALLIGAN et al. 1996). Indeed, intussusception is most frequently and best visualized at the end of evacuation when the rectum is empty and this is when it should be graded. If the apex of the prolapsing folds enters the anal canal then this is termed intraanal intussusception, which is classed as a high-grade phenomenon (Fig. 6.1.5).

Intraanal intussusception is recognized by anal canal splaying as a consequence of the folds entering the canal. However, this may not always be most visible in the conventional lateral view because the rectal folds are coronal. Consequently, it may be worthwhile asking the subject to strain whilst in the anterior-posterior position, a position in which the intussusception is most visible (MCGEE and BARTRAM 1993). Complete rectal prolapse is diagnosed when the full thickness of the rectal wall is extruded through the anal canal (Fig. 6.1.6). Care should be taken not to confuse this with the eversion of the anal margin that sometimes accompanies forceful straining. Anterior mucosal prolapse is diagnosed when only the anterior rectal wall appears to be infolding during rectal evacuation (Fig. 6.1.7). It is commonly seen in association with a rectocele and most likely represents collapse of the rectocele as it empties.

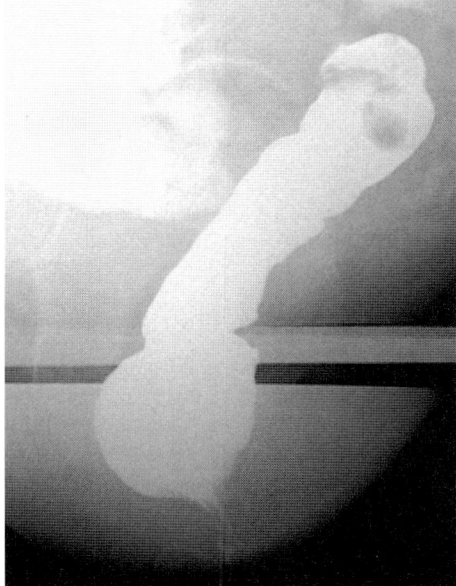

Fig. 6.1.3. In this case, lateral proctography reveals circumferential rectal infolding during evacuation, diagnosing intussusception. The folds remain high in the rectum and are not particularly thick. Such low-grade intussusception is a common finding

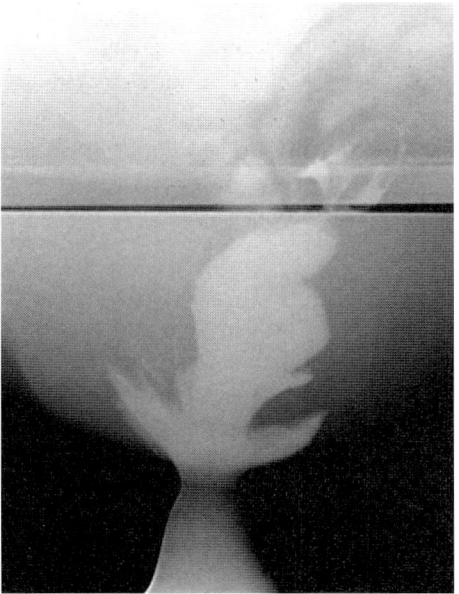

Fig. 6.1.4. Lateral proctography reveals circumferential rectal infolding during evacuation. The folds are thick and prominent and travel towards the distal rectum, typical of high-grade intussusception

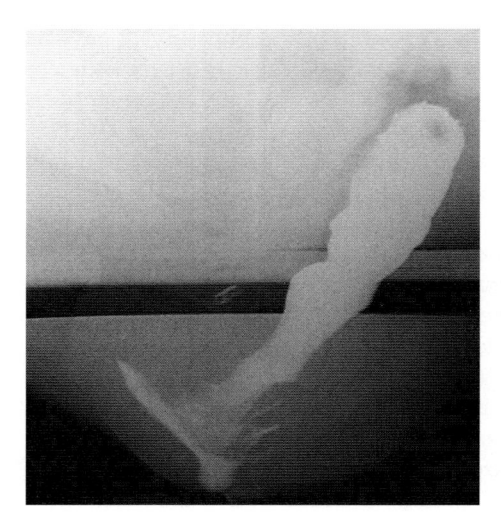

Fig. 6.1.5. The apex of the prolapsing folds enters the anal canal in this patient, diagnosing intraanal intussusception

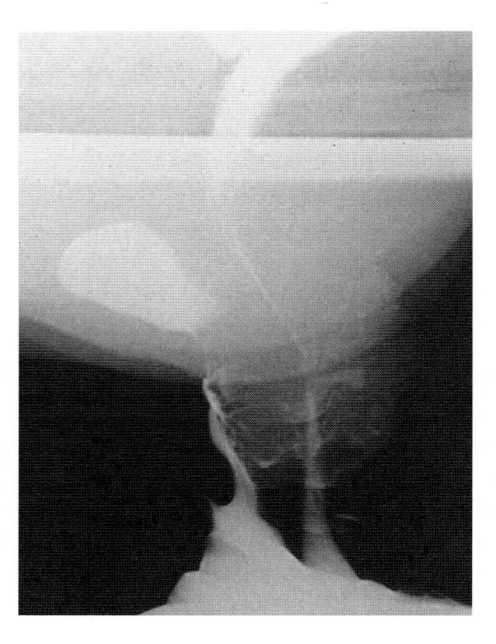

Fig. 6.1.6. Lateral proctography shows complete rectal prolapse, evidenced by extrusion of all rectal wall layers through the anus. There is also retained contrast within a rectocele

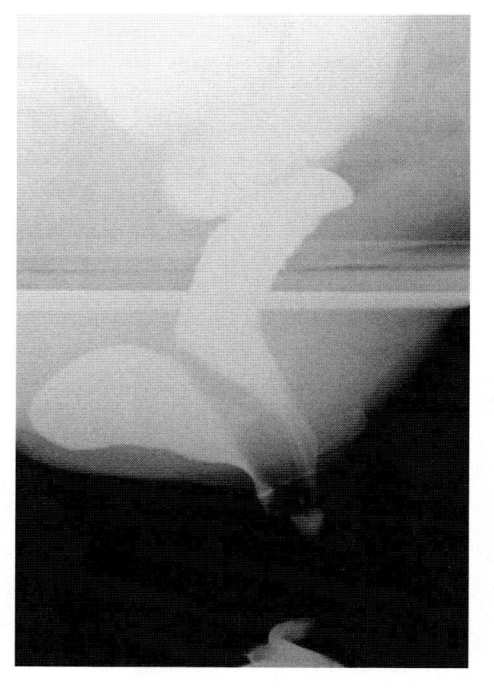

Fig. 6.1.7. In this woman the anterior rectal wall has prolapsed into the anal canal towards the end of evacuation. Note that the process is confined to the anterior rectal wall and is not circumferential so that the diagnosis is anterior mucosal prolapse rather than intussusception. Note that the prolapse also walls off contrast within a rectocele

An association between intussusception and constipation has long been recognized, with several authors hypothesizing that the prolapsing folds obstruct the rectal lumen and are thus the cause of incomplete evacuation (IHRE 1990). Because of this, proctographic diagnosis of intussusception has attracted considerable attention. Moreover, the clear implication is that once diagnosed, surgical obliteration of the prolapse will ameliorate symptoms (HOFFMAN et al. 1984). However, the role of intussusception remains unclear. Whilst some authors report excellent symptomatic results following surgery (JOHANSSON et al. 1985; LIBERMAN et al. 2000), others have had less success despite proof that the prolapse has been cured (CHRISTIANSEN et al. 1992; HALLIGAN et al. 1995a; ORROM et al. 1991). Indeed, by definition, intussusception occurs only when the rectum collapses, and it only collapses when it is emptying! It is most likely that high-grade intussusception creates a sensation of incomplete evacuation, but does not in itself cause mechanical rectal blockage.

Much of this uncertainty may be explained by the fact that the mechanism of intussusception remains poorly understood in most cases. Some believe that intussusception inevitably progresses to complete rectal prolapse with time (HOFFMAN et al. 1984), whilst others believe there is no evidence to support this in longitudinal studies (MELLGREN et al. 1997), raising the possibility that they are different syndromes. It has also been suggested that rectal hypersensitivity, which encourages the subject to void small volumes repeatedly, in combination with a weak sphincter mechanism provides the ideal conditions for prolapse into the anal canal, and that this is the mechanism for all forms of rectal prolapse (Sun et al. 1989). Perhaps the most prevalent current theory is that rectal intussusception is merely a secondary response to prolonged and chronic straining because of an underlying functional disorder (Eu and Seow-Choen 1997). Supporting this, surgical series where underlying functional disorder has been preoperatively excluded report excellent symptomatic outcomes (van Tets and Kuijpers 1995). Moreover, symptoms thought characteristic of intussusception, such as perineal and rectal digitation, are now known to be strongly associated with functional disorders (Halligan and Bartram 1996). Furthermore, intussusception is easy to demonstrate in asymptomatic individuals, which also queries its significance as the primary cause of constipation; Shorvon and co-workers found proctographic intussusception in 22 (50%) of 44 normal volunteers (Shorvon et al. 1989).

The solitary rectal ulcer syndrome is a well-recognized diagnosis that describes a combination of rectal prolapse and functional abnormality. The condition is characterized by repeated fruitless straining, often accompanied by the passage of blood and mucus. Proctoscopy usually reveals rectal inflammation and ulceration which is accompanied by specific histopathological changes within the prolapsing mucosa (Halligan et al. 1995b). Although the precise aetiology remains obscure, it is widely believed that ulceration is a direct result of mucosal ischaemia secondary to repeated straining (Womack et al. 1987). Proctographic abnormalities are common and many patients exhibit high-grade rectal intussusception or complete rectal prolapse (Halligan et al. 1995b) (Fig. 6.1.8).

6.1.4.2
Pelvic Floor Descent

By relating the position of the anorectal junction to a landmark, such as the ischial tuberosities or commode seat, proctography provides a simple method to determine the position of the pelvic floor at rest and how far it descends during evacuation. It is generally accepted that proctography provides the most accurate estimate of pelvic floor position and descent because clinical methods using a perineometer measure movement of the anal verge during maximum straining and not to the point of anal canal opening (Oettle et al. 1985). Parks described a clinical syndrome where the main finding was excessive pelvic floor descent, defined as more than 3–4 cm, coupled with a low resting level of more than 3 cm below the pubococcygeal line (Fig. 6.1.9) (Parks et al. 1966). Of a series of 100 consecutive patients attending a rectal clinic, 12 displayed these characteristics, 10 of whom (83%) strained excessively at stool compared with only 20 (23%) of the remaining 88. Because of this, Parks suggested that the underlying abnormality was likely due to irreparable pudendal nerve traction neuropathy as a consequence of chronic stretching (Parks et al. 1966). It has been estimated that the pudendal nerves may be stretched by as much as 20% over time (Henry et al. 1982).

It is clear that excessive pelvic floor descent is frequently found in patients referred for evacuation proctography (Skomorowska et al. 1988), and is often seen in combination with perineal ballooning, rectocele, intussusception and impaired evacuation. Furthermore, there is no doubt that straining stresses the pudendal nerves. A study of asymptomatic individuals found that voluntary excessive straining temporarily slowed pudendal nerve latency when measured immediately afterwards (Engel and Kamm 1994). However, whether the pelvic floor ballooning that accompanies the syndrome is responsible for symptoms of constipation is uncertain. Indeed, many patients with pudendal neuropathy and pelvic floor descent are incontinent. In an attempt to explain this, it has been suggested that chronic straining, precipitated by an underlying functional disorder, causes pudendal neuropathy, the ultimate expression of which is sphincter denervation and subsequent incontinence (Henry et al. 1982). The

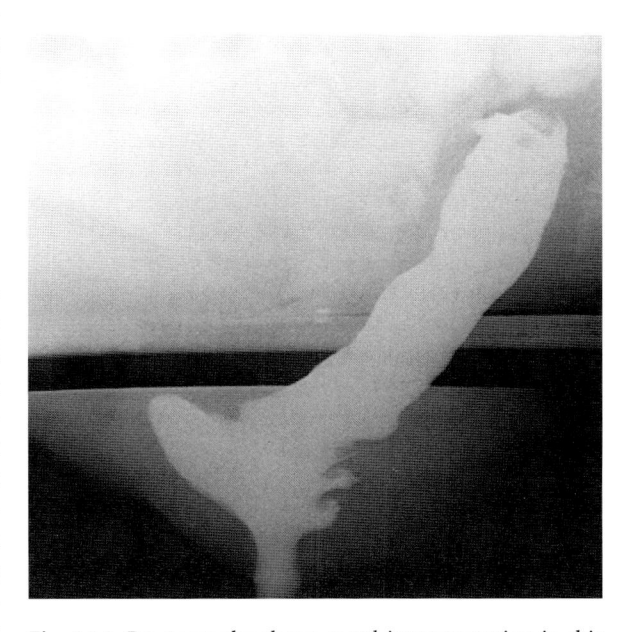

Fig. 6.1.8. Proctography shows rectal intussusception in this woman known to have solitary rectal ulcer syndrome (SRUS)

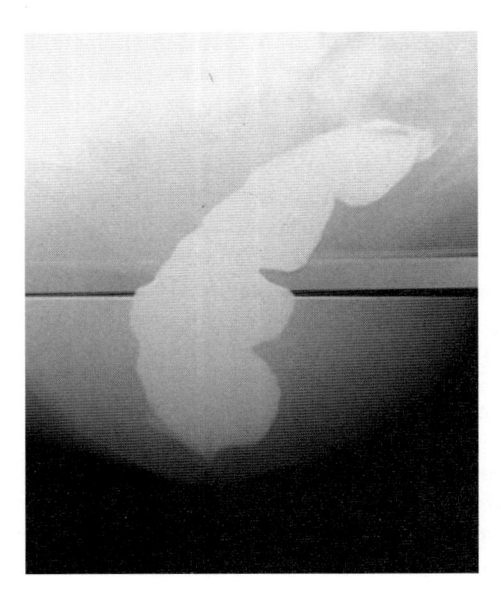

Fig. 6.1.9. Lateral proctography shows gross pelvic floor descent at rest, evidenced by the distance of the anorectal junction below the commode seat

pelvic floor may also be weakened by childbirth, which can also cause perineal descent. Thus, the finding probably reflects a multifactorial spectrum of pelvic floor injury rather than indicating a specific syndrome or aetiology. Supporting this, a prospective proctographic study of 213 patients found no correlation between pudendal neuropathy and perineal descent (JORGE et al. 1993a). Surgery directed specifically at restoration of normal pelvic floor configuration is highly contentious and unlikely to be helpful, but behavioural therapy may help selected patients (HAREWOOD et al. 1999).

6.1.4.3
Rectocele

A rectocele is an anterior rectal wall bulge that is usually most evident during evacuation (Fig. 6.1.10). Rectoceles are common in women because the vagina creates an opening in the perineal membrane not present in men and are likely to be a normal variant: Shorvon and co-workers found a "rectocele" in 96% of asymptomatic women studied (SHORVON et al. 1989). However, there is an undoubted association between a large rectocele and difficult rectal evacuation. Patients, usually women, describe a specific constellation of symptoms: the urge to defaecate is normal but voiding is obstructed, often with a lump appearing at the introitus. Proctography is frequently requested for diagnosis and a large rectocele may be defined as one deeper than 4 cm (KELVIN et al. 1992). It is frequently believed that the need to use the fingers to elevate the rectocele to facilitate emptying signifies functional significance (HALLIGAN and BARTRAM 1995). Pushing lateral or dorsal to the anus are nonspecific. Similarly, contrast retention within the rectocele at the end of evacuation is also thought to be important (HALLIGAN and BARTRAM 1995).

It is likely that aetiology is multifactorial. Two main groups seem to emerge: those in whom the rectovaginal septum has been damaged following childbirth, and those in whom the rectocele is the consequence of chronic straining at stool, most likely due to a functional disorder of evacuation. Surgery aims to restore rectovaginal support and postoperative proctography is able to demonstrate technical success in most

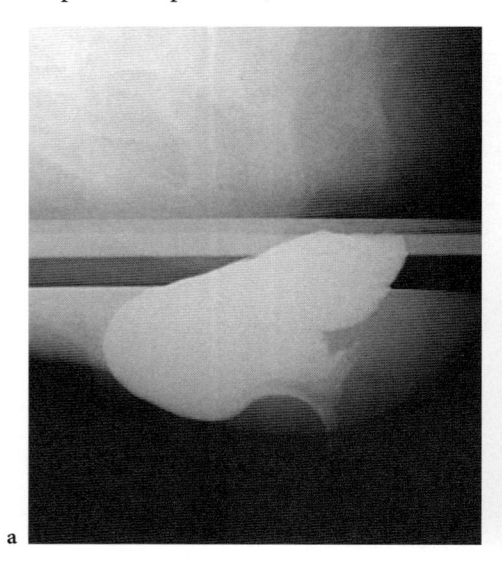

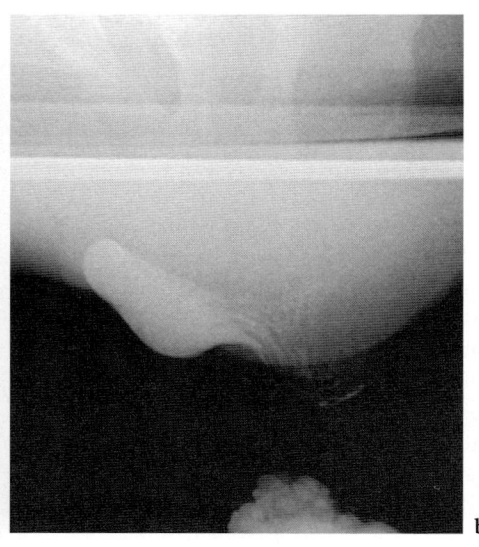

Fig. 6.1.10. Proctography during evacuation reveals a large anterior rectocoele in this woman. Contrast is retained in the rectocoele after evacuation: "barium trapping"

patients (LODER et al. 1996). However, symptomatic failure is common (ARNOLD et al. 1990), possibly because any underlying functional disorder is not treated. Consequently, there has been considerable interest in using proctography not only for diagnosis, for which it is the gold-standard test, but also to predict symptomatic outcome. This has not been simple, and results are confusing. For example, whilst some have found proctographic contrast retention within the rectocele to reliably predict good symptomatic outcome (MURTHY et al. 1996), others have not: a study of 74 patients found no relationship between the size of the rectocele and ability to evacuate, and surgical outcome (VAN DAM et al. 2000). It seems likely that outcome is confounded by the presence or absence of underlying functional disorder, which is often neglected once attention has been drawn towards a large rectocele. For example, a study of 41 patients with difficult evacuation initially ascribed to rectocele found underlying functional disorder in 29 (71%) (JOHANSSON et al. 1992). Supporting this, surgery is successful if functional disorder has been excluded preoperatively (TJANDRA et al. 1999). Indeed, behavioural therapy (biofeedback) alone may ameliorate symptoms (MIMURA et al. 2000) and continued manual elevation of the rectocele is an option. Because rectoceles are commonest in middle-aged women, a plethora of other factors may contribute to symptoms, in addition to the size of the rectocele itself (LAARHOVEN et al. 1999).

It should also be noted that rectoceles might also rarely be posterior in position (Fig. 6.1.11). However, in contrast to the anterior type, these are not due to a midline weakness. Rather, imaging in the frontal plane reveals that they are lateralized to one side of the pelvic floor and are actually due to rectal herniation through the levator plate musculature (HALLIGAN 1994). Thus, a more correct term is probably "posterior perineal hernia". In contrast to anterior rectocele, men are equally affected and the aetiology is most likely chronic straining (CAVALLO et al. 1993) or sometimes a penetrating injury to the levator plate itself.

6.1.4.4
Functional Disorder

Ever since evacuation proctography first visualized the dynamics of rectal evacuation, there has been an understandable focus on abnormalities of rectal configuration, with many investigators believing these responsible for obstructive symptoms. Surprisingly, proctographic estimates of the rate and completeness of rectal evacuation have received relatively little attention. However, rectal evacuation is a functional event, requiring coordination between voluntary and involuntary nervous pathways, and smooth and striated muscles. It has long been recognized that some patients experience difficulties with rectal evacuation simply because of an inability to coordinate this necessarily complex series of events. Given this, the configuration the rectum adopts when emptying may be irrelevant if the patient can empty without effort. Conversely, abnormalities of rectal configuration may actually occur secondary to chronic straining rather than be the primary abnormality.

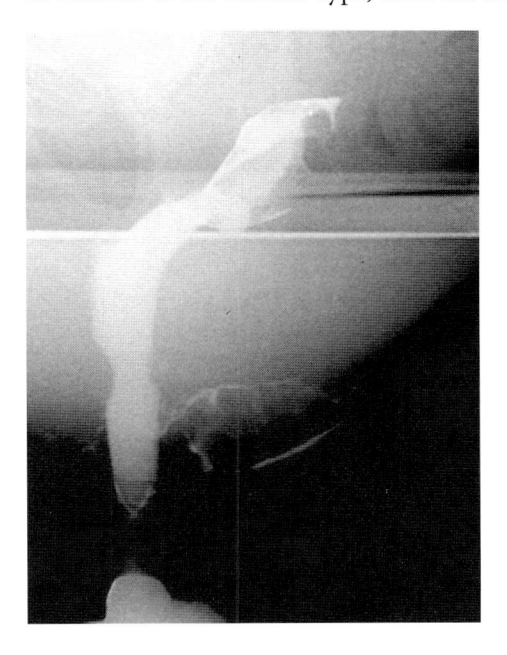

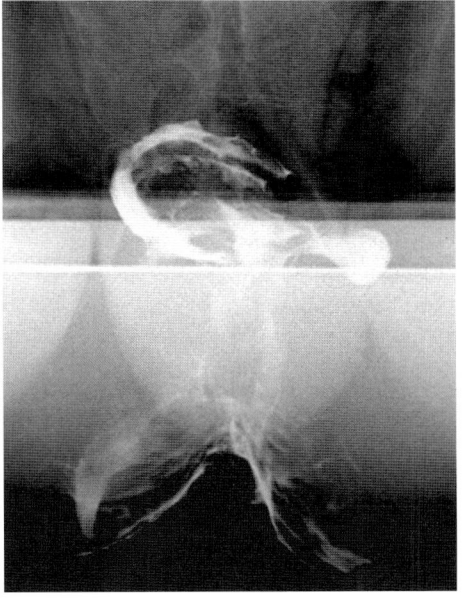

Fig. 6.1.11. Posterior perineal hernia or "posterior rectocele". The lateral proctogram during evacuation suggests a well-defined posterior rectal wall bulge in this 50-year-old man. Screening in the AP position during straining reveals that the bulge is a left-sided posterior perineal hernia

Some patients cannot void without inappropriate effort, even when the rectum is only full of fluid (ALSTRUP et al. 1997). Why is this? Normally, striated pelvic floor musculature is in a state of tonic contraction. This contraction is inhibited during defaecation so that the pelvic floor relaxes to allow stool passage. In contrast, simultaneous electromyography of pelvic floor musculature has shown that some constipated patients fail to relax their pelvic floor when attempting to evacuate. Indeed, many inappropriately contract their muscles above baseline levels: a study of 15 constipated women revealed that the puborectalis and external sphincter muscles contracted forcefully when the subject attempted to evacuate a rectal balloon (PRESTON and LENNARD-JONES 1985). There is therefore no primary structural abnormality as such, rather a disorder of functional integration.

This syndrome has been termed "anismus" because it may be analogous to the type of muscular spasm seen in vaginismus. Because the puborectalis muscle is physiologically accessible, it was the first muscle in which unexpected contraction during evacuation was demonstrated, hence alternative terms such as "non-relaxing puborectalis syndrome" (FLESHMAN et al. 1992) and "paradoxical puborectalis contraction syndrome" (JONES et al. 1987) have been suggested. Indeed, Wasserman was the first to notice the role of this muscle and named it "puborectalis syndrome" (WASSERMAN 1964). However, it is increasingly recognized that the problem is unlikely to be confined to a single muscle and a more general term such as "pelvic floor incoordination" may be preferable since it does not identify any particular muscular group or necessarily imply inappropriate contraction (HALLIGAN and BARTRAM 1998). The latter is important because some patients fail to relax, whereas others do not generate adequate intrarectal pressure (HALLIGAN et al. 1995c). In any event, the cause is a functional disorder and the result is the same: failure to evacuate.

The aetiology remains obscure, but anismus is likely to be a learned inappropriate response. For example, there is an association with pelvic surgery and previous sexual abuse (LEROI 1995). Although anismus can be found in both normal and incontinent patients (JONES et al. 1987), and may disappear when investigations are made away from the hospital environment (DUTHIE and BARTOLO 1992), there is a clear association with constipation and the diagnosis is worthwhile, not least because pelvic floor behavioural therapy using biofeedback has been very successful (BLEIJENBERG and KUIJPERS 1987). This approach also avoids unnecessary surgical treatment of secondary phenomena such as rectocele where this is unnecessary.

Because the puborectalis was the first muscle implicated, diagnosis has historically focused on demonstrating inappropriate puborectalis contraction during attempted evacuation. Using evacuation proctography for diagnosis, workers have drawn attention to the finding of a prominent puborectal impression posterior to the anorectal junction (Fig. 6.1.12). Kuijpers and Bleijenberg suggested that the anorectal angle directly reflects puborectalis activity after finding failure of the anorectal angle to open in 12 patients subsequently found to have paradoxical puborectalis contraction on electromyography (KUIJPERS and BLEIJENBERG 1986). However, although subsequently frequently cited as a sign of anismus, more recent evidence suggests that this finding is only weakly associated with functional disorder: a proctographic study of 24 patients with physiologically proven anismus found that a prominent puborectal impression and anorectal angle configuration during attempted evacuation was unable to differentiate patients from asymptomatic control subjects (HALLIGAN et al. 1995d). Supporting this, simultaneous proctography and puborectal electromyography reveals no correlation between muscular activity and anorectal junction configuration (THORPE et al. 1993).

Instead, the major proctographic difference between patients with and without anismus is intuitively obvious: patients with anismus cannot easily empty their

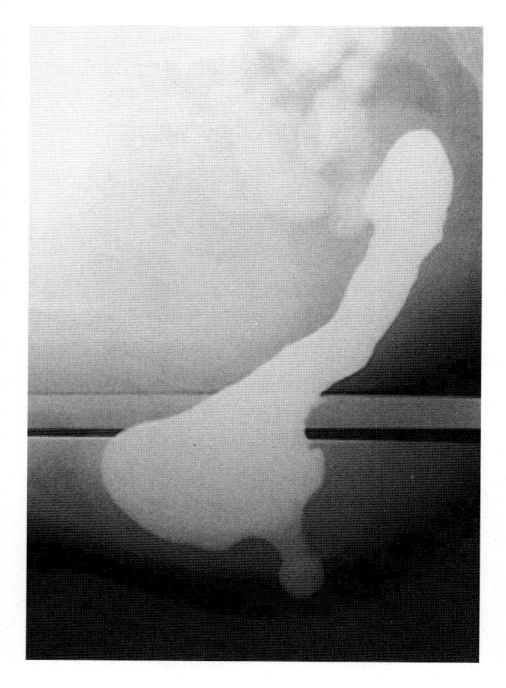

Fig. 6.1.12. Evacuation was very prolonged in this woman, suggesting anismus. Note the posterior rectal wall impression, presumed to be due to paradoxical puborectalis contraction

rectum. Evacuation studies in normal volunteers show that they rapidly and completely empty their rectum (Kamm et al. 1989) whereas, in complete contrast, patients with anismus exhibit prolonged and incomplete evacuation, or no evacuation at all. The rate and completeness of rectal evacuation are easily determined using evacuation proctography (Halligan et al. 1994), and it seems sensible to base a proctographic diagnosis of anismus on evacuation failure. Using these criteria Halligan and co-workers found abnormally prolonged and/or incomplete contrast evacuation in 20 of 24 patients (83%), a phenomenon not found in any of the controls (Halligan et al. 1995d). Furthermore, anorectal angle measurements were nonspecific. Moreover, when the authors applied their findings prospectively in a continuous, unselected group of constipated patients, the positive predictive value of impaired proctographic evacuation for diagnosis of anismus was in excess of 90% (Halligan et al. 2001). Using 120 ml of rectal contrast, evacuation times greater than 30 s accurately predicted functional disorder (Halligan et al. 2001). The time taken to initiate anal canal opening and the rate of evacuation are more important for diagnosis than the final percentage of contrast voided because most patients, even those with severe anismus, will eventually fully empty their rectum if given enough time to do so and if they strain forcefully enough. Proctography is as good as electromyography for diagnosis (Jorge et al. 1993b). There have also been attempts to use proctography to determine who will benefit from subsequent biofeedback, which implies that those with moderate symptoms do better than those who are severely affected (McKee et al. 1999).

Anismus is characterized by chronic, excessive, prolonged straining, a practice that probably weakens the pelvic floor and encourages pelvic floor descent, intussusception and prolapse. Because of this, patients with anismus often have associated structural pelvic floor abnormalities by the time they come to be investigated (Fig. 6.1.13). It is highly likely that many surgical disappointments happen because an underlying diagnosis of anismus was neglected. For example, a study of 41 patients whose constipation had been ascribed to rectocele, found underlying anismus disorder in 29 (71%) (Johansson et al. 1992), whilst another study found it in 34 of 56 (60%) (Mellgren et al. 1998).

The same may apply to intussusception. A proctographic study of patients treated for intussusception found that symptoms persisted if there was underlying functional disorder (Orrom et al. 1991). Furthermore, a study of patients with solitary rectal ulcer syndrome found that preoperative proctographic features of impaired evacuation predicted persistent postoperative symptoms in the face of objective evidence that the prolapse itself had been successfully treated (Halligan et al. 1995a). These studies suggest that intussusception in some patients may merely be an epiphenomenon. When prolonged and incomplete contrast evacuation is encountered during proctography, a diagnosis of functional pelvic floor incoordination should be considered whatever the rectal configuration. Supporting this, a proctographic study of 58 constipated patients found that the only significant difference from controls was a prolongation of evacuation time and failure to fully empty the rectum, clearly suggesting that functional measurements of emptying are more important than changes in rectal configuration (Turnbull et al. 1988). It also seems that abnormalities of rectal configuration occurring secondary to incoordination do not prejudice the success of subsequent behavioural therapy (Lau et al. 2000).

6.1.5
Summary

Although evacuation proctography has been widely practised for several years, debate concerning its clin-

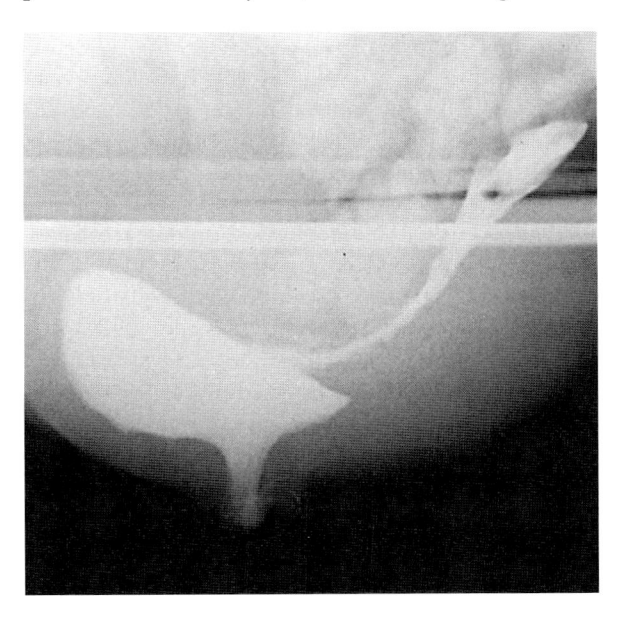

Fig. 6.1.13. Evacuation proctography in this 39-year-old woman reveals a large rectocoele, pelvic floor descent and ballooning, and enterocele. However, evacuation was prolonged and subsequent physiological testing found anismus, raising the possibility that the structural abnormalities demonstrated by imaging merely reflect functional disorder

ical relevance continues. Whilst, no one would argue against the central role of anal endosonography in characterizing the cause of incontinence, the place of proctography is less certain. Much of this derives from the excessive attention that has been devoted to the detailed and complex anatomical measurements that are possible during the procedure. Any rectal configuration occurring during emptying, other than that of a symmetrically collapsing tube, has been considered abnormal in the face of conflicting evidence. The gradual realization that many patients are actually suffering from functional disorders, coupled with an increasing emphasis on proctographic assessment of function, may help redress this. Proctography will probably always be controversial because severely constipated patients are so difficult to treat, not least because the precise aetiology of their affliction frequently remains obscure and the patients' perception of their disability varies. It is highly likely that patients are heterogeneous and the disorder is multifactorial. For example, some have heightened rectal awareness, which may lead to sensations of incomplete evacuation ignored by others. Others complain of sensations of rectal fullness despite proctographic evidence that the rectum is empty (HALLIGAN et al. 1996).

The main value of proctography lies with its ability to simultaneously diagnose both structural and functional abnormalities, and determine which is most likely to be relevant in each individual case. Problems with interpretation most often occur when anatomical findings are given undue emphasis. Generally, impaired evacuation raises the possibility of a functional disorder, whatever the rectal configuration, and biofeedback should be tried first. It is less invasive than surgery, more likely to be effective, and does not preclude a subsequent surgical option.

Some workers have attempted to assess the clinical impact of evacuation proctography (HILTUNEN et al. 1994; OTT et al. 1994) but these studies have attracted fierce criticism from advocates of the technique (HALLIGAN 1995; KELVIN et al. 1995). Evaluation of imaging techniques is fraught with difficulty, especially because the effects of treatment are usually included in assessment of outcomes. This especially disadvantages proctography because constipation is a functional disorder and treatment is so often ineffective. As stated in the introduction to this chapter, the main role of proctography is to place patients into clinically defined groups. With this in mind, a prospective study of 50 consecutive patients referred for evacuation proctography sought to determine the effect of imaging on clinical understanding and management: using a pre- and postintervention design, the authors found that evacuation proctography has considerable diagnostic and therapeutic effect, and significantly increases diagnostic confidence (HARVEY et al. 1999). Indeed, 44 of 47 (94%) requesting clinicians generally found proctography of "major" or "moderate" benefit (HARVEY et al. 1999). Diagnostic confidence rose significantly after evacuation proctography (mean 7.0 before vs 8.4 after, $P=0.0006$). The lead diagnosis changed in nine patients (18%). Intended surgical management became nonsurgical after evacuation proctography in seven (14%) patients, and intended nonsurgical therapy became surgical in two (4%). Surgery remained likely management in 15 patients but its nature changed in five (10%).

Presently, there is a trend towards expanding the basic proctographic examination to encompass the entire pelvic floor (KELVIN and MAGLINTE 1997), an approach that probably has most appeal to the urogynaecologist. Dynamic pelvic MR imaging has obvious application in this arena (LIENEMANN et al. 1997) but has also been specifically employed to image constipated patients (HEALY et al. 1997). Nevertheless, for the reasons described above, evaluation of rectal evacuation will remain central to meaningful assessment. Although this can be performed in the supine position, few investigators have access to the more practical vertical configuration machines (SCHOENBERGER et al. 1998). It is also clear that, like conventional proctography, MR imaging also reveals supposed abnormalities in asymptomatic subjects (GOH et al. 2000). Whilst further investigation of MR imaging is undoubtedly warranted, the anatomical possibilities offered should not detract from what is more often a functional diagnosis in the constipated patient.

References

Alstrup N, Ronholt C, Fu C, et al (1997) Viscous fluid expulsion in the evaluation of the constipated patient. Dis Colon Rectum 40:580–584

Arnold MW, Stewart WR, Aguilar PS (1990) Rectocele repair: four years experience. Dis Colon Rectum 33:684–687

Bernini A, Madoff RD, Lowry AC, et al (1998) Should patients with combined colonic inertia and nonrelaxing pelvic floor undergo subtotal colectomy? Dis Colon Rectum 41: 1363–1366

Bleijenberg G, Kuijpers HC (1987) Treatment of the spastic

pelvic floor syndrome with biofeedback. Dis Colon Rectum 30:108–111
Bouchard C (1906) Lectures on auto-intoxication in disease or self-poisoning of the individual. Davis, Philadelphia
Broden B, Snellman B (1968) Procidentia of the rectum studied with cineradiography: a contribution to the discussion of the causative mechanism. Dis Colon Rectum 11:330–347
Cavallo G, Salzano A, Grassi R, et al (1993) Functional intraperineal pouch of rectal wall (posterior rectocele). Dis Colon Rectum 36:179–181
Chaussade S, Khyari A, Roche H, et al (1989) Determination of total and segmental colonic transit time in constipated patients: results in 91 patients with a new simplified method. Dig Dis Sci 34:1168–1172
Christiansen J, Zhu BW, Rasmussen OO, et al (1992) Internal rectal intussusception: results of surgical repair. Dis Colon Rectum 35:1026–1029
Drossman DA (1994) Idiopathic constipation: definition, epidemiology and behavioural aspects. In: Kamm M, Lennard-Jones J (eds) Constipation. Wrightson Biomedical, Petersfield, pp 11–17
Duthie GS, Bartolo DC (1992) Anismus: the cause of constipation? World J Surg 16:831–835
Ebbell BB (ed) (1937) The papyrus Ebers. Levin and Munksgaard, Copenhagen
Engel AF, Kamm MA (1994) The acute effect of straining on pelvic floor neurological function. Int J Colorectal Dis 9:8–12
Eu KW, Seow-Choen F (1997) Functional problems in adult rectal prolapse and controversies in surgical management. Br J Surg 84:904–911
Fleshman JW, Dreznik Z, Cohen E, et al (1992) Balloon expulsion test facilitates diagnosis of pelvic floor outlet obstruction due to nonrelaxing puborectalis muscle. Dis Colon Rectum 35:1019–1025
Gattuso JM, Kamm MA (1997) Clinical features of idiopathic megarectum and idiopathic megacolon. Gut 41:93–99
Glia A, Lindberg G (1998) Antroduodenal manometry findings in patients with slow-transit constipation. Scand J Gastroenterol 33:55–62
Goh V, Halligan S, Kaplan G, et al (2000) Dynamic MR imaging of the pelvic floor in asymptomatic subjects. AJR Am J Roentgenol 174:661–666
Halligan S (1994) Posterior perineal hernia or posterior rectocele? Clin Radiol 49:219
Halligan S (1995) The benefits or otherwise of evacuation proctography. Abdom Imaging 20:280
Halligan S, Bartram CI (1995) Is barium trapping in rectoceles significant? Dis Colon Rectum 38:764–768
Halligan S, Bartram CI (1996) Is digitation associated with proctographic abnormality? Int J Colorectal Dis 11:167–171
Halligan S, Bartram CI (1998) Anismus: fact or fiction? Dis Colon Rectum 41:1070–1071
Halligan S, McGee S, Bartram CI (1994) Quantification of evacuation proctography. Dis Colon Rectum 37:1151–1154
Halligan S, Nicholls RJ, Bartram CI (1995a) Proctographic changes following rectopexy for solitary rectal ulcer syndrome and preoperative predictive factors for a successful outcome. Br J Surg 82:314–317
Halligan S, Nicholls RJ, Bartram CI (1995b) Evacuation proctography in patients with solitary rectal ulcer syndrome: anatomic abnormalities and frequency of impaired emptying and prolapse. AJR Am J Roentgenol 164:91–95
Halligan S, Thomas J, Bartram CI (1995c) Intrarectal pressures and balloon expulsion related to evacuation proctography. Gut 31:100–104
Halligan S, Bartram CI, Park HY, et al (1995d) The proctographic features of anismus. Radiology 197:679–682
Halligan S, Bartram C, Hall C, et al (1996) Enterocele revealed by simultaneous evacuation proctography and peritoneography: does "defecation block" exist? AJR Am J Roentgenol 167:461–466
Halligan S, Malouf A, Bartram CI, et al (2001) Predictive value of impaired proctographic evacuation for diagnosis of anismus. AJR Am J Roentgenol 177:633–636
Harewood GC, Coulie B, Camilleri M, et al (1999) Descending perineum syndrome: audit of clinical and laboratory features and outcome of pelvic floor retraining. Am J Gastroenterol 94:126–130
Harvey C, Halligan S, Bartram CI, et al (1999) Evacuation proctography: a prospective study of diagnostic and therapeutic impact. Radiology 211:223–227
Heaton KW, Ghosh S, Braddon FEM (1991) How bad are the symptoms and bowel dysfunction of patients with the irritable bowel syndrome? A prospective controlled study with emphasis on stool form. Gut 32:73–79
Healy JC, Halligan S, Reznek RH, et al (1997) Dynamic magnetic resonance imaging of the pelvic floor in patients with obstructed defecation. Br J Surg 84:1555–1558
Henry MM, Parks AG, Swash M (1982) The pelvic floor musculature in the descending perineum syndrome. Br J Surg 69:470–472
Hiltunen KM, Kolehmainen H, Matikainen M (1994) Does defaecography help in diagnosis and clinical decision making in defecation disorders? Abdom Imaging 19:355–358
Hinton JM, Lennard-Jones JE, Young AC (1969) A new method for studying gut transit times using radio-opaque markers. Gut 10:842–847
Hoffman MJ, Kodner IJ, Fry RD (1984) Internal intussusception of the rectum: diagnosis and surgical management. Dis Colon Rectum 27:435–441
Ihre T (1990) Intussusception of the rectum and the solitary rectal ulcer syndrome. Ann Med 22:419–423
Johanson JF, Sonnenberg A, Koch TR (1989) Clinical epidemiology of chronic constipation. J Clin Gastroenterol 11:525–536
Johansson CJ, Ihre T, Ahlback SO (1985) Disturbances in the defecation mechanism with special reference to intussusception of the rectum. Dis Colon Rectum 28:920–924
Johansson C, Nilsson BY, Holmstrom B, et al (1992) Association between rectocele and paradoxical sphincter response. Dis Colon Rectum 35:503–509
Jones PN, Lubowski DZ, Swash M, et al (1987) Is paradoxical contraction of puborectalis muscle of functional importance? Dis Colon Rectum 30:667–670
Jorge JMN, Wexner SD, Ehrenpreis ED, et al (1993a) Does perineal descent correlate with pudendal neuropathy? Dis Colon Rectum 36:475–483
Jorge JM, Wexner SD, Ger GC, et al (1993b) Cinedefecography and electromyography in the diagnosis of non-relaxing puborectalis syndrome. Dis Colon Rectum 36:668–676
Kamm MA, Hawley PR, Lennard-Jones JE (1988) Outcome

of colectomy for severe idiopathic constipation. Gut 29:969–973

Kamm MA, Bartram CI, Lennard-Jones JE (1989) Rectodynamics – quantifying rectal evacuation. Int J Colorectal Dis 4:161–163

Kelvin FM, Maglinte DDT (1997) Dynamic cystoproctography of female pelvic floor defects and their interrelationships. AJR Am J Roentgenol 169:769–774

Kelvin FM, Maglinte DDT, Hornback JA, et al (1992) Pelvic prolapse: assessment with evacuation proctography (defecography). Radiology 184:547–551

Kelvin FM, Maglinte DDT, Benson JT, et al (1995) Re: The role of defecography in clinical practice. Abdom Imaging 20:279–280

Klauser AG, Voderholzer WA, Heinrich CA, et al (1990) Behavioural modification of colonic function: can constipation be learned? Dig Dis Sci 35:1271–1275

Knowles CH, Scott SM, Wellmer A, et al (1999) Sensory and autonomic neuropathy in patients with idiopathic slow transit constipation. Br J Surg 86:54–60

Kuijpers HC, Bleijenberg G (1986) The spastic pelvic floor syndrome: a cause of constipation. Dis Colon Rectum 28:669–672

Laarhoven CJHM, Kamm MA, Bartram CI, et al (1999) Relationship between anatomic and symptomatic long-term results after rectocele repair for impaired defecation. Dis Colon Rectum 42:204–211

Lane WA (1913) An address on chronic intestinal stasis. BMJ ii:1126

Lau CW, Heymen S, Alabaz O, et al (2000) Prognostic significance of rectocele, intussusception and abnormal perineal descent in biofeedback treatment for constipated patients with paradoxical puborectalis contraction. Dis Colon Rectum 43:478–482

Leroi AM (1995) Anismus as a marker of sexual abuse: consequences of abuse on anorectal motility. Dig Dis Sci 40:1411–1416

Liberman H, Hughes C, Dippolito A (2000) Evaluation and outcome of the delorme procedure in the treatment of rectal outlet obstruction. Dis Colon Rectum 43:188–192

Lienemann A, Anthuber C, Baron A, et al (1997) Dynamic MR colpocystorectography assessing pelvic floor descent. Eur Radiol 7:1309–1317

Loder P, Watson S, Halligan S, et al (1996) Transperineal repair of symptomatic rectocele with Marlex mesh: a clinical, physiological and radiological assessment of treatment. J Am Coll Surg 183:257–261

McGee SG, Bartram CI (1993) Intra-anal intussusception: diagnosis by posteroanterior stress proctography. Abdom Imaging 2:136–140

McKee RF, McEnroe L, Anderson JH, et al (1999) Identification of patients likely to benefit from biofeedback for outlet obstruction constipation. Br J Surg 86:355–359

Mellgren A, Schultz I, Johansson C, et al (1997) Internal rectal intussusception seldom develops into total rectal prolapse. Dis Colon Rectum 40:817–820

Mellgren A, Lopez A, Schultz I, et al (1998) Rectocele is associated with paradoxical anal sphincter reaction. Int J Colorectal Dis 13:13–16

Mimura T, Roy AJ, Storrie JB, et al (2000) Treatment of impaired defecation associated with rectocele by behavioural retraining (biofeedback). Dis Colon Rectum 43:1267–1272

Murthy VK, Orkin BA, Smith LE, et al (1996) Excellent outcome using selective criteria for rectocele repair. Dis Colon Rectum 39:374–378

Oettle GJ, Roe AM, Bartolo DC, et al (1985) What is the best way of measuring perineal descent? A comparison of radiographic and clinical methods. Br J Surg 72:999–1001

Orrom WJ, Bartolo DCC, Miller R, et al (1991) Rectopexy is an ineffective treatment for obstructed defecation. Dis Colon Rectum 34:41–46

Ott DJ, Donati DL, Kerr RM, et al (1994) Defecography: results in 55 patients and impact on clinical management. Abdom Imaging 9:349–354

Parks AG, Porter NH, Hardcastle JD (1966) The syndrome of the descending perineum. Proc R Soc Med 59:477–482

Preston DM, Lennard-Jones JE (1985) Anismus in chronic constipation. Dig Dis Sci 30:413–418

Preston DM, Lennard-Jones JE (1986) Severe chronic constipation of young women: idiopathic slow transit constipation. Gut 27:41–48

Prior A, Maxton DG, Whorwell JP (1990) Anorectal manometry in irritable bowel syndrome: differences between diarrhoea and constipation predominant subjects. Gut 31:458–462

Probert CSJ, Emmett PM, Cripps HA, et al (1994) Evidence for the ambiguity of the term constipation: the role of the irritable bowel syndrome. Gut 35:1455–1458

Read NW (1989) Tests of anorectal function: summary and conclusions. In: Read NW (ed) Gastrointestinal motility: which test? Wrightson Biomedical, Petersfield, pp 277–282

Read NW, Timms JM, Bannister JJ, et al (1986) Impairment of defecation in young women with severe constipation. Gastroenterology 90:53–60

Rex DR, Lappas JC, Goutet RC, et al (1992) Selection of constipated subjects as subtotal colectomy candidates. J Clin Gastroenterol 15:212–217

Sandler RS, Drossman DA (1987) Bowel habits in young adults not seeking health care. Dig Dis Sci 32:841–845

Schoenberger AW, Debatin JF, Guldenschuh I, et al (1998) Dynamic MR defecography with a superconducting, open-configuration MR system. Radiology 206:641–646

Shorvon PJ, McHugh S, Diamant NE, et al (1989) Defecography in normal volunteers: results and implications. Gut 30:1737–1749

Skomorowska E, Hegedus V, Christiansen J (1988) Evaluation of perineal descent by defaecography. Int J Colorectal Dis 3:191–194

Sun WM, Read NW, Donnelly TC, et al (1989) A common pathophysiology for full thickness rectal prolapse, anterior mucosal prolapse and solitary rectal ulcer. Br J Surg 76:290–295

Talley NJ, Weaver AL, Zinmeister AR, et al (1993) Functional constipation and outlet delay: a population based study. Gastroenterology 105:781–790

Thompson WG, Dotevall G, Drossman DA, et al (1989) Irritable bowel syndrome: guidelines for the diagnosis. Gastroenterol Int 2:92–95

Thorpe AC, Williams NS, Badenoch DF, et al (1993) Simultaneous electromyographic proctography and cystometrography. Br J Surg 80:115–120

Tjandra JJ, Ooi BS, Tang CL, et al (1999) Transanal repair of rectocele corrects obstructed defecation if it is not associated with anismus. Dis Colon Rectum 42:1544–1550

Turnbull GK, Bartram CI, Lennard-Jones JE (1988) Radiologic

studies of rectal evacuation in adults with idiopathic constipation. Dis Colon Rectum 31:190–197

Tuttle JP (1903) A treatise on the diseases of the anus, rectum and pelvic colon. Appleton, New York London

van Dam JH, Hop WC, Schouten WR (2000) Analysis of patients with poor outcome of rectocele repair. Dis Colon Rectum 43:1556–1560

van Tets WF, Kuijpers JHC (1995) Internal rectal intussusception – fact or fancy? Dis Colon Rectum 38:1080–1083

Wasserman IF (1964) Puborectalis syndrome (rectal stenosis due to anorectal spasm). Dis Colon Rectum 7:87–98

Whorton J (2000) Civilisation and the colon: constipation as the «disease of diseases». BMJ 321:1586–1589

Womack NR, Williams NS, Holmfield JHM, et al (1987) Pressure and prolapse: the cause of the solitary rectal ulcer syndrome. Gut 28:1228–1233

6.2 Faecal Incontinence

C. I. Bartram

CONTENTS

6.2.1 Introduction 159
6.2.2 The Aetiology of Incontinence 160
6.2.3 Neurological Damage 160
6.2.4 Congenital Anomalies 162
6.2.5 Sphincter Injury 162
6.2.6 Conclusions 163
References 163

6.2.1 Introduction

Anal incontinence may be categorized into an inability to control flatus, liquid or solid stool, and faecal leakage divided into minor when there is just some staining of underwear or bedding, or major where there is definite soiling. The prevalence of some degree of faecal incontinence in the general population is about 2% (Nelson et al. 1995) rising to 7% in the elderly (Kamm 1998). Faecal incontinence has a considerable impact on quality of life. It is a socially embarrassing problem that inhibits up to a third of sufferers from seeking medical attention.

A number of questionnaires have been devised to quantify anal incontinence. The initial system by Browning and Parks (1983) simply categorized what the patient was incontinent to, i.e. flatus, liquid or solid stool. The Wexner questionnaire is perhaps one of most widely used scoring systems (Jorge and Wexner 1993). A major advantage is that it combines an estimation of leakage frequency, with the need to wear a pad and the overall effect on lifestyle (Table 6.2.1). Using this system a score of 0 indicates perfect continence, and 20 complete incontinence.

Faecal incontinence is complex in causation, and radiologists should not oversimplify the aetiology by just concentrating on mechanical damage to the sphincter. There are many factors involved, and the relationship between these underlies the paradox of how some patients, with neurological damage but intact sphincters or damaged sphincters but intact neurology, remain continent. Incontinence may be divided into "passive", where leakage is the main problem, and "urge" where stool cannot be held back (Engel et al. 1995). The former is more likely to be due to internal, and the latter to external, sphincter damage.

Table 6.2.1. The Wexner score (Jorge and Wexner 1993)

Type of incontinence	Frequency				
	Never	Rarely (<1 per month)	Sometimes (<1 per week, >1 per month)	Usually (<1 per day, >1 per week)	Always (>1 per day)
Solid	0	1	2	3	4
Liquid	0	1	2	3	4
Gas	0	1	2	3	4
Wears pad	0	1	2	3	4
Lifestyle alteration	0	1	2	3	4

C. I. Bartram, FRCS, FRCP, FRCR
Intestinal Imaging, Level 4V, St Mark's Hospital, Northwick Park, Harrow, HA1 3UJ, UK

6.2.2
The Aetiology of Incontinence

There are many causes of incontinence that may act independently or in conjunction to compromise continence. The speed and volume of colonic contents reaching the rectum are critical. Anyone with severe diarrhoea may be incontinent. With a normal stool delivery, rectal compliance, capacity and sensation are essential. If the patient is unaware of stool entering the rectum, none of the protective mechanisms may be evoked, and the patient incontinent despite an intact sphincter. Episodes of incontinence become more common if the ability to differentiate between gas and stool is lost. Leakage will be a problem if the sphincters and pelvic floor are not providing an adequate sphincter closure pressure, or the closure pressure may be adequate, but the final seal by the anal cushions or subepithelium incomplete due excision of tissue at surgery. Many factors must therefore work in coordination to achieve continence. These include:

- stool delivery
  - adequate consistency and volume
- rectal function
  - compliance
  - sensation
  - contractility
- anorectal responses
  - recto-anal inhibitory reflex and anal sampling
- anal sphincters
  - sphincters intact
  - good sphincter function and muscle bulk
  - coordinated contraction

Disorders of these components may be neuropathic or structural, which includes congenital anomalies.

6.2.3
Neurological Damage

This may involve the pudendal nerve that supplies the pelvic floor and anal sphincter, or the autonomic supply to the rectum.

Childbirth is the commonest cause of pudendal nerve injury. As the foetal head pushes downwards on the pelvic floor to dilate the introitus, the branches of the pudendal nerve to the anal sphincter and levator ani will be stretched. Nerve damage from pelvic sidewall compression is now extremely rare, being really a complication of chronically obstructed labour. Epi-siotomy may reduce the degree of stretching required for the baby's head to pass through the introitus, but a reduction of nerve damage has not be demonstrated. Following vaginal delivery the pudendal nerve motor terminal latencies are increased for about 6 months, but even when these return to normal, some underlying damage remains as there is a fall in squeeze pressure after vaginal delivery, irrespective of sphincter damage. At 9 months after a first vaginal delivery, 1% of women had faecal incontinence, and 26% involuntary passage of flatus (ZETTERSTROM et al. 1999). Nerve damage appears to be cumulative, whereas direct sphincter damage is most likely in the first delivery. Sphincter injury suffered during the first delivery may be insufficient to compromise continence, but when combined with progressive nerve damage from a second delivery may be sufficient to produce overt incontinence (FYNES et al. 1999).

Diabetes mellitus may be associated with a profound autonomic neuropathy leading to dysfunction of the colorectum and sphincters. Low anterior resection also compromises the autonomic supply with loss of the inferior mesenteric ganglion leading to minor incontinence, and more major incontinence with damage to the hypogastric plexus (RAO et al. 1996).

Abnormal thinning of the internal sphincter with passive incontinence (VAIZEY et al. 1997) is common and of unknown aetiology. Changes in the ultrastructure of the internal sphincter with neurogenic incontinence have been described with an increased collagen content (SPEAKMAN et al. 1995), though the relationship to sphincter thickness has not been documented. Thinning of the internal sphincter, associated with the onset of faecal incontinence, has been described in systemic sclerosis (Fig. 6.2.1) (ENGEL et al. 1994).

Disorders of rectal motor complexes are common with autonomic neuropathy. There may be high-pressure contractions that exceed sphincter tone, or the absence of compensatory increases of tone in the sphincter. With pudendal neuropathy the resting and squeeze pressures are reduced. Transient internal sphincter relaxations, a normal feature of anal sampling, become more profound and longer so that normal rectal pressures may often exceed sphincter tone, again leading to incontinence.

Pelvic floor descent may be measured at rest and during straining. Clinical measurement of the perineal descent is on straining, as it is measured with the patient recumbent. The same applies to dynamic MRI studies. It is only when the patient is seated for proctography that the weight of the abdominal contents stresses the pelvic floor to reveal the abnormal

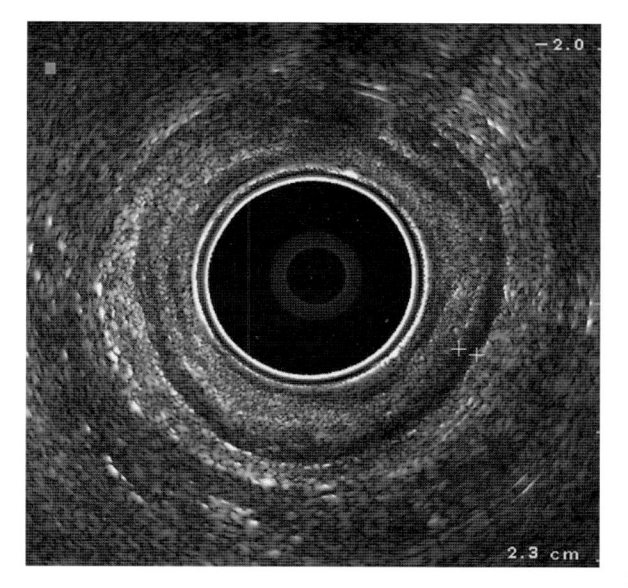

Fig. 6.2.1. Thin internal sphincter (1.5 mm between markers in a middle-aged woman) in systemic sclerosis associated with faecal incontinence

- normal
- slight atrophy – some decrease in muscle mass compared to the puboviceralis
- moderate atrophy – some muscle fibres present
- severe atrophy – no muscle fibres remaining and only fascia identifiable.

Gross atrophy is easily recognized (Fig. 6.2.5). Less obvious though still functional significant atrophy is more difficult to recognize.

position of the pelvic floor at rest (Fig. 6.2.2). Descent is common with advanced age. It may be secondary to prolonged straining, and the condition has been considered to cause primary damage to the pudendal nerves by stretching (PARKS et al. 1966). It is a marker of pelvic floor weakness, as it implies fascial stretching secondary to weakness of the support muscles, which is usually neuropathic in origin.

Leakage of contrast at rest on evacuation proctography (Fig. 6.2.3) is also a good indication of sphincter weakness (REX and LAPPAS 1992), and is found only in patients with overt faecal incontinence. This does depend on how much contrast is injected. If the rectum is filled to maximum tolerated capacity this may invoke the rectoanal reflex and cause leakage.

External sphincter atrophy is difficult to recognize on endosonography, as the outer border of the external sphincter is lost, so that the sphincter thickness cannot be measured (see Chapter 4). The criteria on endocoil MRI are not clearly established. A relationship between cross-sectional area of the sphincter, fat content and squeeze pressure has been established (WILLIAMS et al. 2001), but is too time consuming for routine use. Based on single-fibre electromyography, a template for normal, intermediate (Fig. 6.2.4) and advanced atrophy has been validated. An alternative grading system (BRIEL et al. 1999; BRIEL et al. 2000) may be used to quantify atrophy:

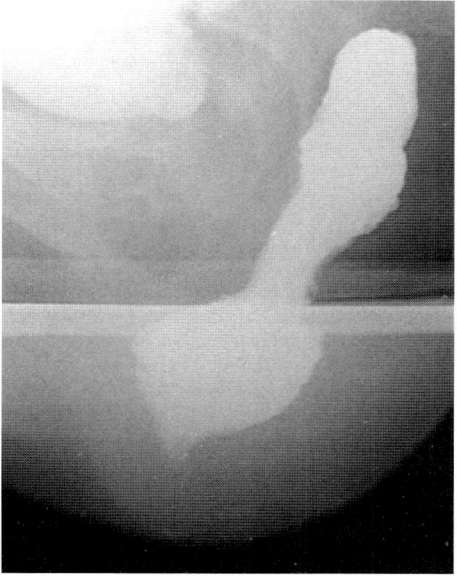

Fig. 6.2.2. Evacuation proctography showing marked pelvic floor descent at rest with the anorectal junction considerably below the ischial tuberosity level (normal <1 cm below)

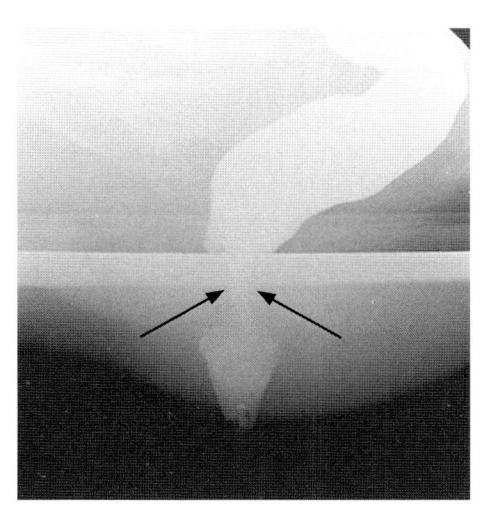

Fig. 6.2.3. The anal canal (*between arrows*) is open at rest, indicating significant sphincter weakness

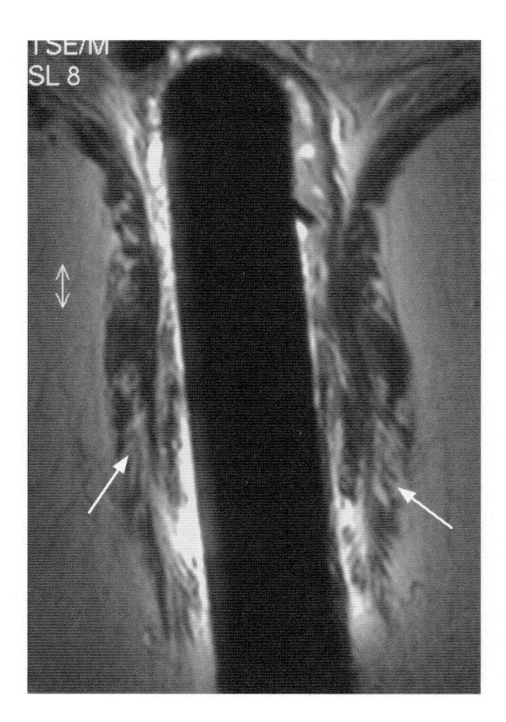

Fig. 6.2.4. MRI endocoil in coronal plane showing intermediate atrophy with excess fat between residual muscle fibres (*arrows*)

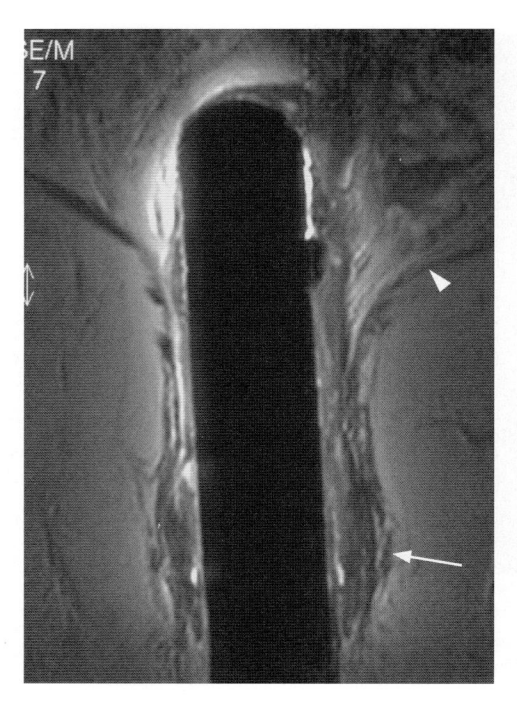

Fig. 6.2.5. MRI endocoil in axial plane showing gross atrophy of the external sphincter (*arrow*) and levator ani (*arrowhead*)

6.2.4
Congenital Anomalies

Low lesions involve a membranous covering to the canal. The sphincteric mechanism is largely intact, so that simply cutting the membrane has good results, although about a half will have some bowel function problem as adults. High anomalies, requiring pull-throughs, have much greater anatomical derangement. There is no internal sphincter with a pull through. The external sphincter and puborectalis may be patchy and may be ectopic. Endocoil MRI is ideal to show residual muscle around the canal and ectopic placement (DESOUZA et al. 1999) (Fig. 6.2.6). Endosonography also shows residual sphincter around the canal, but does not detect displaced muscle so clearly.

6.2.5
Sphincter Injury

The function of the anal sphincter is to exert a background of constant pressure with intermittent increases to maintain the mucosal seal despite wide fluctuations of rectal pressure. Sphincter function is impaired if there is a break in the ring of the sphincter, as then the sphincter is effectively lengthened and for a given fibre contraction the pressure generated in the centre is reduced. Likewise, if the unit strength of the muscle fibres in the sphincters is reduced, the effective closing pressure will also decrease.

Endosonography is the optimum examination to show damage to the internal sphincter, either with general thinning as found in internal sphincter degeneration, or from focal breaks in the sphincter from any cause of trauma, but particularly from surgical procedures such as anal stretch, lateral internal anal sphincterotomy, fistulotomy for fistula, or as part of generalized sphincter trauma from childbirth. The thickness of the internal sphincter has a more complex relationship to function. It is not correct to relate thickness to strength, as the internal sphincter is very thin in young patients but very effective. In the elderly an increase in thickness does not correlate with more smooth muscle, but an increase in collagen (HAAS and FOX 1980; SPEAKMAN et al. 1995). Possibly this increase compensates for the decrease in smooth muscle, so that the thin internal sphincter in an elderly patient represents a failure of this process, which is associated with a reduction in resting pressure (VAIZEY et al. 1997).

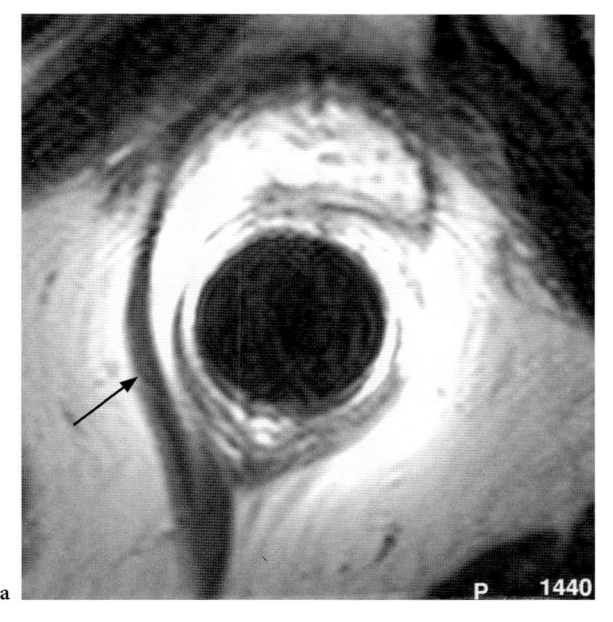

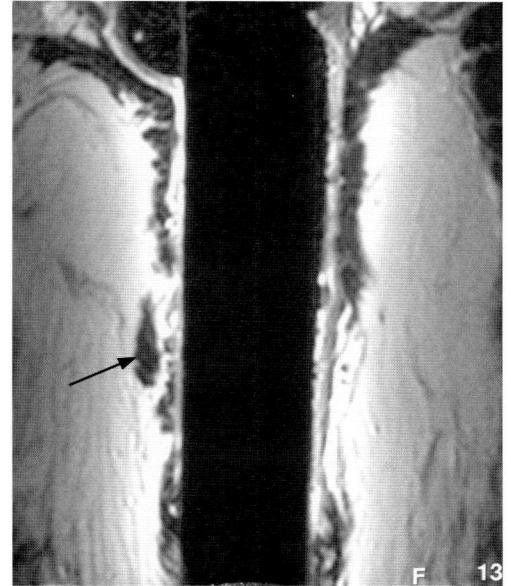

Fig. 6.2.6a, b. Axial (a) and coronal (b) MRI endocoil images after a pull through with only a little puborectalis on the right side (*arrows*) and no external sphincter

Tears in the external sphincter are also well defined by endosonography, but any overall loss of striated muscle fibres from denervation is difficult to determine and endocoil MRI is required for this.

6.2.6
Conclusions

Faecal incontinence is often multifactorial. Clinical examination may not detect the cause in about 25% of patients, although a surgically correctable aetiology is less likely to be missed (KEATING et al. 1997). MRI is a powerful tool to investigate weakness of the pelvic floor generally and atrophy of the external sphincter. Endosonography is valuable as a screening procedure to pick up sphincter tears amenable to surgical correction. Proctography may demonstrate pelvic floor and sphincter weakness by abnormal descent at rest and anal leakage, but, unless there is a concomitant problem such as prolapse, is not indicated routinely.

References

Briel JW, Stoker J, Rociu E, et al (1999) External anal sphincter atrophy on endoanal magnetic resonance imaging adversely affects continence after sphincteroplasty. Br J Surg 86:1322–1327

Briel JW, Zimmerman DD, Stoker J, et al (2000) Relationship between sphincter morphology on endoanal MRI and histopathological aspects of the external anal sphincter. Int J Colorectal Dis 15:87–90

Browning GG, Parks AG (1983) Postanal repair for neuropathic faecal incontinence: correlation of clinical result and anal canal pressures. Br J Surg 70:101–104

deSouza NM, Ward HC, Williams AD, et al (1999) Transanal MR imaging after repair of anorectal anomalies in children: appearances in pull-through versus posterior sagittal reconstructions. AJR Am J Roentgenol 173:723–728

Engel AF, Kamm MA, Talbot IC (1994) Progressive systemic sclerosis of the internal anal sphincter leading to passive faecal incontinence. Gut 35:857–859

Engel AF, Kamm MA, Bartram CI, et al (1995) Relationship of symptoms in faecal incontinence to specific sphincter abnormalities. Int J Colorectal Dis 10:152–155

Fynes M, Donnelly V, Behan M, et al (1999) Effect of second vaginal delivery on anorectal physiology and faecal continence: a prospective study. Lancet 354:983–986

Haas PA, Fox TA Jr (1980) Age-related changes and scar formations of perianal connective tissue. Dis Colon Rectum 23:160–169

Jorge JM, Wexner SD (1993) Etiology and management of fecal incontinence. Dis Colon Rectum 36:77–97

Kamm MA (1998) Faecal incontinence. BMJ 316:528–532

Keating JP, Stewart PJ, Eyers AA, et al (1997) Are special investigations of value in the management of patients with fecal incontinence? Dis Colon Rectum 40:896–901

Nelson R, Norton N, Cautley E, et al (1995) Community-based prevalence of anal incontinence. JAMA 274:559–561

Parks AG, Hardcastle JD, Hardcastle JD (1966) The syndrome of the descending perineum. Proc R Soc Med 59:477–482

Rao GN, Drew PJ, Lee PW, et al (1996) Anterior resection syndrome is secondary to sympathetic denervation. Int J Colorectal Dis 11:250–258

Rex DK, Lappas JC (1992) Combined anorectal manometry and defecography in 50 consecutive adults with fecal incontinence. Dis Colon Rectum 35:1040–1045

Speakman CT, Hoyle CH, Kamm MA, et al (1995) Abnormal internal anal sphincter fibrosis and elasticity in fecal incontinence. Dis Colon Rectum 38:407–410

Vaizey CJ, Kamm MA, Bartram CI (1997) Primary degeneration of the internal anal sphincter as a cause of passive faecal incontinence. Lancet 349:612–615

Williams AB, Bartram CI, Modhwadia D, et al (2001) Endocoil magnetic resonance imaging quantification of external anal sphincter atrophy. Br J Surg 88:853–859

Zetterstrom JP, Lopez A, Anzen B, et al (1999) Anal incontinence after vaginal delivery: a prospective study in primiparous women. Br J Obstet Gynaecol 106:324–330

6.3 Surgical Management of Faecal Incontinence

C. J. Vaizey and C. I. Bartram

CONTENTS

6.3.1 Introduction 165
6.3.2 Sphincter Repair 165
6.3.2.1 Postanal Repair 167
6.3.3 Neosphincters 167
6.3.3.1 Dynamic Graciloplasty 167
6.3.3.2 The Artificial Anal Sphincter 168
6.3.3.3 Sphincter Augmentation
   with Injectable Biomaterials 168
6.3.3.4 Sacral Nerve Stimulation 169
6.3.4 Biofeedback 169
6.3.5 Conclusions 169
   References 170

6.3.1 Introduction

Surgical innovation by Park's in the 1970's established a role for surgery in the management of faecal incontinence. The techniques he pioneered were the overlapping repair for sphincter trauma (Parks and McPartlin 1971) and the post anal repair for sphincter weakness (Parks 1967). Of equal importance was his scientific investigation of faecal incontinence that led to a greater understanding of its aetiology (Neill et al. 1981; Parks et al. 1966). Since then other procedures have been developed, but as with some of Parks' original operations, these have not stood the test of long-term follow-up and have been replaced by newer techniques.

Imaging has become closely involved in patient selection for surgery, and for the investigation of operative complication or poor outcome.

C. J. Vaizey, MD, FRCS(Gen), FCS(SA)
Consultant Colorectal Surgeon, Colorectal Surgical Unit, The Middlesex Hospital, Mortimer St, London W1T 3AA, UK
C. I. Bartram, FRCS, FRCP, FRCR
Intestinal Imaging, Level 4V, St Mark's Hospital, Northwick Park, Harrow, HA1 3UJ, UK

6.3.2 Sphincter Repair

The objectives of sphincter repair are to restore sphincter continuity with a complete ring of external sphincter with no interposed fibrous tissue. Although this may be achieved with an end-to-end abuttal, technically the overlapping repair seems to work better. This may in part be due to tightening of the sphincter ring, which will reduce slightly the sphincter radius. LaPlace's law states that the internal pressure in a tube equals the wall tension divided by the radius. Given that the wall tension from muscle fibre resting tone and contraction is constant whatever the means of repair, reducing the radius will increase the pressure in the anal canal and may help achieve more complete closure.

With the patient in the lithotomy or prone jack-knife position an arced incision is made around the anus at the site of the defect (Fig. 6.3.1), the scar tissue divided and the cut ends of the external and internal sphincters mobilized from the underlying subepithelium (Fig. 6.3.2). The scar tissue is usually retained to help anchor the sutures. The ends are overlapped and sutured together (Figs. 6.3.3, 6.3.4).

The benefit from sphincter repair has been reported as 60–80%, with poor results due to a persistent defect

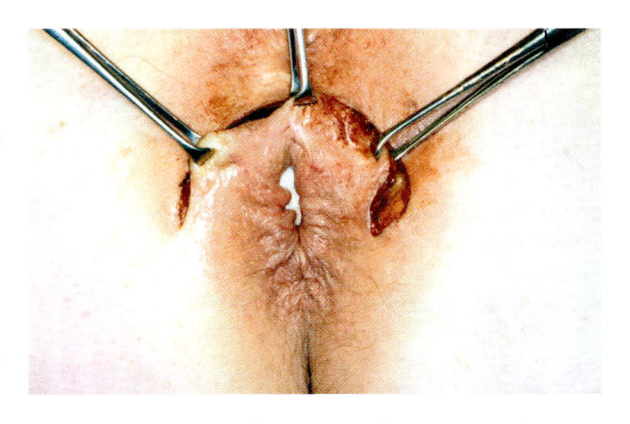

Fig. 6.3.1. Skin incision for anterior sphincter repair (courtesy of Professor R.K.S. Phillips, St Mark's Hospital)

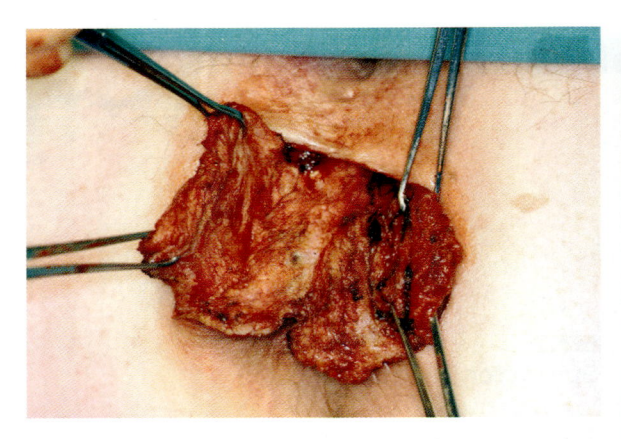

Fig. 6.3.2. Sphincter ends mobilized (courtesy of Professor R.K.S. Phillips, St Mark's Hospital)

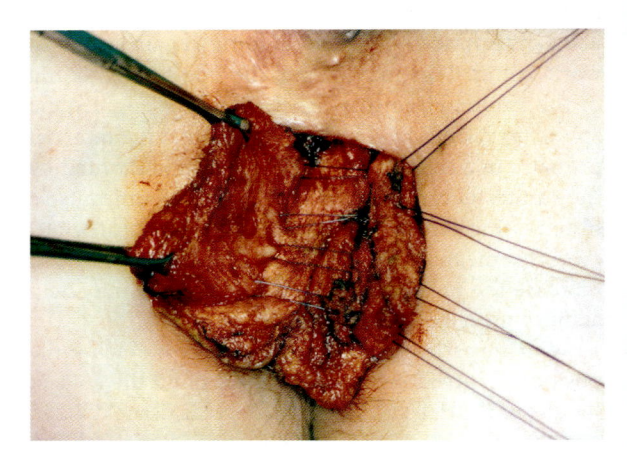

Fig. 6.3.3. Start of overlapping suturing to complete repair (courtesy of Professor R.K.S. Phillips, St Mark's Hospital)

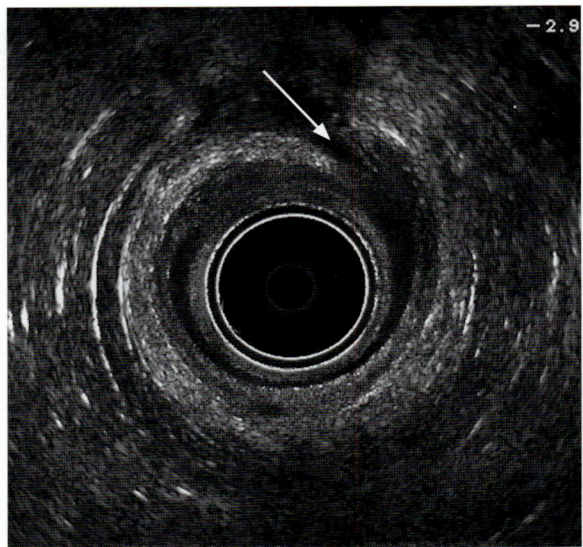

Fig. 6.3.4. Endoanal ultrasound of a satisfactory anterior sphincter repair. Note the way the internal sphincter (*arrow*) overlaps the external sphincter with no intervening segment of scarring

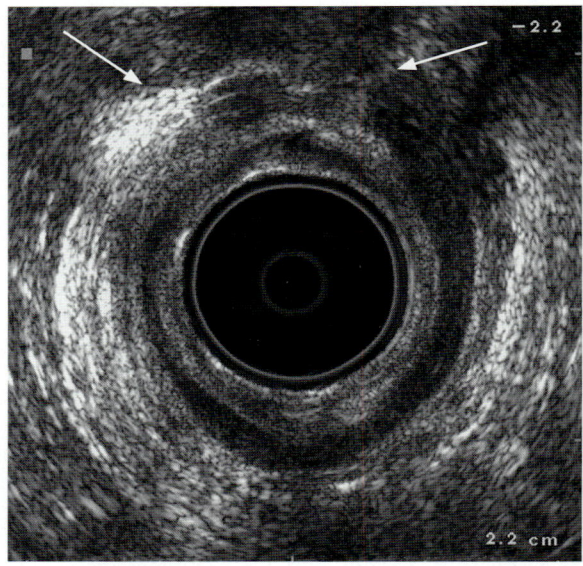

Fig. 6.3.5. Endoanal ultrasound of an incomplete repair with a segment of scarring between the sphincter ends (*arrows*)

(ENGEL et al. 1994) (Fig. 6.3.5). A recent long-term follow-up of these patients suggests that the initial good results were not maintained (MALOUF et al. 2000). Although bias from different methods of continence assessment may explain some of these findings, there are grounds for concern as to the long-term benefit. In those patients in whom a primary repair fails, a secondary sphincteroplasty is possible, and its success, as in a primary repair, relates to restoration of an intact sphincteric ring (PINEDO et al. 1999).

An important consideration is the quality of the sphincteric muscle being repaired. The easiest and simplest way to assess this is just to get the patient to contract the sphincter during digital examination. A good squeeze indicates that the striated sphincteric muscle is adequate for a satisfactory repair. The role of endocoil MRI has yet to be clarified fully, though there is good evidence of its value in assessing external sphincter atrophy. Based on MRI thinning of the muscle fibres or fatty infiltration of the external sphincter, atrophy (Fig. 6.3.6) was diagnosed in 40% of patients undergoing sphincter repair in one series (BRIEL et al. 1999) (see Chapter 4.4). The area of the sphincter, including both external and internal, measured in a mid-canal

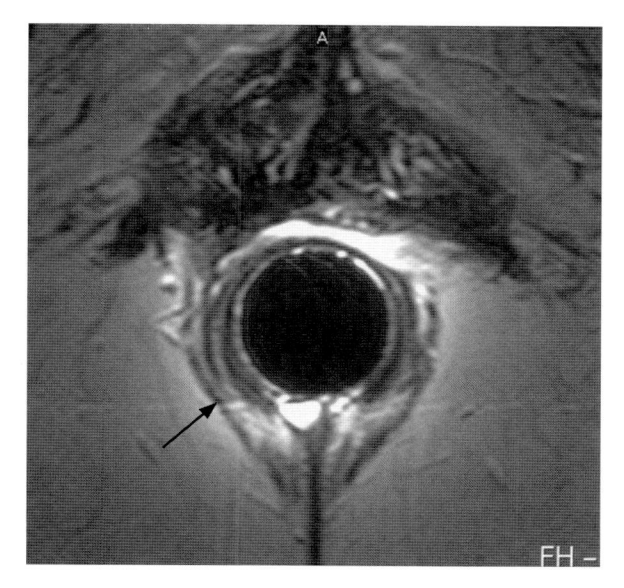

Fig. 6.3.6. Axial MRI with an endocoil showing very thin sphincter in a 51-year-old female with gross atrophy (*arrow* abnormally thin external sphincter) and no sphincter tear

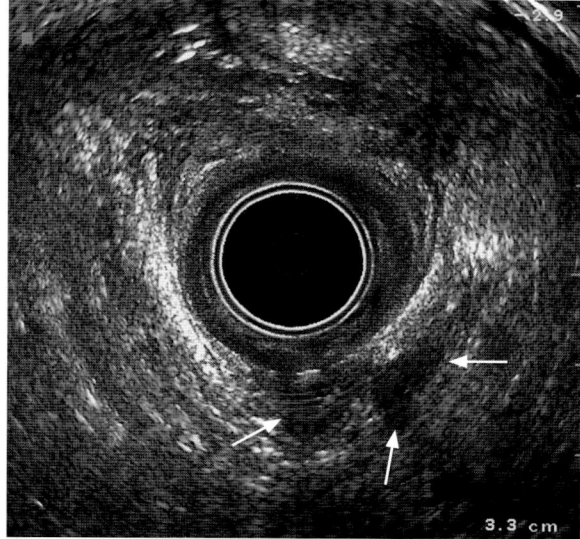

Fig. 6.3.7. Endoanal ultrasound at the level of the puborectalis. Scarring is seen within the muscle (*arrows*) as a result of the postanal repair. The puborectalis and upper external sphincter may be seen to be pinched together from the repair

axial slice, proved to be a significant prognostic factor for outcome. All the patients with an area >360 mm² regained continence, whereas seven of ten with an area <360 mm² did not. Imaging is complementary in this situation with endosonography being a simple cheap test for sphincter tears to select patients for sphincteroplasty, with specialized endocoil MRI needed to exclude significant atrophy in cases where there is doubt clinically as to external sphincter function.

6.3.2.1
Postanal Repair

The rationale for this now outdated procedure was the restoration of an acute anorectal junction angle that Parks believed maintained continence. The procedure also lengthened and tightened the anal canal, with an increase in resting and squeeze pressures. The operation was usually performed in the lithotomy position, with a posterior paraanal incision. The intersphincteric space was opened up, and then the levator ani, puborectalis and external sphincter pulled together and sutured in separate layers to tighten and elongate the anal canal along its posterior aspect. These changes are visible on endosonography (Fig. 6.3.7).

The initial results were most encouraging, with 83% regaining continence (BROWNING and PARKS 1983), but later results unfortunately did not support this earlier enthusiasm. Also, difficulty in evacuation despite an uncomplicated repair could occur. Recent reports suggest only a 35% success rate, with no assessment criteria to determine outcome (MATSUOKA et al. 2000). Postanal repair is seldom performed due to the absence of any defined selection criteria and the poor overall results.

6.3.3
Neosphincters

6.3.3.1
Dynamic Graciloplasty

This is a complex procedure where the gracilis is mobilized and wrapped scarf-like around the anus to be inserted into the opposing ischial tuberosity or tethered to the skin (Fig. 6.3.8). The gracilis contains mainly type-2 fast-twitch fibres, unlike the slow-twitch fibres of the external sphincter. It is possible to transform skeletal muscle, and the second part of the operation is to implant an electrical stimulator into the anterior abdominal wall and connect this to the nerve supply of the gracilis. A programme of incremental stimulation over several weeks converts the fast twitch to fatigue-resistant slow-twitch fibres.

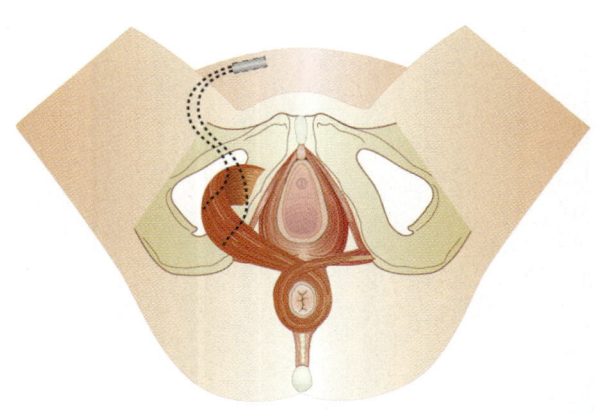

Fig. 6.3.8. Diagrammatic representation of graciloplasty wrap around the anus and insertion into the opposite ischial tuberosity with stimulator in place

Although there have been some specialist centres reporting continence rates of up to 76% (Baeten et al. 2001), its acceptability has been limited due to operative complexity and high morbidity. In two multicentre studies the incidence of severe operative related complications was 42–74% with a reintervention rate of 40% (Baeten et al. 2000; Matzel et al. 2001).

6.3.3.2
The Artificial Anal Sphincter

Artificial sphincter technology was developed for urinary incontinence, and with some minor modification similar devices may be used for anal incontinence.

The hydraulic cuff is implanted circumferentially around the anus, the balloon reservoir into the preperitoneal space just above the inguinal ligament, and the valve placed into the scrotum or labia. Fully implanted siliconized tubing connects the three main components, and the device is filled with a water-soluble contrast agent for radiographic visibility (Fig. 6.3.9). Squeezing the valve deflates the cuff, temporarily transferring fluid into the reservoir to allow defaecation. Passive fluid transfer back from the reservoir slowly reinflates the cuff to restore continence.

The major complication is sepsis, and although the neosphincter may work well (Vaizey et al. 1998), this risk is currently limiting the implantation of devices.

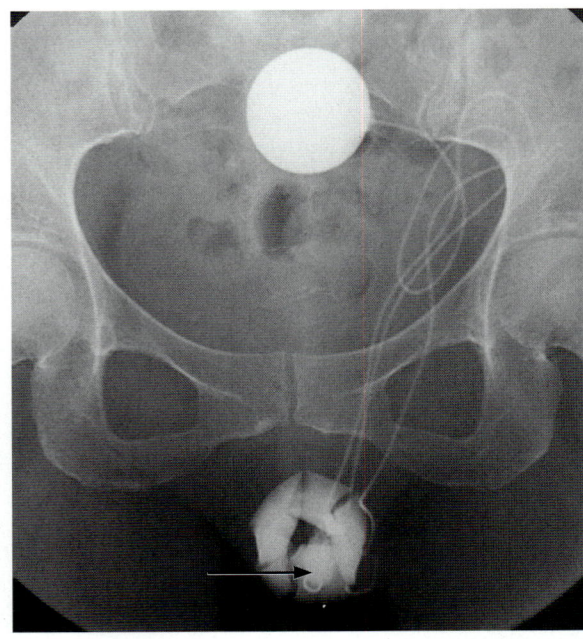

Fig. 6.3.9. Radiograph of an artificial anal sphincter in a woman. The cuff (*C*) is wrapped around the anorectal level. The connections to the reservoir (*R*) and valve in the labium (*arrow*) are clearly outlined by the presence of contrast medium

6.3.3.3
Sphincter Augmentation with Injectable Biomaterials

This is another technology borrowed from urology, where collagen or silicone-based materials are injected around the bladder neck for the treatment of stress incontinence.

Injections into the subepithelial tissues of the anal canal bulk up the cushion effect and aid canal closure. This has proved helpful where there is leakage from an internal sphincter defect or sphincter weakness (Malouf et al. 2001). A recent study (Kenefick et al. 2002) has shown that the median resting pressure rose 63%, with a rise of 45% in the squeeze pressure, though the cause for the latter is uncertain. The optimum injection site is just above the dentate line, so that the injections are pain free, and below the puborectalis to keep the material within the upper anal canal (Fig. 6.3.10). One failure was attributed to migration of the material above the puborectalis. The carrier gel is excreted in a few days, with the silicone particles becoming emeshed in collagen fibrils after 6 weeks to form a permanent bulking agent.

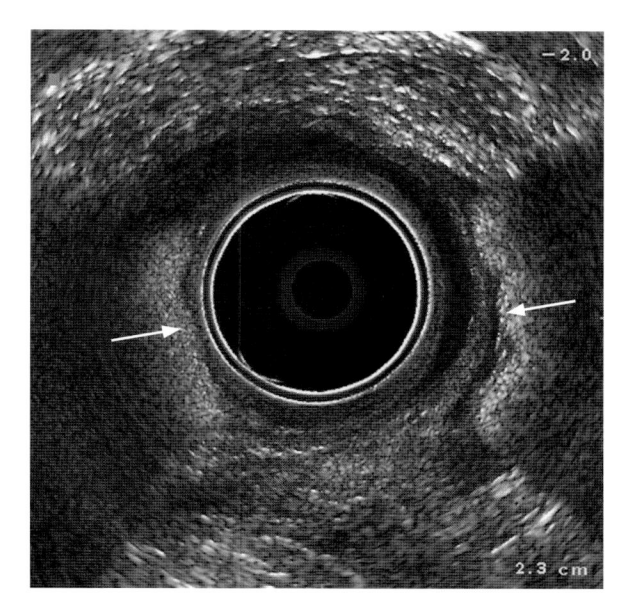

Fig. 6.3.10. Endoanal ultrasound of injected biomaterial. The material creates a dense acoustic shadow so that only the inner edge of the material is visible (*arrows*). The material is in the upper canal just below the puborectalis

6.3.3.4
Sacral Nerve Stimulation

Sacral nerve stimulation is based on the use of modified cardiac pacemakers, and may be suitable for patients in whom other surgical interventions are not applicable or have failed to restore incontinence.

The procedure is performed in three stages with the patient in the prone position:
1. An initial test is undertaken by inserting an insulated needle into the third sacral foramen, and assessing the response to nerve stimulation using a handheld neurostimulator. Stimulation of the S3 root causes anal sphincter contraction with lifting of part of the pelvic floor – the bellows action, and flexion of the big toe.
2. Once the needle has been optimally positioned, a percutaneous stimulator lead is inserted using the needle as a conduit, the needle removed and the lead connected to a small portable external neurostimulator. The patient then keeps an incontinence diary over 2 weeks to assess clinical benefit.
3. If this temporary stimulation produces a marked reduction in incontinence episodes, a permanent and fully implanted electrode and pacemaker are placed in the sacral foramen and buttock.

This is a relatively minor procedure, with a low risk of sepsis or other complication, that works surprisingly well (MALOUF et al. 2001; ROSEN et al. 2001). Quite why is uncertain, and it has been suggested that this may be due to modification of sacral reflexes and stabilization of rectal contractility, as much as any direct effect on the external sphincter (MALOUF et al. 2001). This may explain why it may also have a use in refractory idiopathic constipation, where it has been shown to increase bowel frequency, alter rectal sensation and normalize colonic transit (KENEFICK et al. 2002).

6.3.4
Biofeedback

Surgical techniques must be evaluated by comparison to noninvasive procedures. Pelvic floor retraining using biofeedback techniques is well established in the management of constipation, but also helps faecal incontinence. A systematic review of 46 studies (KAMM 2001; NORTON and KAMM 2001) indicated that 72% received significant benefit from biofeedback and pelvic floor exercises, suggesting that conservative management may help many patients with faecal incontinence.

6.3.5
Conclusions

Decision-making becoming more dependent on meta-analysis and cost effectiveness studies, which have practical difficulties in this condition. The different aetiology of faecal incontinence, difficulty in standardization, evolution of devices, patient choice and need for long-term follow-up limit the possibility of randomized controlled studies (MALOUF et al. 2001). However, studies using new continence scoring systems and quality of life assessment do allow meaningful comparison, and the surgical management of faecal incontinence is undergoing constant development as new techniques become available, and older procedures are reassessed from long-term outcome. Sphincter atrophy and general pelvic floor weakness remain underlying problems limiting the efficacy of primary surgical repairs. Sacral nerve stimulation is a novel procedure that reveals both the complexity of faecal incontinence and a potential method to compensate for the neurological damage. The indications and contraindications of many of these new procedures have yet to be determined.

References

Baeten CG, Bailey HR, Bakka A, et al (2000) Safety and efficacy of dynamic graciloplasty for fecal incontinence: report of a prospective, multicenter trial. Dynamic Graciloplasty Therapy Study Group. Dis Colon Rectum 43:743–751

Baeten CG, Uludag OO, Rongen MJ (2001) Dynamic graciloplasty for fecal incontinence. Microsurgery 21:230–234

Briel JW, Stoker J, Rociu E, et al (1999) External anal sphincter atrophy on endoanal magnetic resonance imaging adversely affects continence after sphincteroplasty. Br J Surg 86:1322–1327

Browning GG, Parks AG (1983) Postanal repair for neuropathic faecal incontinence: correlation of clinical result and anal canal pressures. Br J Surg 70:101–104

Engel AF, Kamm MA, Sultan AH, et al (1994) Anterior anal sphincter repair in patients with obstetric trauma. Br J Surg 81:1231–1234

Kenefick NJ, Nicholls RJ, Cohen RG, et al (2002) Permanent sacral nerve stimulation for treatment of idiopathic constipation. Br J Surg 89:882–888

Kenefick NJ, Vaizey CJ, Malouf AJ, et al (2002) Injectable silicone biomaterial for faecal incontinence due to internal anal sphincter dysfunction. Gut 51:225–228

Malouf AJ, Norton CS, Engel AF, et al (2000) Long-term results of overlapping anterior anal-sphincter repair for obstetric trauma. Lancet 355:260–265

Malouf AJ, Chambers MG, Kamm MA (2001) Clinical and economic evaluation of surgical treatments for faecal incontinence. Br J Surg 88:1029–1036

Malouf AJ, Vaizey CJ, Norton CS, et al (2001) Internal anal sphincter augmentation for fecal incontinence using injectable silicone biomaterial. Dis Colon Rectum 44:595–600

Matsuoka H, Mavrantonis C, Wexner SD, et al (2000) Postanal repair for fecal incontinence – is it worthwhile? Dis Colon Rectum 43:1561–1567

Matzel KE, Madoff RD, LaFontaine LJ, et al (2001) Complications of dynamic graciloplasty: incidence, management, and impact on outcome. Dis Colon Rectum 44:1427–1435

Neill ME, Parks AG, Swash M (1981) Physiological studies of the anal sphincter musculature in faecal incontinence and rectal prolapse. Br J Surg 68:531–536

Norton C, Kamm MA (2001) Anal sphincter biofeedback and pelvic floor exercises for faecal incontinence in adults – a systematic review. Aliment Pharmacol Ther 15:1147–1154

Parks AG (1967) Post-anal perineorrhaphy for rectal prolapse. Proc R Soc Med 60:920–921

Parks AG, McPartlin JF (1971) Late repair of injuries of the anal sphincter. Proc R Soc Med 64:1187–1189

Parks AG, Hardcastle JD, Hardcastle JD (1966) The syndrome of the descending perineum. Proc R Soc Med 59:477–482

Pinedo G, Vaizey CJ, Nicholls RJ, et al (1999) Results of repeat anal sphincter repair. Br J Surg 86:66–69

Rosen HR, Urbarz C, Holzer B, et al (2001) Sacral nerve stimulation as a treatment for fecal incontinence. Gastroenterology 121:536–541

Vaizey CJ, Kamm MA, Gold DM, et al (1998) Clinical, physiological, and radiological study of a new purpose-designed artificial bowel sphincter. Lancet 352:105–109

Subject Index

A

Anal sphincter
- age related changes 23, 24
- anatomy 20–24
- congenital anomalies 162
- nerve supply 24
- sex differences 72, 83
- transvaginal ultrasound 77
- ultrasound 69–78

Anismus
- associated features 153
- definition 152
- proctographic diagnosis 153

Anorectal angle
- definition 47
- relationship to puborectalis activity 152

Ano-rectal physiology 101–106
- anorectal sensation 104
- clinical examination 101
- electromyography (EMG) of anal sphincters 103
- functional anal canal length 103
- pudendal nerve terminal motor latency (PNTML) 103, 104
- resting and squeeze pressures 102
- vector manometry 103

Anterior mucosal prolapse 147

Arcus tendineus fascia pelvis 5, 6, 12, 17, 31, 108, 114

B

Biofeedback
- faecal incontinence 169
- urinary incontinence 133

Bladder
- anatomy 10–12
- beaking of urethrovesical junction 97
- diary 90
- diverticula 97
- emptying 95
- hypermobile outlet 97
- residual volume 95

Bladder neck
- hypermobile on fluoroscopy 97
- mobility, on clinical examination 130
- mobility, perineal ultrasound 97

C

Cloaca 2
Coccygeus muscle 4, 7, 8, 25, 62
Colonic transit with radio-opaque markers 105
Constipation 143–146
- aetiology 144
- autointoxication 143
- definition 143
- evacuation proctography in 146
- idiopathic slow transit 145
- incidence 143, 144
- obstructed defaecation 145, 146
- outlet obstruction 146
- rectal sensory perception in 146
- slow transit, relationship to defaecation 144–146
- water soluble contrast in 145

Cystocele 57, 114
- anterior colporraphy 115, 116
- dynamic cystoproctography 52, 54, 57
- graft placement 115
- incidence on DCP compared to clinical 111
- MRI 61
- paravaginal repair 115
- repair 115, 134
- support, loss of 30, 31
- triphasic examination to diagnose 54, 57, 112

Cystourethrocele 31

D

Defecation block 55
Detrusor muscle anatomy 10–12
Dynamic cystoproctography, fluoroscopic 51–58
- prolapse, grading 53
- synonyms 51
- technique 52, 53
- triphasic 112

Dynamic graciloplasty 167, 168
Dynamic MR imaging pelvic floor 58–65
- fluoroscopy comparison 65, 66
- prolapse 60–65
- technique 58–60

E

Electromyography single fibre 161
Endopelvic fascia 7, 27–29
- interaction with pelvic floor 32, 35
- tears 62

Enterocele
- aetiology 54, 120
- defecation block and 55
- detection by dynamic endosonography 55
- dynamic cystoproctography 51
- grading 53
- incidence on DCP compared to clinical 57, 111
- MRI dynamic 65
- post-hysterectomy 54
- radiological significance 110
- relationship to peritoneocele 56
- surgery 121
- value triphasic examination in diagnosis 52, 54, 61
- widening rectovaginal septum in 63

Evacuation proctography 45–50
- clinical relevance, discussion 154
- compared to scintigraphy 49
- frontal imaging 48
- leakage at rest 161
- normal findings 46–48
- prolonged evacuation 48
- puborectalis impression 48
- radiation dose 46
- stress views 48
- technique 45–46
- with intraperitoneal contrast 49, 56, 66

External anal sphincter
- age related changes 24
- anatomy 21–23
- atrophy 59, 76, 83, 84, 166
- congenital anomalies 162
- embryology 3, 4
- endosonography 70, 71
- MRI 82, 83
- MRI: endosonography diagnosis tears 87
- post partum changes 76
- sex differences 72
- sphincteroplasty 165, 166
- squeeze pressure 102
- tears 74, 84, 85
- tears, incidence post partum 75
- tears, occult 76
- urge faecal incontinence 101

F
Faecal Incontinence 159–164
- aetiology 160
- autonomic neuropathy 160
- incidence 159
- internal sphincter thinning 160
- scoring, Parks & Wexner systems 159
- surgical management 165–170
- types, passive and urge 159

Flap valve
- in vagina 28
- theory of anal continence 47

H
Hirschsprung's disease 145

I
Iliococcygeus 8, 25, 60, 108
Incontinence dual urinary and faecal 130
Internal anal sphincter
- abnormal thickness 72, 84
- age related changes 72, 162
- anatomy 19–21
- dilatation from sexual abuse 74
- endosonography 70
- hereditary myopathy 75
- idiopathic degeneration 84, 160
- lateral internal anal sphincterotomy 73
- MRI 82
- passive faecal incontinence 159
- sex differences 72
- stretch procedures 73
- tears 84
- transvaginal ultrasound 77

International Continence Society
- definition incontinence 125
- grading prolapse 110
- website 90

Intersphincteric space
- anatomy 21, 71, 82
- surgical plane 20

Intra-anal intussusception 147
- digitation 149
- progression to rectal prolapse 148, 149
- relationship to constipation 148

Irritable bowel syndrome Rome criteria 146
Ischioanal fossa 18

K
Kegel's exercises pelvic floor muscle training, and 132

L
Levator ani
- anatomy 5, 7, 8, 28, 32, 34, 35
- defects 63
- effects contraction 15, 31, 108, 109
- embryology 3
- MRI 60

Levator ani muscle
- functional anatomy 32, 34, 35, 110
- localised defects 63
- MRI 60
- prolapse, in 35, 109–111, 113

Longitudinal layer
- anus, anatomy 8, 17, 20, 21, 24
- – sex differences 24
- – age related changes 24
- – –endosonography 70, 71
- – –MRI 80, 81
- bladder 11
- rectum 19
- urethra 13, 37

M
Megacolon, idiopathic 145
Megarectum, idiopathic 145
Midpubic line hymenal ring reference on MRI 64
MRI, endoanal 81–87
- and abnormal thickness 85, 86
- and atrophy 85, 86
- atrophy, comparison
- comparisons with endosonography 85, 87
- disruption, internal anal sphincter 84
- endosonography 87
- external anal sphincter, normal
- fibrous scars, signal 85
- indications 87
- internal anal sphincter, normal
- longitudinal muscle 82, 83
- normal findings 82–85
- pitfalls 82, 83
- role of 87
- sequences 82
- sex differences in anal sphincter 83
- tears, comparison to
- tears, external anal sphincter 85
- technique 81, 82
- to endosonography 85

Subject Index

– transverse perineii 83
Muscularis submucosae ani 21
– endosonography 70
– MRI 82

N
Neuropathy, pudendal 42, 43
– childbirth and, 150
– electromyography 103
– nerve traction in pelvic floor descent 149
– pudendal nerve terminal latency 103, 104
– vaginal delivery 160

O
Obstetric trauma
– external anal sphincter tears, incidence 75
– occult tears 75

P
Pelvic floor
– anatomy 1–26
– clinical syndrome 149
– denervation 42–44
– descent 160, 161
– embryology 3–5
– endopelvic fascia 7, 28, 32
– functional anatomy 27–38
– functional support 27–35
– innervation, autonomic 41, 42
– innervation, somatic 39–41
– layers 6
– levator ani, attachments 4–8
– prolapse, movement in 28
– sensory 42
– tendineus arcs 5, 15
Pelvic floor, prolapse
– clinico-radiological comparisons 111
– co-existing urinary incontinence 113, 114
– etiology 109
– grading system, International continence Society 110
– levator ani dysfunction and 109
– MRI, cost in 113
– MRI, 3D in 109
– repair, surgical approach 113
– surgery and clinical imaging 107–121
Perianal connective tissue 18
Perineal body
– anatomy 18, 19, 23, 32, 33
– confusion with tears 83
– detachment 111
– endosonography 72
– graft 119
– membrane 8, 35
– surgical support 116, 117
Perineal body thickness 77
Perineal ultrasound 77, 78
Perineum
– detachment from levator ani and prolapse 33
– embryology 4
– perineal body 32, 33, 108
Peritoneocele 56
– MRI detection 65
– peritoneography 56, 66

Peritoneography 49, 56
Periurethral ligament 15
Puboanalis
– anatomy 22
– endosonography 70, 71
– tears 75
Pubovisceralis anatomy 1, 4, 8, 23
Puboccygeal line
– definition 63
– „HMO" classification 63
– pelvic organ prolapse, reference point 63
Pubococcygeal line
– "HMO" classification 63
– reference point, prolapse 53, 56, 57, 63
– – pelvic floor descent 149
Puborectalis 8, 23, 24, 34
– anismus 150
– ano-rectal angle 17
– asymmetry 60
– congenital anomalies 162
– endosonography 70, 71
– MRI 80
– post anal repair 165
– syndromes, non-relaxing & Paradoxical contraction 152

R
Rectal prolapse 146–150
– complete 147
– grading on evacuation proctography 147
– internal intussusception 147
– types 146
Rectocoele 53, 54
– aetiology 150
– definition 150
– functional disorders and significance of 151
– graft placement 119
– posterior 151
– rectal wall imbrication 119, 120
– repair of rectovaginal defect 119
– repair, posterior colporraphy 119
– repair, trans-anal 120
Rectovaginal fascia
– anatomy 17, 29, 108
– defects of 61, 63, 65
Rectovaginal septum
– histology 108
– normal depth 110
Rectum anatomy 19, 20

S
Sacral nerve stimulation
– aecal incontinence 169
– detrusor instability 137
Sigmoidocele 56, 112
Solitary rectal ulcer syndrome 149
– internal anal sphincter, thickened in 72
Sphincter, repair
– anterior sphincteroplasty 165–167
– artificial 168
– atrophy, endocoil MRI in 166
– augmentation 168, 169
– postanal 167

Stress incontinence
- aetiology 31, 94
- bladder diary in 91
- decision analysis 134
- prevalence 127, 128
- suburethral sling 135
- tension free vaginal tape 136
- transvaginal ultrasound and 77
- treatment, Cochrane database reviews and 132
- urodynamics 90, 91
- urodynamics, indications 90

T
Transverse perineii
- anatomy 8–10
- endoanal MRI 83
- endoanal ultrasound 71
- obstetric tears 75
- sex differences 83

U
Ultrasound, endoanal 69–78
- external anal sphincter 71
- interface reflections 70
- internal anal sphincter 70
- normal 4 layer pattern 70, 71
- puboanalis 71
- subepithelium 70
- technique 69, 70
Ultrasound, transvaginal anal sphincters 77
Urethra
- anatomy 3, 11, 12–16, 35–37
- diverticula 60, 61
- dynamic MRI 60, 61
- external sphincter 13, 14
- functional anatomy 35–37, 93
- glands 37
- leak pressures 93–95
- mobility, dynamic MRI 60
- mobility, ultrasound 60
- MRI 60, 61
- sphincter 37
- support 14–16, 30, 31
- support mechanisms 31, 114
- surgery 136, 137
Urethrovaginal sphincter 16
Urinary incontinence
- abdominal retropubic urethropexy 135
- artificial urethral sphincter 137
- bladder outlet disorders 128
- blue dye test for 129
- bulking agents for urethra 137, 138
- causes, of 127–129
- clinical evaluation 129–131
- Cochrane database
- colporraphy, anterior 134, 115
- definition 125, 126
- detrusor abnormalities 128
- incontinence impact questionnaire 130
- needle urethropexy (colposuspension) 134
- pelvic floor muscle training 132
- pharmacological treatment 133
- prevalence 126, 127
- reviews for treatment of 132

- risk factors, for 127
- stress 92, 128
- suburethral sling 135, 136
- surgical and clinical considerations 125–141
- surgical management 133–138
- tension free tape 136
- urge 128
- urogenital distress inventory 130
- vesico-vaginal fistula, methylene
Urodynamics 89–99
- bladder diary 90–92
- cystometry,
- cystometry, ambulatory 92, 93
- cystometry, simple 91
- definition 89, 90
- guidelines, for 90
- multichannel (subtracted) 91, 92
- residual volume 95
Uroflometry
- combined with pressure flow 96
- complex 96
- electromyography 96
- fluoroscopy 96, 97
- perineal ultrasound 97
- simple 95, 96
Uterovaginal
- apical prolapse 30, 57
- levels of support 29, 30
- paracolpium 29
- prolapse, MRI 61
- uterosacral ligaments 29
Utero-vaginal prolapse surgery for 118
Uterovaginal support
- concepts 28
- mechanisms 29
- prolapse 30
- surgery 116
- utero-sacral and cardinal ligaments in 4, 7, 15, 17, 29, 57, 108
Uterus
- anatomy 16–18
- embryology 3, 4
- prolapse 30, 61
- support structures 29, 30, 35
Uterus anatomy and support 16–18

V
Vagina
- abdominal sacral colpopexy 116
- anatomy 16–18
- dynamic MRI 60–61
- embryology 3
- mechanisms and levels of support 28–33, 108
- opacification
- – fluoroscopic 51, 53
- – MRI 58
- – Dynamic ultrasound 77
- paravaginal tears, MRI 61
- prolapse 30, 57, 60, 61, 110
- sacrospinous vault suspension 117
- utero-sacral ligament
- vault suspension 118
- vault prolapse 116–118

List of Contributors

CLIVE I. BARTRAM, FRCS, FRCP, FRCR
Consultant Radiologist, St. Mark's Hospital
Northwick Park
Harrow HA1 3UJ
UK
and
Professor of Gastrointestinal Radiology
Imperial College Faculty of Medicine, London

J. THOMAS BENSON, MD, FACOG
Clinical Professor, Obstetrics and Gynecology
Director, Female Pelvic Medicine & Reconstructive Surgery
Methodist/Indiana University Hospital
Indiana University
Diplomate American Board of Electrodiagnostic Medicine
1633 North Capitol Avenue, Suite 436
Indianapolis, IN 46202-1227
USA

JOHN O.L. DELANCEY, MD
Norman F. Miller Professor of Gynecology
Department of Obstetrics and Gynecology
L 4000 Women's Hospital
1500 E. Medical Center Dr.
Ann Arbor, MI 48109-0276
USA

ANTON V. EMMANUEL, MD, MRCP
Physiology Unit
St. Mark's Hospital
Northwick Park
Watford Road
Harrow, Middlesex HA1 3UJ
UK

DOUGLAS S. HALE, FACOG
Associate Director, Female Pelvic Medicine
& Reconstructive Surgery Fellowship
Methodist/Indiana University Hospital
1633 N Capitol Ave, Suite 436
Indianapolis, IN 46202
USA

STEVE HALLIGAN, MD, MRCP, FRCR
Intestinal Imaging Centre
Level 4V
St. Mark's Hospital
Watford Road
Northwick Park
Harrow, Middx.HA1 3UJ
UK

FREDERICK M. KELVIN, MD
Department of Radiology
Methodist Hospital of Indiana
Clinical Professor of Radiology
Indiana University School of Medicine
1701 North Senate Boulevard
Indianapolis, IN 46202
USA

HARPREET K. PANNU, MD
Assistant Professor of Radiology
The Russell H. Morgan Department
of Radiology and Radiological Science
Johns Hopkins Medical Institutions
600 North Wolfe Street, Room 100
Baltimore, MD 21287
USA

ELENA ROCIU, MD
Department of Radiology
Academic Medical Center
University of Amsterdam
P.O. Box 22700
1100 DE Amsterdam
The Netherlands

JAAP STOKER, MD, PhD
Department of Radiology
Academic Medical Center
University of Amsterdam
P.O. Box 22700
1100 DE Amsterdam
The Netherlands

KRIS STROHBEHN, MD, FACOG, FACS
Associate Professor, Dartmouth Medical School
Department of Obstetrics and Gynecology
Director, Division of Urogynecology/Reconstructive
Pelvic Surgery
Dartmouth-Hitchcok Medical Center
One Medical Center Drive
Lebanon, NH 03756
USA

CAROLYNNE J.VAIZEY, MD, FRCS(Gen), FCS(SA)
Consultant Colorectal Surgeon
Colorectal Surgical Unit
The Middlesex Hospital
Mortimer St
London W1T 3AA
UK

MEDICAL RADIOLOGY Diagnostic Imaging and Radiation Oncology
Titles in the series already published

DIAGNOSTIC IMAGING

Innovations in Diagnostic Imaging
Edited by J. H. Anderson

Radiology of the Upper Urinary Tract
Edited by E. K. Lang

The Thymus - Diagnostic Imaging, Functions, and Pathologic Anatomy
Edited by E. Walter, E. Willich, and W. R. Webb

Interventional Neuroradiology
Edited by A. Valavanis

Radiology of the Pancreas
Edited by A. L. Baert, co-edited by G. Delorme

Radiology of the Lower Urinary Tract
Edited by E. K. Lang

Magnetic Resonance Angiography
Edited by I. P. Arlart, G. M. Bongartz, and G. Marchal

Contrast-Enhanced MRI of the Breast
S. Heywang-Köbrunner and R. Beck

Spiral CT of the Chest
Edited by M. Rémy-Jardin and J. Rémy

Radiological Diagnosis of Breast Diseases
Edited by M. Friedrich and E.A. Sickles

Radiology of the Trauma
Edited by M. Heller and A. Fink

Biliary Tract Radiology
Edited by P. Rossi

Radiological Imaging of Sports Injuries
Edited by C. Masciocchi

Modern Imaging of the Alimentary Tube
Edited by A. R. Margulis

Diagnosis and Therapy of Spinal Tumors
Edited by P. R. Algra, J. Valk, and J. J. Heimans

Interventional Magnetic Resonance Imaging
Edited by J. F. Debatin and G. Adam

Abdominal and Pelvic MRI
Edited by A. Heuck and M. Reiser

Orthopedic Imaging
Techniques and Applications
Edited by A. M. Davies and H. Pettersson

Radiology of the Female Pelvic Organs
Edited by E. K.Lang

Magnetic Resonance of the Heart and Great Vessels
Clinical Applications
Edited by J. Bogaert, A. J. Duerinckx, and F. E. Rademakers

Modern Head and Neck Imaging
Edited by S. K. Mukherji and J. A. Castelijns

Radiological Imaging of Endocrine Diseases
Edited by J. N. Bruneton
in collaboration with B. Padovani and M.-Y. Mourou

Trends in Contrast Media
Edited by H. S. Thomsen, R. N. Muller, and R. F. Mattrey

Functional MRI
Edited by C. T. W. Moonen and P. A. Bandettini

Radiology of the Pancreas
2nd Revised Edition
Edited by A. L. Baert
Co-edited by G. Delorme and L. Van Hoe

Emergency Pediatric Radiology
Edited by H. Carty

Spiral CT of the Abdomen
Edited by F. Terrier, M. Grossholz, and C. D. Becker

Liver Malignancies
Diagnostic and Interventional Radiology
Edited by C. Bartolozzi and R. Lencioni

Medical Imaging of the Spleen
Edited by A. M. De Schepper
and F. Vanhoenacker

Radiology of Peripheral Vascular Diseases
Edited by E. Zeitler

Diagnostic Nuclear Medicine
Edited by C. Schiepers

Radiology of Blunt Trauma of the Chest
P. Schnyder and M. Wintermark

Portal Hypertension
Diagnostic Imaging-Guided Therapy
Edited by P. Rossi
Co-edited by P. Ricci and L. Broglia

Recent Advances in Diagnostic Neuroradiology
Edited by Ph. Demaerel

Virtual Endoscopy and Related 3D Techniques
Edited by P. Rogalla,
J. Terwisscha Van Scheltinga, and B. Hamm

Multislice CT
Edited by M. F. Reiser, M. Takahashi, M. Modic, and R. Bruening

Pediatric Uroradiology
Edited by R. Fotter

Transfontanellar Doppler Imaging in Neonates
A. Couture and C. Veyrac

Radiology of AIDS
A Practical Approach
Edited by J.W.A.J. Reeders and P.C. Goodman

CT of the Peritoneum
Armando Rossi and Giorgio Rossi

Magnetic Resonance Angiography
2nd Revised Edition
Edited by I. P. Arlart, G. M. Bongratz, and G. Marchal

Pediatric Chest Imaging
Edited by Javier Lucaya and Janet L. Strife

Applications of Sonography in Head and Neck Pathology
Edited by J. N. Bruneton in collaboration with C. Raffaelli and O. Dassonville

Imaging of the Larynx
Edited by R. Hermans

3D Image Processing
Techniques and Clinical Applications
Edited by D. Caramella and C. Bartolozzi

Imaging of Orbital and Visual Pathway Pathology
Edited by W. S. Müller-Forell

Pediatric ENT Radiology
Edited by S. J. King and A. E. Boothroyd

Radiological Imaging of the Small Intestine
Edited by N. C. Gourtsoyiannis

Imaging of the Knee
Techniques and Applications
Edited by A. M. Davies
and V. N. Cassar-Pullicino

Perinatal Imaging
From Ultrasound to MR Imaging
Edited by Fred E. Avni

Radiological Imaging of the Neonatal Chest
Edited by V. Donoghue

Diagnostic and Interventional Radiology in Liver Transplantation
Edited by E. Bücheler, V. Nicolas, C. E. Broelsch, X. Rogiers, and G. Krupski

Radiology of Osteoporosis
Edited by S. Grampp

Imaging and Intervention in Abdominal Trauma
Edited by R. F. Dondelinger

Imaging of the Foot and Ankle
Techniques and Applications
Edited by A. M. Davies, R. W. Whitehouse, and J. P. R. Jenkins

Interventional Radiology in Cancer
Edited by A. Adam, R. F. Dondelinger, and P. R. Mueller

Imaging of the Pancreas
Cystic and Rare Tumors
Edited by C. Procassi and A. J. Megibow

Intracranial Vascular Malformations and Aneurysms
From Diagnostic Work-Up to Endovascular Therapy
Edited by M. Forsting

Imaging Pelvic Floor Disorders
Edited by C. I. Bartram and J. O. L. DeLancey
Associate Editors: S. Halligan, F. M. Kelvin, and J. Stoker

High Resolution Sonography of the Peripheral Nervous System
Edited by S. Peer and G. Bodner

Radiology Imaging of the Ureter
Edited by F. Joffre, Ph. Otal, and M. Soulie

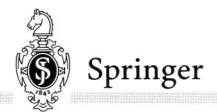

Springer

MEDICAL RADIOLOGY Diagnostic Imaging and Radiation Oncology
Titles in the series already published

RADIATION ONCOLOGY

Lung Cancer
Edited by C.W. Scarantino

Innovations in Radiation Oncology
Edited by H. R. Withers and L. J. Peters

Radiation Therapy of Head and Neck Cancer
Edited by G. E. Laramore

Gastrointestinal Cancer – Radiation Therapy
Edited by R.R. Dobelbower, Jr.

Radiation Exposure and Occupational Risks
Edited by E. Scherer, C. Streffer, and K.-R. Trott

Radiation Therapy of Benign Diseases
A Clinical Guide
S.E. Order and S. S. Donaldson

Interventional Radiation Therapy Techniques – Brachytherapy
Edited by R. Sauer

Radiopathology of Organs and Tissues
Edited by E. Scherer, C. Streffer, and K.-R. Trott

Concomitant Continuous Infusion Chemotherapy and Radiation
Edited by M. Rotman and C. J. Rosenthal

Intraoperative Radiotherapy – Clinical Experiences and Results
Edited by F. A. Calvo, M. Santos, and L.W. Brady

Radiotherapy of Intraocular and Orbital Tumors
Edited by W. E. Alberti and R. H. Sagerman

Interstitial and Intracavitary Thermoradiotherapy
Edited by M. H. Seegenschmiedt and R. Sauer

Non-Disseminated Breast Cancer
Controversial Issues in Management
Edited by G. H. Fletcher and S.H. Levitt

Current Topics in Clinical Radiobiology of Tumors
Edited by H.-P. Beck-Bornholdt

Practical Approaches to Cancer Invasion and Metastases
A Compendium of Radiation Oncologists' Responses to 40 Histories
Edited by A. R. Kagan with the Assistance of R. J. Steckel

Radiation Therapy in Pediatric Oncology
Edited by J. R. Cassady

Radiation Therapy Physics
Edited by A. R. Smith

Late Sequelae in Oncology
Edited by J. Dunst and R. Sauer

Mediastinal Tumors. Update 1995
Edited by D. E. Wood and C. R. Thomas, Jr.

Thermoradiotherapy and Thermochemotherapy
Volume 1:
Biology, Physiology, and Physics
Volume 2:
Clinical Applications
Edited by M.H. Seegenschmiedt, P. Fessenden, and C.C. Vernon

Carcinoma of the Prostate
Innovations in Management
Edited by Z. Petrovich, L. Baert, and L.W. Brady

Radiation Oncology of Gynecological Cancers
Edited by H.W. Vahrson

Carcinoma of the Bladder
Innovations in Management
Edited by Z. Petrovich, L. Baert, and L.W. Brady

Blood Perfusion and Microenvironment of Human Tumors
Implications for Clinical Radiooncology
Edited by M. Molls and P. Vaupel

Radiation Therapy of Benign Diseases
A Clinical Guide
2nd Revised Edition
S. E. Order and S. S. Donaldson

Carcinoma of the Kidney and Testis, and Rare Urologic Malignancies
Innovations in Management
Edited by Z. Petrovich, L. Baert, and L.W. Brady

Progress and Perspectives in the Treatment of Lung Cancer
Edited by P. Van Houtte, J. Klastersky, and P. Rocmans

Combined Modality Therapy of Central Nervous System Tumors
Edited by Z. Petrovich, L. W. Brady, M. L. Apuzzo, and M. Bamberg

Age-Related Macular Degeneration
Current Treatment Concepts
Edited by W. A. Alberti, G. Richard, and R. H. Sagerman

Radiotherapy of Intraocular and Orbital Tumors
2nd Revised Edition
Edited by R. H. Sagerman, and W. E. Alberti

Clinical Target Volumes in Conformal and Intensity Modulated Radiation Therapy
A Clinical Guide to Cancer Treatment
Edited by V. Grégoire, P. Scalliet, and K. K. Ang

Biological Modification of Radiation Response
Edited by C. Nieder, L. Milas, and K. K. Ang

Palliative Radiation Oncology
R. G. Parker. N. A. Janjan, and M. T. Selch

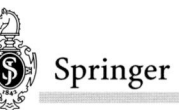

Springer